T0250951

Bayesian Designs for Phase I–II Clinical Trials

Ying Yuan

The University of Texas
MD Anderson Cancer Center
Houston, Texas, USA

Hoang Q. Nguyen

The University of Texas
MD Anderson Cancer Center
Houston, Texas, USA

Peter F. Thall

The University of Texas
MD Anderson Cancer Center
Houston, Texas, USA

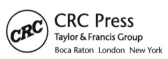

CRC Press
Taylor & Francis Group
Boca Raton London New York

CRC Press is an imprint of the
Taylor & Francis Group, an **informa** business

A CHAPMAN & HALL BOOK

Chapman & Hall/CRC Biostatistics Series

Published Titles

Adaptive Design Methods in Clinical Trials, Second Edition
Shein-Chung Chow and Mark Chang

Adaptive Designs for Sequential Treatment Allocation
Alessandro Baldi Antognini
and Alessandra Giovagnoli

Adaptive Design Theory and Implementation Using SAS and R, Second Edition
Mark Chang

Advanced Bayesian Methods for Medical Test Accuracy
Lyle D. Broemeling

Applied Biclustering Methods for Big and High-Dimensional Data Using R
Adetayo Kasim, Ziv Shkedy,
Sebastian Kaiser, Sepp Hochreiter,
and Willem Talloen

Applied Meta-Analysis with R
Ding-Geng (Din) Chen and Karl E. Peace

Basic Statistics and Pharmaceutical Statistical Applications, Second Edition
James E. De Muth

Bayesian Adaptive Methods for Clinical Trials
Scott M. Berry, Bradley P. Carlin,
J. Jack Lee, and Peter Muller

Bayesian Analysis Made Simple: An Excel GUI for WinBUGS
Phil Woodward

Bayesian Designs for Phase I–II Clinical Trials
Ying Yuan, Hoang Q. Nguyen,
and Peter F. Thall

Bayesian Methods for Measures of Agreement
Lyle D. Broemeling

Bayesian Methods for Repeated Measures
Lyle D. Broemeling

Bayesian Methods in Epidemiology
Lyle D. Broemeling

Bayesian Methods in Health Economics
Gianluca Baio

Bayesian Missing Data Problems: EM, Data Augmentation and Noniterative Computation
Ming T. Tan, Guo-Liang Tian,
and Kai Wang Ng

Bayesian Modeling in Bioinformatics
Dipak K. Dey, Samiran Ghosh,
and Bani K. Mallick

Benefit-Risk Assessment in Pharmaceutical Research and Development
Andreas Sashegyi, James Felli,
and Rebecca Noel

Published Titles

Benefit-Risk Assessment Methods in Medical Product Development: Bridging Qualitative and Quantitative Assessments
Qi Jiang and Weili He

Biosimilars: Design and Analysis of Follow-on Biologics
Shein-Chung Chow

Biostatistics: A Computing Approach
Stewart J. Anderson

Cancer Clinical Trials: Current and Controversial Issues in Design and Analysis
Stephen L. George, Xiaofei Wang, and Herbert Pang

Causal Analysis in Biomedicine and Epidemiology: Based on Minimal Sufficient Causation
Mikel Aickin

Clinical and Statistical Considerations in Personalized Medicine
Claudio Carini, Sandeep Menon, and Mark Chang

Clinical Trial Data Analysis using R
Ding-Geng (Din) Chen and Karl E. Peace

Clinical Trial Methodology
Karl E. Peace and Ding-Geng (Din) Chen

Computational Methods in Biomedical Research
Ravindra Khattree and Dayanand N. Naik

Computational Pharmacokinetics
Anders Källén

Confidence Intervals for Proportions and Related Measures of Effect Size
Robert G. Newcombe

Controversial Statistical Issues in Clinical Trials
Shein-Chung Chow

Data Analysis with Competing Risks and Intermediate States
Ronald B. Geskus

Data and Safety Monitoring Committees in Clinical Trials
Jay Herson

Design and Analysis of Animal Studies in Pharmaceutical Development
Shein-Chung Chow and Jen-pei Liu

Design and Analysis of Bioavailability and Bioequivalence Studies, Third Edition
Shein-Chung Chow and Jen-pei Liu

Design and Analysis of Bridging Studies
Jen-pei Liu, Shein-Chung Chow, and Chin-Fu Hsiao

Design & Analysis of Clinical Trials for Economic Evaluation & Reimbursement: An Applied Approach Using SAS & STATA
Iftekhar Khan

Design and Analysis of Clinical Trials for Predictive Medicine
Shigeyuki Matsui, Marc Buyse, and Richard Simon

Design and Analysis of Clinical Trials with Time-to-Event Endpoints
Karl E. Peace

Design and Analysis of Non-Inferiority Trials
Mark D. Rothmann, Brian L. Wiens, and Ivan S. F. Chan

Difference Equations with Public Health Applications
Lemuel A. Moyé and Asha Seth Kapadia

DNA Methylation Microarrays: Experimental Design and Statistical Analysis
Sun-Chong Wang and Arturas Petronis

DNA Microarrays and Related Genomics Techniques: Design, Analysis, and Interpretation of Experiments
David B. Allison, Grier P. Page, T. Mark Beasley, and Jode W. Edwards

Dose Finding by the Continual Reassessment Method
Ying Kuen Cheung

Dynamical Biostatistical Models
Daniel Commenges and Hélène Jacqmin-Gadda

Elementary Bayesian Biostatistics
Lemuel A. Moyé

Empirical Likelihood Method in Survival Analysis
Mai Zhou

Exposure–Response Modeling: Methods and Practical Implementation
Jixian Wang

Published Titles

Frailty Models in Survival Analysis
Andreas Wienke

Fundamental Concepts for New Clinical Trialists
Scott Evans and Naitee Ting

Generalized Linear Models: A Bayesian Perspective
Dipak K. Dey, Sujit K. Ghosh, and Bani K. Mallick

Handbook of Regression and Modeling: Applications for the Clinical and Pharmaceutical Industries
Daryl S. Paulson

Inference Principles for Biostatisticians
Ian C. Marschner

Interval-Censored Time-to-Event Data: Methods and Applications
Ding-Geng (Din) Chen, Jianguo Sun, and Karl E. Peace

Introductory Adaptive Trial Designs: A Practical Guide with R
Mark Chang

Joint Models for Longitudinal and Time-to-Event Data: With Applications in R
Dimitris Rizopoulos

Measures of Interobserver Agreement and Reliability, Second Edition
Mohamed M. Shoukri

Medical Biostatistics, Third Edition
A. Indrayan

Meta-Analysis in Medicine and Health Policy
Dalene Stangl and Donald A. Berry

Mixed Effects Models for the Population Approach: Models, Tasks, Methods and Tools
Marc Lavielle

Modeling to Inform Infectious Disease Control
Niels G. Becker

Modern Adaptive Randomized Clinical Trials: Statistical and Practical Aspects
Oleksandr Sverdlov

Monte Carlo Simulation for the Pharmaceutical Industry: Concepts, Algorithms, and Case Studies
Mark Chang

Multiregional Clinical Trials for Simultaneous Global New Drug Development
Joshua Chen and Hui Quan

Multiple Testing Problems in Pharmaceutical Statistics
Alex Dmitrienko, Ajit C. Tamhane, and Frank Bretz

Noninferiority Testing in Clinical Trials: Issues and Challenges
Tie-Hua Ng

Optimal Design for Nonlinear Response Models
Valerii V. Fedorov and Sergei L. Leonov

Patient-Reported Outcomes: Measurement, Implementation and Interpretation
Joseph C. Cappelleri, Kelly H. Zou, Andrew G. Bushmakin, Jose Ma. J. Alvir, Demissie Alemayehu, and Tara Symonds

Quantitative Evaluation of Safety in Drug Development: Design, Analysis and Reporting
Qi Jiang and H. Amy Xia

Quantitative Methods for Traditional Chinese Medicine Development
Shein-Chung Chow

Randomized Clinical Trials of Nonpharmacological Treatments
Isabelle Boutron, Philippe Ravaud, and David Moher

Randomized Phase II Cancer Clinical Trials
Sin-Ho Jung

Sample Size Calculations for Clustered and Longitudinal Outcomes in Clinical Research
Chul Ahn, Moonseong Heo, and Song Zhang

Published Titles

Sample Size Calculations in Clinical Research, Second Edition
Shein-Chung Chow, Jun Shao, and Hansheng Wang

Statistical Analysis of Human Growth and Development
Yin Bun Cheung

Statistical Design and Analysis of Clinical Trials: Principles and Methods
Weichung Joe Shih and Joseph Aisner

Statistical Design and Analysis of Stability Studies
Shein-Chung Chow

Statistical Evaluation of Diagnostic Performance: Topics in ROC Analysis
Kelly H. Zou, Aiyi Liu, Andriy Bandos, Lucila Ohno-Machado, and Howard Rockette

Statistical Methods for Clinical Trials
Mark X. Norleans

Statistical Methods for Drug Safety
Robert D. Gibbons and Anup K. Amatya

Statistical Methods for Immunogenicity Assessment
Harry Yang, Jianchun Zhang, Binbing Yu, and Wei Zhao

Statistical Methods in Drug Combination Studies
Wei Zhao and Harry Yang

Statistical Testing Strategies in the Health Sciences
Albert Vexler, Alan D. Hutson, and Xiwei Chen

Statistics in Drug Research: Methodologies and Recent Developments
Shein-Chung Chow and Jun Shao

Statistics in the Pharmaceutical Industry, Third Edition
Ralph Buncher and Jia-Yeong Tsay

Survival Analysis in Medicine and Genetics
Jialiang Li and Shuangge Ma

Theory of Drug Development
Eric B. Holmgren

Translational Medicine: Strategies and Statistical Methods
Dennis Cosmatos and Shein-Chung Chow

CRC Press
Taylor & Francis Group
6000 Broken Sound Parkway NW, Suite 300
Boca Raton, FL 33487-2742

First issued in paperback 2021

Version Date: 20160309

ISBN 13: 978-1-03-224264-4 (pbk)
ISBN 13: 978-1-4987-0955-2 (hbk)

DOI: 10.1201/b21600

Publisher's Note
The publisher has gone to great lengths to ensure the quality of this reprint but points out that some imperfections in the original copies may be apparent.

Library of Congress Cataloging-in-Publication Data

Names: Yuan, Ying (Professor of biostatistics) | Nguyen, Hoang Q., author. | Thall, Peter F., author.
Title: Bayesian designs for phase I-II clinical trials / Ying Yuan, Hoang Q. Nguyen, and Peter F. Thall.
Description: Boca Raton : Taylor & Francis, 2016. | Includes bibliographical references and index.
Identifiers: LCCN 2016004874 | ISBN 9781498709552 (alk. paper)
Subjects: LCSH: Clinical trials--Statistical methods. | Drugs--Testing--Statistical methods. | Bayesian statistical decision theory.
Classification: LCC R853.C55 Y83 2016 | DDC 615.5072/4--dc23
LC record available at http://lccn.loc.gov/2016004874

Visit the Taylor & Francis Web site at
http://www.taylorandfrancis.com

and the CRC Press Web site at
http://www.crcpress.com

This book is dedicated to all the patients who suffered more than they should have, or who died sooner than they might have, because they were given suboptimal treatments.

To my wife Suyu and daughter Selina.

Ying Yuan

To the Lord our God who made it all possible.

Hoang Nguyen

I am grateful to Ying for inviting me to collaborate on this book.

Peter Thall

Contents

Preface   xiii

1   Why Conduct Phase I–II Trials?   1

    1.1   The Conventional Paradigm 1
    1.2   The Continual Reassessment Method 5
    1.3   Problems with Conventional Dose-Finding Methods 8
       1.3.1   3+3 Algorithms 8
       1.3.2   Some Comparisons 10
       1.3.3   Problems Going from Phase I to Phase II 18
       1.3.4   Consequences of Ignoring Information 19
       1.3.5   Late-Onset Outcomes 22
       1.3.6   Expansion Cohorts 23
       1.3.7   Guessing a Schedule 25
       1.3.8   Patient Heterogeneity 26

2   The Phase I–II Paradigm   29

    2.1   Efficacy and Toxicity 29
    2.2   Elements of Phase I–II Designs 30
    2.3   Treatment Regimes and Clinical Outcomes 31
    2.4   Sequentially Adaptive Decision Making 33
    2.5   Risk–Benefit Trade-Offs 35
    2.6   Stickiness and Adaptive Randomization 37
    2.7   Simulation as a Design Tool 41

3   Establishing Priors   43

    3.1   Pathological Priors 43
    3.2   Prior Effective Sample Size 46
    3.3   Computing Priors from Elicited Values 50
       3.3.1   Least Squares Algorithm 54
       3.3.2   Pseudo Sampling Algorithm 55

4 Efficacy–Toxicity Trade-Off-Based Designs   **59**

  4.1   General Structure 59
  4.2   Probability Model 60
  4.3   Dose Admissibility Criteria 62
  4.4   Trade-Off Contours 63
  4.5   Establishing a Prior 64
  4.6   Steps for Constructing a Design 67
  4.7   Illustration 69
  4.8   Sensitivity to Target Contours 71
  4.9   Sensitivity to Prior ESS 71
  4.10   Trinary Outcomes 74
  4.11   Time-to-Event Outcomes 79

5 Designs with Late-Onset Outcomes   **89**

  5.1   A Common Logistical Problem 89
  5.2   Late-Onset Events as Missing Data 91
  5.3   Probability Model 96
  5.4   Imputation of Delayed Outcomes 97
  5.5   Illustration 99

6 Utility-Based Designs   **105**

  6.1   Assigning Utilities to Outcomes 105
  6.2   Subjectivity of Utilities 111
  6.3   Utility-Based Sequential Decision Making 113
      6.3.1   Utility Elicitation 113
      6.3.2   Computing Mean Utilities 114
      6.3.3   Regime Acceptability Criteria 115
      6.3.4   Design Evaluation Criteria 116
      6.3.5   Utility Sensitivity Analyses 117
      6.3.6   More Elaborate Utilities 118
  6.4   Optimizing Radiation Dose for Brain Tumors 119

7 Personalized Dose Finding   **129**

  7.1   The EffTox Design with Covariates 129
  7.2   Biomarker-Based Dose Finding 138

8 Combination Trials   **149**

  8.1   Bivariate Binary Outcomes 150
  8.2   Bivariate Ordinal Outcomes 159
      8.2.1   Generalized Continuation Ratio Model 159
      8.2.2   Generalized Aranda–Ordaz Link Model 160

8.2.3 An mTOR Inhibitor Chemo Combination Trial 166
8.2.4 Parametric Dose Standardization 168
8.2.5 mTOR Inhibitor Trial Design 173
8.2.6 Alternative Models 177

9 Optimizing Molecularly Targeted Agents   179

9.1 Features of Targeted Agents 179
9.2 One Targeted Agent 180
9.3 Combining Targeted and Cytotoxic Agents 186
9.4 Combining Two Molecularly Targeted Agents 195

10 Optimizing Doses in Two Cycles   203

10.1 The Two-Cycle Problem 203
10.2 A Two-Cycle Model 205
10.3 Decision Criteria 209
10.4 Illustration 212
10.5 Simulation Study 215

11 Optimizing Dose and Schedule   223

11.1 Schedule-Dependent Effects 223
11.2 Trinary Outcomes 224
11.3 Event Times Outcomes 231

12 Dealing with Dropouts   245

12.1 Dropouts and Missing Efficacy 245
12.2 Probability Model 246
12.3 Dose-Finding Algorithm 248
12.4 Simulations 249

13 Optimizing Intra-Arterial tPA   253

13.1 Rapid Treatment of Stroke 253
13.2 Probability Model 254
13.3 Decision Criteria and Trial Conduct 259
13.4 Priors 260
13.5 Simulations 261

14 Optimizing Sedative Dose in Preterm Infants   267

14.1 Respiratory Distress Syndrome in Neonates 267
14.2 Clinical Outcomes and Probability Model 270
14.3 Prior and Likelihood 273

xii

14.4 Decision Criteria 274
14.5 Simulations 277

Bibliography   **283**

Index   **301**

Preface

This book is about Bayesian designs for clinical trials of experimental treatment regimes being given to humans for the first time. A regime's components may be the dose of a single agent, the dose pair of a two-agent combination, the doses of an agent given in two successive cycles, the schedule of administration, or a (dose, schedule) combination. The regime may comprise the entire therapy given to the patient, or it may be combined with other agents that are given at fixed doses and schedules, or possibly with a procedure such as surgery. The scientific goals of these trials are to explore, refine, and, ideally, optimize the regime. All of the designs that we will discuss include sequentially adaptive treatment decisions for small, successive cohorts of patients, based on very small amounts of regime-outcome data from previous patients. The need to make decisions sequentially in this way is motivated by the ethical concern that some of the treatment regimes being studied may be unsafe due to excessive Toxicity. Consideration of Efficacy along with Toxicity motivates the additional concern that some regimes may be ineffective in terms of anti-disease effect. If this were not the case, then one could proceed much more simply by randomizing patients among the regimes, possibly imposing a restriction to balance the sample sizes of the regimes.

Chapter 1 gives a variety of simple examples that show why the conventional paradigm used for early phase clinical trials is just plain wrong. Chapter 2 explains the general structure of phase I–II designs, which use both Efficacy and Toxicity to evaluate experimental treatment regimes. These first two chapters are written so that they can be understood by nonstatisticians seeking enlightenment or entertainment. Chapter 3, which is about how one actually constructs prior distributions in practice to apply Bayesian models, is more technical. It also gives some useful examples of how smart people may make stupid mistakes without realizing it. The rest of the book, Chapters 4–14, describes specific designs, and these chapters are full of Greek symbols and mathematical formulas. If you are a physician and you wish to avoid such technicalities, we suggest that you read Chapters 1 and 2 in detail, but look only at the general structures of the specific designs that follow. If this convinces you to use a particular design given in these later chapters for one of your trials, just show it to your statistician and explain what you want.

Although we will cover a fair number of different phase I–II designs, this book is neither a survey nor a comprehensive review. The existing literature is far too large to do that in this book. Many different designs can be classified as phase I–II, in the sense that they combine aspects of conventional phase I and phase II designs. As one might expect, we will focus primarily on designs that we have developed. Because methodological developments have run far ahead of the process of writing user-friendly computer programs, there is a great need for a comprehensive software package that provides a basis for simulating and implementing the designs. A challenging project would be to write such a software package, including a graphical user interface. For those designs that do have reasonably user-friendly computer software, we will indicate where it can be obtained.

In practice, every clinical trial has its own idiosyncrasies, in terms of treatment regimes, entry criteria, patient heterogeneity, ethical constraints, how clinical outcomes are defined, observed, and recorded, accrual rate, scientific goals, safety and futility monitoring rules, patient compliance, administrative issues, regulatory requirements, and financial constraints. In virtually any application, the reality of medical practice is far too complex to model all of its aspects and account for them in a clinical trial design. To apply any existing design, inevitably one must make simplifying assumptions. Much of the art of the clinical trial design process is in deciding how simple a design may be without throwing out the baby with the bathwater, so to speak. In Chapter 1 we will provide numerous examples of wonderfully simple, intuitively appealing clinical trial methods that are used widely but are deeply flawed. If one wishes to avoid the unhappy consequences of oversimplification, it may appear that a solution is to create a detailed model that accounts for all observable variables. These might include long lists of qualitatively different Toxicities, early clinical Efficacy outcomes, biological outcomes, pharmacokinetic and pharmacodynamic variables, longitudinal values of some of these variables, as well as disease progression time and survival time, all as functions of treatment regime doses and schedules, patient baseline prognostic covariates, and possibly genomic variables. This exercise may seem to be scientifically honest and ethically appealing, and it may even result in an impressive paper published in a statistical journal. However, such a model probably would be far too unwieldy for use as the basis for an actual adaptive early phase trial design.

Practical clinical trial designs lie somewhere between the two extremes of oversimplification and unrealistic elaboration. In many cases, an extension of an existing design may be developed to accommodate a more general or slightly different problem than that addressed by an existing design. This was how each of the designs discussed in this book originated. At this writing, many open problems remain, and some are areas of active research. If you are a medical statistician and you listen carefully to the research physicians and scientists with whom you collaborate, you will discover many such problems that have not yet been solved. If you are a physician doing clinical research and your statistician does not understand phase I–II designs or keeps giving you the same off-the-shelf solutions to every clinical trial design or data analysis problem that you come up with, find a new statistician.

1

Why Conduct Phase I–II Trials?

CONTENTS

1.1	The Conventional Paradigm	1
1.2	The Continual Reassessment Method	5
1.3	Problems with Conventional Dose-Finding Methods	8
	1.3.1 3+3 Algorithms	8
	1.3.2 Some Comparisons	10
	1.3.3 Problems Going from Phase I to Phase II	18
	1.3.4 Consequences of Ignoring Information	19
	1.3.5 Late-Onset Outcomes	22
	1.3.6 Expansion Cohorts	23
	1.3.7 Guessing a Schedule	25
	1.3.8 Patient Heterogeneity	26

"The conventional view serves to protect us from the painful job of thinking."

John Kenneth Galbraith

1.1 The Conventional Paradigm

In its simplest form, the conventional clinical trial paradigm for evaluating effects of a new agent or agents in humans has three phases. In phase I, the goal is to determine an acceptably safe dose based on Toxicity. For a single agent, a set of doses to be explored is specified. If two agents given in combination are to be studied, then a set of dose pairs is specified, either as a rectangular grid or a staircase-shaped set where only one of the two doses increases with each step. In some phase I trials, doses are chosen from a continuum, either an interval for one agent or a rectangular set for a pair of agents (Thall et al., 2003; Huo et al., 2012). Phase I is conducted by treating small cohorts of patients, most commonly of size 3, 2, or 1. The dose, or dose pair, of each successive cohort is chosen adaptively based on the dose-Toxicity data of previous cohorts. Depending on the method used, each cohort's dose may be above, below, or the same as that of the previous cohort. The final chosen dose often is called the "maximum tolerated (or tolerable) dose" (MTD). Conventional phase I designs do not use Efficacy in the dose-finding algorithm, but usually record it as a secondary outcome. In some phase I trials, a so-called "expansion cohort" of some specified number of additional patients is treated at the chosen MTD in order to obtain a more reliable estimator of the probability of Toxicity at that dose. While, intuitively, the idea of enrolling an expansion cohort at the MTD may seem very sensible, some very undesirable problems that are likely to arise from this common practice will be discussed below.

Phase I trials originated with evaluation of new cytotoxic agents, "chemotherapy," for cancer. The underlying motivation is the assumption that, as dose is increased, the probabilities of both Toxicity and Efficacy must increase. The latter assumption is implicit, however, since Efficacy is not used for making decisions in conventional phase I trials. Logical flaws and undesirable consequences of making this implicit assumption and determining an MTD based on Toxicity while ignoring Efficacy will be discussed below.

Once an MTD has been determined in phase I, conventionally, treatment Efficacy is evaluated in phase II. Most phase II designs are based on a binary indicator of Efficacy, with secondary aims to estimate a variety of other outcomes, such as pharmacokinetic or pharmacodynamic variables. The rationale for using early Efficacy alone for phase II treatment evaluation has three components. The first is that, if the Efficacy event is achieved, this increases the probability of long-term patient benefit, such as extending survival time. The second is that, in early treatment evaluation, it often is impractical to wait to observe long-term events. The third is that, since an MTD has been determined in phase I, safety is no longer a major concern. Severe flaws with this third assumption, and their consequences, will be discussed below.

In oncology, most phase II trials of a new experimental treatment are single-arm, without randomization against a standard treatment. While randomized phase II trials are used more commonly in other disease areas, in oncology a culture of single arm phase II trials continues to persist. In phase II cancer trials, most commonly, Simon's two-stage design (Simon, 1989) is used. This design includes an early stopping rule after its first stage. It has two versions, one optimized to minimize expected sample size and the other to minimize the maximum sample size, each subject to specified Type I and Type II error probability constraints. The Simon design is very simple and very easy to implement using a freely available computer program. It allows one to specify fixed null and alternative response probabilities and Type I and Type II error probabilities and, given these four input values, quickly compute sample sizes and decision cut-offs for the two stages. There are numerous other phase II designs, and a very large literature exists. More complex phase II designs may include more than one interim decision (Fleming, 1982), delayed Efficacy (Cai et al., 2014a), and they may monitor both Efficacy and Toxicity (Thall et al., 1995; Thall and Sung, 1998; Conaway and Petroni,

1995; Bryant and Day, 1995; Thall and Cheng, 1999). As noted earlier, while randomization is more common in phase II trials outside oncology, the use of randomization is very limited in phase II cancer trials. In phase II oncology settings where multiple experimental treatments must be screened, Simon et al. (1985) proposed the idea of using randomization in phase II cancer trials to obtain unbiased treatment comparisons. At that time, this proposal was considered controversial. Unfortunately, despite the great advances of statistical knowledge over the past 30 years, randomization in phase II oncology trials remains controversial (Rubinstein et al., 2005; Sharma et al., 2011; Gan et al., 2010).

If it is concluded based on a phase II trial that an experimental treatment is promising, in that its Efficacy probability is sufficiently high compared to some standard, this may motivate conduct of a confirmatory phase III trial. A typical phase III design is based on survival time or some other long-term outcome, randomizes patients between the experimental treatment and a standard therapy, uses a group sequential testing procedure to decide whether there is a significant treatment difference, controls the overall false positive decision probability to be $\leq .05$, and has specified power, usually .80 or .90, to detect a specified treatment effect difference. Most phase III trials are very large, often last many years, cost millions of dollars, involve multiple medical centers, dozens of physicians, nurses, and other medical and administrative support personnel, and enroll hundreds or thousands of patients. While we will not explore phase III designs here, some useful references are Lan and DeMets (1983); Friedman et al. (2010); Jennison and Turnbull (1999).

Phase II–III designs are a separate topic, but they are quite important and thus worth mentioning. These designs hybridize phase II screening and confirmatory phase III into a single trial. While phase II–III designs certainly are not conventional, they provide practical solutions to severe problems ignored by the conventional clinical trial design paradigm. Unfortunately, phase II–III designs seldom are used in practice. The underlying idea for phase II–III trials was given initially by Ellenberg and Eisenberger (1985), although they did not formalize the methodology. Thall et al. (1988) provided the first formal definition of a phase II–III design, in the context of binary outcomes. This paper included the ideas of combining selection and testing in successive stages of a single trial while controlling overall Type I error, and "generalized power," which is the probability of first correctly selecting and then correctly identifying a single best treatment in a final comparative test. Schaid et al. (1990) addressed the problem in the context of event time outcomes. Their design allows more than one treatment to be selected in the first stage for confirmatory evaluation in a second stage, and it controls pairwise power rather than generalized power. The subsequent literature on phase II–III designs is extensive, including papers by Bauer and Kieser (1999); Stallard and Todd (2003); Liu and Pledger (2005); Bretz et al. (2006); Stallard and Friede (2008), among many others. Reviews of phase II–III designs are given by Thall (2008); Parmar et al. (2008); Korn et al. (2012).

Since most of our experiences with early phase clinical trials have been in oncology, most of the book is oriented around cancer trials. This will be reflected in the way that we present general concepts, our terminology, many of our illustrative examples, and the specific models and decision algorithms that we will discuss. In cancer therapy the main treatment modalities are chemotherapy (chemo), radiation therapy (RT), surgery, stem cell transplantation (SCT), and immunotherapy. Each modality has its own particular forms of Efficacy and Toxicity. We will describe many of these in detail in our illustrative applications. There also are many areas of medicine other than oncology where the designs may be applied usefully. For example, we will present designs to optimize treatment for rapid treatment of acute ischemic stroke, and to optimize the sedative dose given to premature infants being treated for respiratory distress syndrome.

We will refer to the family of designs that we will discuss in this book as "phase I–II" because they combine elements of conventional phase I and phase II trials. There are many different phase I–II designs, with structures motivated by the particular clinical setting, scientific goals, and both ethical and practical constraints. Such trials often are motivated by the fact that the conventional clinical trial paradigm for evaluating new agents or treatment regimes has many logical, scientific, and ethical flaws. Conventional designs do a poor job of optimizing new agents or treatment regimes. It is very likely that, over the years, the failure to reliably optimize new regimes at the start of clinical evaluation in humans has had disastrous consequences. This is because a promising new agent may be crippled quite easily if it is administered at a poorly chosen dose or schedule that is ineffective, unsafe, or effective and safe but substantively suboptimal. A new treatment regime that would have been successful if it had been properly optimized in the early phase of its clinical development, but that instead is given unknowingly at a suboptimal dose or schedule, is more likely to be rejected in a later, large-scale trial. When this sort of false negative occurs, the efforts of medical researchers who have devoted many years to developing new agents are wasted, and people suffering from the disease who would have benefited are denied a treatment advance. It is very likely that the widespread failure to properly optimize doses or schedules of new agents, which preclinical data suggested were very promising, has contributed to the large number of large-scale trials with negative results. Of course, the magnitude of this problem cannot be quantified. Given the importance of reliably optimizing a new agent or treatment regime early in its clinical development, however, the problem should be obvious.

For some new agents, no combination of dose and schedule that is both safe and effective in humans exists. Unfortunately, optimism arising from exciting preclinical results seen in cells or animal models often does not translate into actual clinical advances in humans. In this case, it is critically important to determine this unfortunate fact reliably as early as possible in the clinical evaluation process, to avoid conducting subsequent clinical trials that are likely to be futile. The widespread failure to do this has resulted in an immense waste of resources on clinical trials that never should have been conducted.

Showing practitioners how to identify and deal with these pervasive problems is our main motivation for writing this book. Our goal is to describe state-of-the-art early phase clinical trial designs that may serve either as a bridge, or as a protective barrier, between preclinical treatment development and large scale confirmatory trials.

1.2 The Continual Reassessment Method

The continual reassessment method (CRM), (O'Quigley et al., 1990) is a model-based sequentially adaptive phase I dose-finding design. The CRM was the first design of its kind proposed for dose–finding in early phase trials. Because it uses Toxicity but not Efficacy, it is not a phase I–II design. The CRM assumes a prior dose-Toxicity curve, and repeatedly updates this curve using the observed accumulating Toxicity outcomes from patients in the trial. Based on the updated dose-Toxicity curve, each new cohort of patients is assigned to the dose having posterior mean Toxicity probability closest to a prespecified fixed target Toxicity probability. Because the CRM uses the observed dose-Toxicity data, assumes a dose-Toxicity model, and has an explicit criterion for selecting doses, the 1990 paper triggered subsequent development of numerous sequentially adaptive designs for early phase clinical trials, including phase I–II designs. For phase I, the CRM is much more efficient and yields substantially better operating characteristics than any so called "3+3" design. The most commonly used 3+3 algorithms will be discussed in Section 1.3.

Let $d_1 < d_2 < \cdots < d_J$ denote a set of J prespecified doses for the drug under investigation, and let $p_1 < p_2 < \cdots < p_J$ be prespecified fixed Toxicity probabilities, the CRM model's "skeleton," at those doses. Let Y_T denote the Toxicity indicator and define $\pi_T(d_j, \alpha) = \Pr(Y_T = 1 | d_j, \alpha)$ for $j = 1, \cdots, J$, with α the model parameter. A variety of different "working" models have been used in the CRM to describe the dose-Toxicity curve, including the logistic model and a single-parameter power model, which is used most commonly. The power model defines the Toxicity probability using the fixed skeleton by assuming

$$\pi_T(d_j, \alpha) = p_j^{\exp(\alpha)} \qquad \text{for} \quad j = 1, \cdots, J. \tag{1.1}$$

An alternative 1-parameter logistic model was used by Goodman et al. (1995). They assumed that $\text{logit}^{-1}\{\pi_T(d_j, \alpha)\} = 3 + \alpha x_j$ where the standardized dose is $x_j = \Phi^{-1}\{(p_j)^{\exp(1)}\}$, denoting the $N(0, 1)$ pdf by Φ, with prior $f(\alpha) = \exp(-\alpha)$ for $\alpha > 0$. Many other models have been used to implement the CRM.

Suppose that, at an interim point during trial conduct, among n_j patients treated at dose level j, m_j have experienced Toxicity, $j = 1, \cdots, J$. The likelihood function of $n = \sum_{j=1}^{J} n_j$ treated patients is

$$\mathcal{L}_n = \prod_{j=1}^{J} \{p_j^{\exp(\alpha)}\}^{m_j} \{1 - p_j^{\exp(\alpha)}\}^{n_j - m_j}.$$

Denote the data from the first n patients by $\mathcal{D}_n = \{(d_{[1]}, Y_1), \cdots, (d_{[n]}, Y_n)\}$, where $d_{[i]}$ denotes the dose administered and $Y_i = \mathrm{I}(\text{Toxicity})$ for the ith patient. Using Bayes' theorem, the Toxicity probabilities $\pi_T(d_j, \alpha)$, for $j = 1, \cdots, J$, can be estimated by their posterior means,

$$\begin{aligned}
\hat{\pi}_{T,n}(d_j, \alpha) &= E\{\pi_T(d_j, \alpha)|\mathcal{D}_n\} \\
&= \int p_j^{\exp(\alpha)} \frac{\mathcal{L}_n f(\alpha)}{\int \mathcal{L}_n f(\beta) d\beta} d\alpha
\end{aligned}$$

where $f(\cdot)$ is a prior distribution for the parameter α. Alternatively (cf. Goodman et al., 1995), the posterior mean $\hat{\alpha}_n = E(\alpha|\mathcal{D}_n)$ may be used as a plug-in estimator to compute the approximation $\pi_T(d_j, \hat{\alpha}_n)$. Typically, the prior is assumed to be a normal distribution $N(0, \sigma_\alpha^2)$, i.e.,

$$f(\alpha) = \frac{1}{\sqrt{2\pi}\sigma_\alpha} \exp\left(-\frac{\alpha^2}{2\sigma_\alpha^2}\right),$$

with the single hyperparameter σ_α^2 fixed at a value near 2.

Let π_T^* denote the target Toxicity probability specified by physicians, and N a specified maximum sample size. The CRM can be described as follows:

1. Patients in the first cohort are treated at the lowest dose d_1, or at a higher starting dose specified by the physician.

2. The posterior estimates of the mean Toxicity probabilities, $\hat{\pi}_{T,n}(d_j, \alpha) = E\{\pi_T(d_j, \alpha)|\mathcal{D}_n\}$ for $j = 1, \cdots, J$, are computed based on the current accumulated data, $\mathcal{D}_n$. The next cohort is treated at the dose level j_n^* having posterior mean Toxicity probability closest to π_T^*, i.e.,

$$j_n^* = \operatorname*{argmin}_{j=1,\cdots,J} \left|\hat{\pi}_{T,n}(d_j, \alpha) - \pi_T^*\right|.$$

3. Once the maximum sample size N is reached, the dose that has posterior mean Toxicity probability $\hat{\pi}_{T,N}(d_j, \alpha)$ closest to π_T^* based on $\mathcal{D}_N$ is selected as the MTD.

In practice, when using the CRM additional safety rules often are added. The first rule is that an untried dose may not be skipped when escalating, as suggested by Goodman et al. (1995), although the original CRM (1990) allows dose skipping. The second safety rule stops the trial if the lowest dose is too toxic, formally if $\Pr(\pi_T(d_1, \alpha) > \pi_T^* | \mathcal{D}_n) > p_U$, with typical cut-off values p_U = .80, .85, .90, or .95.

From a logical viewpoint, a natural question is why it is better to have a dose with Toxicity probability close to a given target π_T^*, rather than simply not treating the patient, which would ensure that $\pi_T = 0$, i.e., that Toxicity is impossible. For example, applying the CRM with $\pi_T^* = .30$ says that it is better to have Toxicity probability .30 than the lower value .10. The answer is that, like any phase I method based on Toxicity alone, the CRM relies on the implicit assumption that there is some Efficacy outcome for which $\pi_E(d)$ = $\Pr(Y_E = 1 | d)$ increases with d, where Y_E indicates Efficacy. For settings where an Efficacy outcome cannot be observed early enough to be included in an adaptive dose-finding decision, Efficacy may be characterized by a longer term outcome, such as progression-free survival (PFS) time. In this case, the implicit assumption is that, on average, PFS time must increase with dose d. This practice arose in the context of evaluating new cytotoxic agents, where it is realistic to assume that the probabilities or mean probabilities of both Toxicity and Efficacy must increase with dose. In practice, if this monotonicity assumption for Efficacy is not true, then it makes no sense to apply the CRM or any other dose escalation method based only on Toxicity for dose-finding. An example is a biologic agent for which the dose-Efficacy curve initially increases but then reaches a plateau where higher doses do not improve Efficacy, but $\pi_T(d)$ still increases with d. This case will be discussed in Chapters 7 and 9.

Many generalizations of the CRM have been proposed to handle more challenging dose-finding settings where the outcome is more complex than a single binary variable observed quickly after the start of treatment. Cheung and Chappell (2000) proposed the time-to-event CRM (TITE-CRM), which utilizes right censored time-to-Toxicity data. The TITE-CRM provides a practical solution to the common logistical problem that Toxicity might not be observed immediately, and must be defined as occurring or not over a given time interval, such as 90 days. This problem arises in trials to study radiation therapy (RT), where late-onset toxicities are commonplace and may occur six months or later from the start of therapy. In such settings, a binary Toxicity indicator cannot be scored as "No Toxicity" until the patient has been followed for the entire interval without Toxicity being observed. Moreover, Toxicity may occur late during the observation interval, so in any case one often must wait a non-trivial amount of time to observe each patient's outcome. This may delay and complicate adaptive decision-making, and it also introduces bias in the estimators of the $\pi_T(d_j)$'s. Braun (2002) extended the CRM to model bivariate competing outcomes. Liu et al. (2013) developed a Bayesian data augmentation CRM to handle late-onset toxicities, thus providing an improved solution to the problem first addressed by Cheung and Chappell (2000). Bekele and Thall (2004) used elicited weights for severity grades of several qualitatively different toxicities to define total Toxicity burden (TTB), with each successive dose chosen to have posterior mean TTB closest to a pre-specified elicited target. This is similar to the CRM, but uses

TTB in place of $\pi_T(d)$ as a decision criterion. Van Meter et al. (2011) extended the CRM to accommodate ordinal Toxicity. A limitation of the CRM is that its behavior is highly dependent on the numerical values of the skeleton, $(p_1, \cdots, p_J)$, which must be pre-specified and fixed in advance. In some cases, assuming a particular skeleton may cause the CRM to behave pathologically (Cheung, 2005). Yin and Yuan (2009b) addressed this problem by proposing the Bayesian model averaging CRM (BMA-CRM), which improves the robustness of the CRM by providing a formal basis for specifying several possible skeletons. For each adaptive decision, the BMA-CRM first uses the data to compute an average model, and then applies this to determine a dose. Pan et al. (2014) extended BMA-CRM to accommodate ordinal Toxicity. A thorough account of the CRM and many of its generalizations is given in the monograph by Cheung (2011), who also provides computer software for implementation.

1.3 Problems with Conventional Dose-Finding Methods

"Common sense is not so common."

Voltaire

1.3.1 3+3 Algorithms

The designs used most commonly for dose-finding in phase I trials are variants of the so-called "3+3 algorithm." This actually is a family of algorithms, and there are numerous versions. Table 1.1 gives a specification of a 3+3 algorithm that is used very commonly as a boilerplate in many phase I protocols. Whatever version of the 3+3 algorithm is used, it almost always is given in a simple form, such as that in Table 1.1, that is very intuitively appealing but in fact is incomplete and does not specify fully what to do in many cases. Consequently, in actual trial conduct, many subjective decisions must be made by physicians or research nurses based on their interpretations of whatever rules are given in the protocol. In addition to their apparent simplicity, a major reason for the popularity of 3+3 algorithms is that they do not require a computer program or a statistician to implement. However, 3+3 algorithms have no explicit criteria for what a good or bad dose may be. They are just decision rules.

To see why the 3+3 algorithm given in Table 1.1 is incomplete, consider the following possibilities.

1. In some cases, an MTD as defined does not exist, and the algorithm does not say what to do or what to conclude. This occurs, for example, if either

TABLE 1.1: A common boilerplate phase I protocol 3+3 algorithm

Number of Patients with a DLT at a Given Dose Level	Escalation Decision Rule
0/3	Enter 3 patients at the next dose level.
1/3	Enter at least 3 more patients at this dose level • If 0 of these 3 patients experience DLT, proceed to the next dose level. • If ≥ 1 of this group suffer DLT, this dose exceeds the MTD and dose escalation is stopped. 3 additional patients will be entered at the next lower dose level if only 3 patients were treated previously at that dose.
≥ 2	Dose escalation will be stopped. This dose level will be declared the maximally administered dose (highest dose administered). Three (3) additional patients will be entered at the next lower dose level if only 3 patients were treated previously at that dose.

<u>MTD</u>: The highest dose at which no more than 1 of 6 evaluable
patients has had a DLT. Six patients should be treated
before the dose is declared as MTD.

2/3 DLTs are seen at the lowest dose level or 0/3 DLTs are observed at the highest dose level.

2. The use of " ≥ 2" in the left-hand column of Table 1.1 is ambiguous because it does not specify a denominator. For example, 2/3, 2/6, and 2/9 DLTs have three very different meanings.

3. The absence of a stopping rule creates ambiguity. For example, suppose that you observe 0/3 DLTs at level 1, 0/3 at level 2, 1/3 + 1/3 at level 3, and so de-escalate to level 2, treat 3 more and observe 0/3, for a total of 0/6 at level 2. It is not specified whether one then should treat 3 more at level 2, or stop and declare level 2 the MTD. If one decides to treat 3 more at level 2, then the data at that level could be 0, 1, 2, or 3 DLTs in 9 patients. It is not specified what the decisions should be for each of these four possibilities.

   Due to the absence of sufficiently specific rules, in actual trial conduct the decision of what dose to give each new patient or cohort often must be made subjectively. Beyond the fact that the above boilerplate for a 3+3 algorithm is incomplete in that it leaves many decisions unspecified, a severe problem is that many oncologists are taught that a decision as important as choosing a dose level in a phase I trial never should be left in the hands of a statistician, but rather should be made by the attending physician based on their clinical judgment. This confuses medical practice with conduct of a clinical trial, which is a scientific experiment. Making dose-finding decisions in a subjective manner that varies from physician to physician is not a clinical trial, and it serves patients poorly. A very important point in this regard is that optimal sequential decisions based on rational and ethical criteria that maximize benefit to the patients in the trial and to future patients often are not intuitively obvious. The main difficulty in specifying statistical designs for early phase clinical trials is that they must produce decision rules that are clinically reasonable, ethical, and rational.

While there are many versions in the family of 3+3 algorithms, Table 1.2 gives completely specified versions of two commonly used forms, both allowing the possibility that the first cohort is treated at a dose level above the lowest. This complete specification allows the behavior of these 3+3 algorithms to be simulated on a computer so that they may be compared to other methods. Even with these complete specifications, however, these 3+3 algorithms suffer from two severe flaws common to all versions of the so-called "3+3 algorithm." The first flaw is that all 3+3 algorithms have short memories, and fail to use all of the available data from previously treated patients when making decisions. The second flaw is that 3+3 algorithms produce phase I trials with very small sample sizes, hence very unreliable results. We will illustrate the consequences of these flaws below.

1.3.2   Some Comparisons

Because most phase I protocols do not fully specify a 3+3 algorithm, as noted above there is insufficient detail to write a computer program to simulate the algorithm actually used in order to study its behavior. We can evaluate the 3+3 algorithms given in Table 1.2, however. To do this usefully, we include the Efficacy–Toxicity (EffTox) trade-off design (Thall and Cook, 2004), which will be presented in detail in Chapter 4, as one of comparators, along with the CRM, 3+3A, and 3+3B designs. While we are getting ahead of ourselves, so to speak, by including EffTox, it is worthwhile to include this phase I–II design in this early comparative example since our purpose, in part, is to motivate you to read the rest of the book. Moreover, many flaws in phase I methods can be seen by comparing them to phase I–II designs. The simulations, given below, show how badly one can go astray in an early phase trial if a bad design, such as the 3+3A or 3+3B, is used, or Efficacy is ignored by using a phase I design.

As general notation for bivariate binary outcomes, let Y_E and Y_T denote indicators of Efficacy and Toxicity, with $Y = (Y_E, Y_T)$. Given the doses $d_1 < d_2 < \cdots < d_J$ to be studied, denote the marginal probabilities

$$\pi_k(d_j, \theta) = \Pr(Y_k = 1 \mid d_j, \theta) \ \text{ for } k = E, T, \ \ j = 1, \cdots, J,$$

with θ the vector of model parameters. When no meaning is lost, we will use the notation $\pi_{k,j}$ or $\pi_{k,j}(\theta) = \pi_k(d_j, \theta)$. Denote the prior means by $\mu_{k,j} =$

TABLE 1.2: Two commonly used phase I trial 3+3 algorithms

General Rules

1. Never re-escalate to a level after de-escalating from that level
2. If the decision is to de-escalate or choose one level lower but current level is lowest, stop and choose no level
3. If decision is to escalate above highest level, stop and choose no level
4. If decision is to stop and choose one level lower, but one level lower has 3 or fewer patients, treat 3 more at that lower level

# toxicities/ # patients	Decision
0/3	Escalate one level, if allowed by General Rule 1, otherwise treat 3 more at current level.
0/3 + [0/3 or 1/3]†	Stop, choose *current* level as MTD
0/3 + 2/3†	<u>3+3 A</u>: Stop, choose *one level lower* as MTD
0/3 + 2/3†	<u>3+3 B</u>: Stop, choose *current level* as MTD
0/3 + 3/3†	Stop, choose *one level lower* as MTD
1/3	Treat 3 more at *current* level
1/3 + 1/3	<u>3+3 A</u>: Stop, choose *one level lower* as MTD
1/3 + 1/3	<u>3+3 B</u>: Stop, choose *current* level as MTD
2/3 or 3/3	De-escalate one level
1/3 + 0/3	Escalate one level if allowed by General Rule 1, otherwise choose *current* level as MTD
1/3 + [2/3 or 3/3]	Stop, choose *one level lower* as MTD

† after de-escalating back to this level from a higher level

$E\{\pi_{k,j}(\theta)\}$, with vectors $\mu_k = (\mu_{k,1}, \cdots, \mu_{k,J})$ for $k = E, T$. We will use π_E and π_T to denote generic marginal probabilities, and $\pi = (\pi_E, \pi_T)$. We will write the joint probabilities as $\pi(a, b) = \Pr(Y_E = a, _T = b)$, for $a, b = 0, 1$.

Briefly, EffTox is a phase I–II design based on either a bivariate binary or a trinary outcome (Thall and Cook, 2004). It relies on a trade-off function, $\phi(\pi) = \phi(\pi_E, \pi_T)$, that is defined for π in the unit square $[0, 1]^2$ in the bivariate binary case, or for π in the triangle where $\pi_E + \pi_T \leq 1$ in the trinary case. The trade-off function $\phi(\pi)$ increases with π_E and decreases with π_T, with higher values of ϕ corresponding to more desirable π pairs. The EffTox design includes two dose acceptability rules, based on a fixed upper limit $\bar{\pi}_T$ on all $\pi_{T,j}(\theta)$ and a fixed lower limit $\underline{\pi}_E$ on all $\pi_{E,j}(\theta)$. Either of these rules may stop the trial early if no dose is acceptable. The EffTox design is applied with a specified cohort size c and maximum sample size N. This design will be described in detail in Chapter 4.

Table 1.3 summarizes simulations that compare the 3+3A and 3+3B algorithms given in Table 1.2, the CRM, and the EffTox design in each of four dose-outcome scenarios, for the case where Y is a bivariate binary outcome. The numerical doses are 100, 200, 300, 400, 500. In these simulations, the EffTox design was implemented with upper probability limit $\bar{\pi}_T = .40$ on Toxicity, lower probability limit $\underline{\pi}_E = .20$ on Efficacy, fixed posterior admissibility probability cut-offs $p_{E,L} = p_{T,L} = .10$, prior means $\mu_T = (.05, .10, .15, .20, .30)$ and $\mu_E = (.20, .30, .45, .60, .70)$, prior effective sample size ESS $= .90$, and target trade-off contour determined by the three (π_E, π_T) pairs $(.50, 0)$, $(1, .70)$, and $(.70, .25)$. The upper limit $\bar{\pi}_T = .40$ is used for a Toxicity safety stopping rule like that given above for the CRM, and the lower limit $\underline{\pi}_E = .20$ is used in a futility stopping rule that requires a dose to have Efficacy probabilities at least .20 in order to be considered acceptable. The improved version of EffTox described by Thall et al. (2014a) was used, with computations done using version 4.0 of the EffTox program. This more recent version of EffTox uses precisely the same structures and principles as that originally given in 2004, but it provides explicit methods and algorithms for the critically important problems of specifying the prior hyperparameters and target trade-off contour. This provides an explicit basis for avoiding specifying a design that may have pathological properties because either the prior or the contour were not calibrated properly. The CRM was simulated with target $\pi_T^* = .30$, fixed skeleton $(p_1, \cdots, p_5) = (.10, .20, .35, .40, .45)$, $\sigma_\alpha^2 = 2$, and the rule to stop the trial early and choose no MTD if $\Pr\{\pi_T(d_1, \alpha) > .30 \mid data_n\} > .90$. This rule says to stop the trial if, based on the interim data, the lowest dose is likely to have Toxicity probability larger than the target .30. Each design was evaluated for cohort size 3, maximum sample sizes $N = 30, 45$, or 60, with 10,000 replications of each combination of design and scenario of true Efficacy and Toxicity probabilities assumed for the simulation.

For each (outcome,dose) index pair (k, j), denote the fixed, assumed "true" value of $\pi_{k,j}(\theta)$ used to simulate each scenario by $\pi_{k,j}^{true}$ or True $\pi_{k,j}$. It is important to note that an assumed fixed value $\pi_{k,j}^{true}$ used in a simulation

TABLE 1.3: Comparison of the 3+3A, 3+3B, CRM, and EffTox design

			Dose Level					
			d_1	d_2	d_3	d_4	d_5	None
Scenario 1	True $\pi_E(d_j)$		.05	.10	.30	.55	.60	
	True $\pi_T(d_j)$		.10	.20	.35	.40	.60	
	Trade-off		34	32	38	58	48	
$N=30$	3+3 A		29	39	16	6	0	11
	3+3 B		19	39	25	11	1	5
	CRM		2	38	45	13	2	0
	EffTox		2	11	25	28	25	9
$N=45$	CRM		0	36	52	10	1	0
	EffTox		1	8	28	37	16	10
$N=60$	CRM		0	34	58	8	0	0
	EffTox		0	7	30	42	10	12
Scenario 2	True $\pi_E(d_j)$		.30	.60	.65	.70	.75	
	True $\pi_T(d_j)$		.20	.25	.45	.60	.70	
	Trade-off		48	81	66	59	57	
$N=60$	3+3 A		30	31	7	0	0	31
	3+3 B		31	38	15	1	0	15
	CRM		9	70	17	0	0	4
	EffTox		14	54	28	3	1	1
Scenario 3	True $\pi_E(d_j)$		.05	.10	.30	.50	.70	
	True $\pi_T(d_j)$		.05	.10	.20	.30	.35	
	Trade-off		37	38	48	61	86	
$N=60$	3+3 A		10	28	31	16	0	15
	3+3 B		5	19	33	24	6	13
	CRM		0	0	21	40	38	0
	EffTox		0	3	14	13	68	1
Scenario 4	True $\pi_E(d_j)$		.01	.02	.04	.06	.07	
	True $\pi_T(d_j)$		.12	.15	.30	.50	.55	
	Trade-off		30	30	24	18	17	
$N=60$	3+3 A		18	38	27	3	0	15
	3+3 B		15	32	38	9	1	6
	CRM		0	13	77	9	0	1
	EffTox		0	0	1	3	3	93

* For each scenario and dose-finding method, the tabled values are the dose selection percentages for each dose level.

study is not the same object as a Bayesian model-based probability, such as $\pi_k(d_j, \theta)$, which is random because θ is random, in order to reflect actual uncertainty in the underlying model used by the design.

In all four scenarios, regardless of the specified maximum N, the 3+3 algorithms produce sample sizes having medians varying from 12 to 18 and maximum 30. In Scenario 1, the true probability of Efficacy jumps between d_3 and d_4, from $\pi_{E,3}^{true} = .30$ to $\pi_{E,4}^{true} = .55$, while $\pi_{T,j}^{true}$ is reasonably low for dose levels $j = 1,...,4$ but then jumps up from $\pi_{T,4}^{true} = .40$ to $\pi_{T,5}^{true} = .60$. This is reflected by the Efficacy–Toxicity trade-off value, which is estimated and used by EffTox but not by the other methods, taking its highest level at d_4. In this scenario, for $N = 30$, the 3+3 algorithms choose the lower doses most often, and choose d_1 or d_2, which are ineffective doses in that they have $\pi_E \leq .10$, 68% and 58% of the time, with 3+3A choosing no dose 11% of the time. The 3+3B algorithm is more likely to pick higher doses than 3+3A, which is the case in general. The CRM with fixed target $\pi_T^* = .30$, does a good job of selecting d_3 using Toxicity alone. Its selection percentages for d_3 increase monotonically with maximum sample size N, with respective selection percentages for d_3 of 45%, 52%, and 58% for $N = 30$, 45, and 60. Since the EffTox method uses both Efficacy and Toxicity, it is more likely to pick d_4, with the selection percentages for d_4 increasing correspondingly with N from 28% to 37% to 42%. The key point illustrated by this scenario is that, by using the trade-off function, EffTox considers the pair $(\pi_{E,4}^{true}, \pi_{T,4}^{true}) = (.55, .40)$ more desirable than the pair $(\pi_{E,3}^{true}, \pi_{T,3}^{true}) = (.30, .35)$, so it considers d_4 best and chooses it most often. In contrast, ignoring Efficacy and using the CRM with target $\pi_T^* = .30$ leads most often to the conclusion that d_3 is best. The CRM and EffTox also were simulated for $N = 45$ and 60 to show that, given their respective criteria, their reliabilities both improve with sample size. Values for the 3+3 algorithms are not shown because they stop so quickly that they simply do not employ these larger sample sizes, hence their properties do not change for $N = 45$ or 60.

Since Scenario 1 illustrates how the four methods' behaviors change with maximum sample size, the comparisons in Scenarios 2, 3, and 4 are given only for maximum sample size 60. In Scenario 2, the jump in π_E occurs at the lowest doses, with $\pi_{E,1}^{true} = .30$ and $\pi_{E,2}^{true} = .60$, and the probabilities of Toxicity at these doses are low but then rapidly increase. Here, the EffTox trade-off is highest at d_2. In this scenario, the 3+3 algorithms again are likely to select lower doses, choosing d_1 or d_2 about 60% to 70% of the time, with 3+3A choosing no dose 31% of the time. The CRM with target $\pi_T^* = .30$ reliably chooses d_2 is best, since $\pi_{T,2}^{true} = .25$ is closest to the target .30. The EffTox method also is most likely to pick d_2, since here d_2 also has the highest trade-off value. Essentially, although the CRM ignores Efficacy, in this scenario it gets lucky.

In Scenario 3, Toxicity is acceptable at all doses levels, while $\pi_{E,j}^{true}$ increases to a very high level $\pi_{E,5}^{true} = .70$ at the highest dose, which has by far the largest trade-off value. Again, the 3+3 algorithms have very disperse dose selection distributions, and have probabilities .15 and .13 of choosing no dose. The CRM selects d_4 most often since $\pi_{T,4}^{true} = .30$, whereas the most desirable dose in terms of the trade-off function is d_5, which is chosen by the EffTox design 68% of the time.

Scenario 4 is very important, because it illustrates what can happen if an agent is ineffective but causes substantial Toxicity, and a phase I design, that by definition ignores Efficacy, is used. In contrast, like any reasonable phase II design, a reasonable phase I–II design will include a futility rule based on the observed Efficacy outcomes that will stop the trial early if the data show convincingly that the agent does not provide some specified minimal level of anti-disease effect. Given the fact that all $\pi_{E,k}^{true} \le .07$ in Scenario 4, ideally one would like to stop the trial and not choose any dose. The EffTox design does this 93% of the time, and on average treats 22 patients before it stops the trial. In this case, the futility stopping rule is determined by the fixed lower limit $\underline{\pi}_E = .20$ used by EffTox, which is the value used most often in phase IIA activity trials. The 3+3 designs choose dose levels 1, 2, or 3, which have Efficacy probabilities .01 to .04, 83% and 85% of the time. The CRM chooses d_3, which has true Toxicity probability $\pi_{T,3}^{true} = .30$, the target, 64% of the time. Since the CRM ignores Efficacy, it does not know that the Efficacy probability at d_3 is only .04, has no provision for stopping if the agent is ineffective, and is almost certain to treat all 60 patients, with on average 16 experiencing Toxicity.

Notice that, since 1 to 3 responses may be expected among 60 patients in Scenario 4, any reasonable futility rule based on the observed response data would be very likely to stop the trial early. Recall that phase I designs, which simply ignore Efficacy, choose a dose using dose-Toxicity data only, by relying on the *implicit* assumption that the true dose-Efficacy curve $(\pi_{E,1}^{true}, \cdots, \pi_{E,J}^{true})$ increases substantially with dose to a level that is promising. However, the conventional paradigm leaves the actual level of Efficacy to be determined later, in a phase II trial conducted at the chosen MTD. Based on Scenario 4, it may be argued generally that a phase I design, which by definition ignores Efficacy, is less ethical than a phase I–II design, since a phase I design risks exposing a large number of patients to Toxicity even when the agent is ineffective, as the CRM does in Scenario 4. By ignoring Efficacy in a case like Scenario 4, one is ignoring data that may show empirically that the rationale underlying the phase I method is false.

The simulations show how the EffTox method uses more of the available information by relying on an explicit trade-off between π_E and π_T and, within limits, it allows higher Toxicity as the price for higher Efficacy. That is, EffTox makes explicit the implicit assumption underlying the CRM and other phase I methods based on Toxicity alone. This illustrates the essential difference between phase I designs that use Toxicity only and phase I–II designs that use both Efficacy and Toxicity. This difference is not simply a matter of taste or opinion, because it may have profound consequences in subsequent clinical development and decision making, as we will explain below. Another important general point illustrated by this example is that optimizing dose based on a bivariate binary outcome is a much harder problem than optimizing dose based on one binary outcome. The phase I–II problem becomes more difficult still when Y_E and Y_T are either ordinal or time-to-event variables. In general, while it is better to use more of the available information, doing sequential decision making becomes harder as Y becomes more complex. This is because, unavoidably, the model for $P(Y \mid d, \theta)$ and decision criteria also must become more complex.

A general conclusion from these simulations is that, compared to either the CRM or EffTox, in terms of average performance both 3+3 algorithms are complete disasters. The 3+3 algorithms produce very disperse dose selection percentage distributions, are likely to choose an ineffective dose, often fail to choose any dose, and always stop with very small sample sizes. As an illustrative example, Table 1.4 gives dose-Toxicity data from a typical phase I trial conducted using a 3+3 algorithm. In this example, a total of 18 patients were treated. The usual claim at the end of such a trial is "The maximum tolerable dose is 30." However, computing posterior credible intervals (ci's) starting with a beta(.50, .50) prior on each $\pi_T(d_j, \theta)$, the 95% posterior ci for $\pi_T(20, \theta)$ at the MTD runs from .00 to .54. In terms of their 95% ci's, all four doses are consistent with a Toxicity probability anywhere between .08 and .54, which says that one knows very little about the dose-Toxicity distribution. If, as an alternative data analysis, a logistic regression model

$$\pi_{T,j}(\alpha, \beta) = \frac{e^{\alpha + \beta \log(d_j)}}{1 + e^{\alpha + \beta \log(d_j)}}$$

is fit to these data to borrow strength between doses, final inferences are improved, but still are not very informative. Assuming non-informative priors $\alpha \sim N(1, 1000)$ and $\log(\beta) \sim N(1, 10)$ and fitting this model to the data, the resulting posterior 95% credible intervals are given in the right-hand column of Table 1.4 and displayed in Figure 1.1, which gives the posterior mean curve and 95% ci bands from the fitted model. These ci's are more narrow due to the assumed model, but they still provide little information. Based on the 95% ci's, the data are consistent with all four doses having Toxicity probabilities between .16 and .25, there is almost no evidence to distinguish reliably between doses 20 and 30, and almost nothing is known about the risk of Toxicity at dose 40. The simple point of this example is that, at the completion of a typical phase I trial using a 3+3 algorithm that produces a final sample of size 18, almost nothing of any practical use is known about the dose-Toxicity curve. Declaring any of the four doses to be "the MTD" based on such data is nonsense.

The problem that conventional phase I dose-finding trials have very small sample sizes that produce very unreliable results is extremely important. In the current culture of clinical trials, it often is considered a good thing to complete phase I trials quickly, with small samples sizes. This is completely contrary to the fundamental statistical principle that the reliability of any

TABLE 1.4: Typical data from a phase I trial after using a 3+3 algorithm

Dose	# Tox/# Pats	Posterior 95% Credible Intervals	
		Independent beta(.5, .5) priors	Logistic regression model
10	0/3	.00 – .54	.00 – .25
20	0/3	.00 – .54	.02 – .29
30	1/6	.02 – .56	.09 – .37
40	2/6	.08 – .71	.16 – .62

valid inference improves monotonically with sample size. This is illustrated in Table 1.3 for both the CRM and EffTox which, unlike a 3+3 algorithm, both may be implemented with any given maximum sample size N, and thus may be used to obtain more reliable results if N is increased.

The issue that small sample sizes give unreliable estimates is very closely related to the issue that phase I dose-finding designs ignore Efficacy. The small sample of Toxicity data in Table 1.4 are consistent with, for example, true Toxicity probabilities (.05, .10, .15, .25) at the four doses, in which case all doses probably would be considered safe. The tabled Toxicity data also are consistent with *any* true Efficacy probabilities, simply because Efficacy data are not given. If the true Efficacy probabilities at the four doses were, say, (.05, .10, .25, .50), then choosing $d = 30$, which has $\pi_{T,3}^{true} = .15$ and $\pi_{E,3}^{true} = .25$, would miss the much larger $\pi_{E,4}^{true} = .50$ at $d = 40$. In this case, which is not at all unlikely in practice, choosing $d = 30$ rather than $d = 40$ would result in a large loss in future patient benefit. The common assumption is that progression-free survival (PFS) and overall survival (OS) time increase substantially if Efficacy is achieved, and they also may increase with dose due to direct treatment effects not mediated through an early Efficacy event. Thus, if $d = 30$ were used in subsequent phase II or phase III evaluation, this likely would reduce the new agent's ability to succeed in these later trials due to the lost benefit in PFS and OS time that could have been achieved if $d = 40$ had been used. That is, the agent has not been optimized.

This simple example, and the fact that a typical dose-finding trial with $N = 18$ patients provides very little information for moving forward sensibly with treatment development, together imply that both Efficacy and Toxicity should be used for dose-finding. The example also implies that the sample sizes of dose-finding trials should be large, not small. A phase I trial is not an obstacle to be overcome quickly. Rather, if possible it should be a phase I–II trial, and that trial should be regarded as an experiment to obtain precious information about how to optimize a new agent. Consequently, it is in the best interests of all, including patients and all those involved in developing and evaluating a potential new anti-disease treatment regime, that a phase

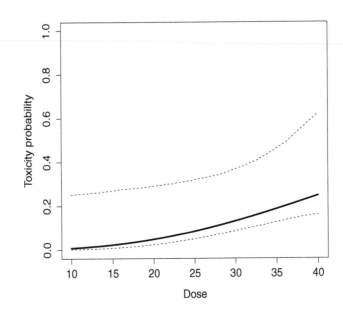

FIGURE 1.1: Logistic regression model-based posterior mean (solid line) and 95 per cent credible interval bands (dashed lines) for $\pi_T(d, \theta)$ as a function of dose d, based on the data in Table 1.4.

I–II trial should be sufficiently large to ensure that the regime optimization is highly reliable.

1.3.3 Problems Going from Phase I to Phase II

A very common problem that arises following a small phase I trial is that the chosen MTD quite easily may turn out to be too toxic in a subsequent phase II trial. For example, if the true Toxicity probabilities giving the data in Table 1.4 were (.25, .35, .40, .60), and the true Efficacy probabilities were (.01, .02, .05, .10), then a dose with $\pi_{E,3}^{true} = .05$ and $\pi_{T,3}^{true} = .40$ has been selected. That is, the chosen MTD is inefficacious and carries a 40% risk of Toxicity. In this case, a two-stage optimal Simon design with null Efficacy probability $p_0 = .05$, targeted value $p_1 = .20$, and Type I and II error probabilities both .10, would require 37 patients to be treated in its first stage. Since about 15/37 patients would be expected to have Toxicity in this case, it is likely that the investigators would find it necessary to violate the Simon design, which does not include any rules involving Toxicity, and stop the trial due to excessive Toxicity for ethical reasons long before reaching the stage 1 sample size. At that point, it might be concluded that some dose below the chosen MTD could be worth investigating, but precisely how one would go about doing that, given the data already obtained, and using either a conventional phase I or phase II design, is unclear. This example illustrates a very likely, very undesirable outcome if Toxicity alone is used in a phase I trial with a small sample size to chose a MTD, and Efficacy alone is used in a subsequent phase II trial to evaluate the treatment at that MTD. In contrast, any reasonable phase I–II design would be very likely to stop early due to the agent being ineffective, aside from its Toxicity. For example, if the EffTox design considered earlier were used, with numerical values corresponding to the previous dose levels 1, 2, 4, and 5 in order to correspond to this example, that design would stop the trial early due to low Efficacy with probability .93, with the conclusion that no dose should be chosen. Essentially, EffTox includes a phase II futility stopping rule formulated in terms of the $\pi_{E,j}$'s, which should be a component of any reasonable phase I–II design.

These examples may be summarized by the following key points for settings where both Efficacy and Toxicity may be observed quickly enough to make adaptive decisions.

1. 3+3 algorithms do a poor job of choosing a MTD.
2. Conventional phase I sample sizes are far too small.
3. It often does not make sense to base dose-finding on Toxicity alone.
4. It does not make sense to design a phase II trial based on Efficacy alone, since safety is an important concern in any clinical trial and the trial must be stopped if excessive Toxicity is observed.
5. The inclusion of a rule based on Efficacy to stop for futility in phase I–II underscores the important point that, at the completion of a phase I–II trial, there is no reason to conduct a conventional phase II trial since it already has been done.

With regard to point 3, important exceptions are settings where either Efficacy or Toxicity are not observed quickly enough to make outcome-adaptive decisions. In such settings, there may be two reasonable practical options. One approach is to do adaptive dose-finding based on time-to-event Efficacy and Toxicity outcomes. A much simpler approach is to take the conventional approach of relying on Toxicity alone for adaptive dose-finding, if this is feasible, while estimating late-onset or longitudinal Efficacy. These cases will be discussed in Chapters 4 and 12.

1.3.4 Consequences of Ignoring Information

The comparative simulation study given in 1.3.2 shows that, if one uses Toxicity alone to choose a dose, the CRM is greatly superior to any 3+3 algorithm. It also shows that, if one uses both Efficacy and Toxicity to choose a dose with EffTox, in cases where $\pi_{E,j}^{true}$ increases sharply with dose the final selected dose is very likely to be higher than that chosen by the CRM. The two methods use different data and different decision criteria and, like any reasonable phase I–II method, EffTox is more complex than the CRM. In order to use Efficacy as well as Toxicity, EffTox employs a trade-off function that allows higher $\pi_{T,j}^{true}$ if sufficiently high $\pi_{E,j}^{true}$ is achieved, which makes explicit the risk–benefit assessment that underlies most clinical decision making. EffTox also has two admissibility criteria that act as gatekeepers to screen out doses that are either inefficacious or too toxic. The simulations provide convincing illustrations of the fact that EffTox is much more likely to select more desirable doses in cases where the CRM cannot because it ignores Efficacy. Thus, the general approach of using Toxicity only while implicitly making the assumption that $\pi_{E,j}^{true}$ increases with dose appears to be inferior to making this assumption explicitly. Put another way, it is better to use relevant available information of treatment Efficacy rather than ignore it. Furthermore, ignoring Efficacy in phase I dose-finding is at odds with the fact that the primary purpose of treatment is to achieve anti-disease effect.

It often is argued that, if Efficacy is observed in phase I at a dose level above the MTD, then this information somehow will be taken into account. In addition to the fact that phase I designs have no formal provisions for how this may be done, it implies that "Toxicity only" phase I designs are inadequate and should account for Efficacy. That is, the implication is that a phase I–II design is needed.

In phase I–II trials with bivariate binary outcome (Y_E, Y_T), one commonly used approach is to base dose-finding on the probability of the best possible event, [Success] $= (Y_E = 1, Y_T = 0)$, Efficacy with no Toxicity. This approach reduces the problem to the one-dimensional case, hence dose-finding may be based on a simple univariate model for Pr(success) as a function of dose. Unfortunately, this approach can lead quite easily to highly flawed conclusions. This is because it treats the three elementary events $(Y_E, Y_T) = (1,1)$, $(0,0)$, and $(0,1)$ as being equivalent "failure" events, when in fact they are very different outcomes. The outcome $(Y_E, Y_T) = (1,1)$ is that both Efficacy and Toxicity occur, while $(Y_E, Y_T) = (0,0)$ is the outcome that neither event occurs, which can be achieved by not treating the patient. In terms of the way that many cytotoxics and other types of agents behave biologically, intensifying therapy by increasing dose very often is likely to increase the probabilities of both Efficacy and Toxicity. That is, the joint probability that both events occur is likely to increase with dose. Thus, optimistically calling $(Y_E = 1, Y_T = 0)$ "success" is unrealistic. Table 1.5 gives an illustrative example where doses d_1 and d_2 have identical marginal Toxicity probabilities .30, and also identical probabilities .25 of the "success" event $(1,0)$. This would seem to imply that d_1 and d_2 are equivalent, since they are equally safe and have the same success probability. A closer examination shows that d_1 has Efficacy probability .30 while d_2 has Efficacy probability .50, essentially because the event $(Y_E = 1, Y_T = 1)$ has much higher probability with d_2. Treating $(Y_E = 1, Y_T = 0)$ as success completely misses this, and it leads to the wrong conclusion. This

TABLE 1.5: Illustration of why all elementary outcomes matter

Distribution for dose d_1			
	$Y_E = 0$	$Y_E = 1$	
$Y_T = 0$	.45	.25	
$Y_T = 1$	.25	.05	.30
		.30	

Distribution for dose d_2			
	$Y_E = 0$	$Y_E = 1$	
$Y_T = 0$	.45	.25	
$Y_T = 1$	.05	.25	.30
		.50	

Distribution for dose d_3			
	$Y_E = 0$	$Y_E = 1$	
$Y_T = 0$	.25	.35	
$Y_T = 1$	.25	.15	.40
		.50	

numerical example shows why considering only $\Pr(Y_E = 1, Y_T = 0 \mid d)$ for dose-finding is just plain wrong.

A more difficult problem is that of comparing d_3 to d_2 in Table 1.5, since marginally both have Efficacy probability .50, but d_3 has higher probabilities of both Toxicity and the "success" event $(Y_E, Y_T) = (1,0)$ compared to d_2. So it is not obvious how to decide between d_3 and d_2. For $d_1 < d_2 < d_3$, one may think of this numerical example as illustrating how increasing dose often has the effect of making the event $(Y_E, Y_T) = (0,0)$ less likely and making one or both of the events $(Y_E, Y_T) = (1,0)$ and $(Y_E, Y_T) = (1,1)$ more likely. Chapter 6, which deals with utility-based designs, provides a rational way to decide between doses based on elementary outcome probabilities.

This toy example illustrates several important practical points for binary outcomes. The first is that combining the three outcomes $(Y_E, Y_T) = (1,1)$, $(0,0)$, and $(0,1)$ as nominal "failure" ignores important information and can easily lead to an incorrect conclusion. The second point is more subtle, but it is extremely important and is central to all of the phase I–II methods that we will discuss. The event $(Y_E, Y_T) = (1,1)$ is both good because $Y_E = 1$, and bad because $Y_T = 1$. For cytotoxic agents, cellular therapies where dose typically is the number of cells infused, either increasing dose or intensifying schedule often has the effect of reducing $\pi_{E,T}(0,0)$ and increasing $\pi_{E,T}(1,1)$. This is because more intensive treatment typically kills more cells, including both cancer cells and normal cells, often for a variety of biological reasons. The hope that more intensive therapy in the form of a higher dose will increase

$\pi_{E,T}(1,0)$ but not $\pi_{E,T}(1,1)$ is optimistic, naive, and ignores the biology of how anti-cancer agents actually behave. Since $\pi_E = \pi_{E,T}(1,1) + \pi_{E,T}(1,0)$ and $\pi_T = \pi_{E,T}(1,1) + \pi_{E,T}(0,1)$, the clinical issue, for both the physician and the patient, is whether the resulting increase in π_E is enough to provide a desirable trade-off for the increase in π_T.

1.3.5   Late-Onset Outcomes

We have argued that both Efficacy and Toxicity should be used for adaptive dose-finding. Logistically, this makes sense if the time periods during which Efficacy and Toxicity are evaluated are short enough, relative to accrual rate, so that outcome-adaptive decision making is feasible. Difficult logistical problems may arise, however. For example, consider a trial where a dose is chosen adaptively for successive cohorts of 3 patients based on all previously treated patients' data, both Efficacy and Toxicity are evaluated within a 28-day period from the start of treatment, Toxicity can occur at any time up to day 28, but Efficacy is evaluated in terms of disease status by imaging or a tissue sample at day 28. Suppose that the first three patients were accrued and their treatments begun at days 5, 20, and 40 of the study. For patient 1, if Toxicity occurs 17 days from the start of treatment, at day 5+17 = 22 of the study, then at that time it is known that patient 1 has $Y_T = 1$. In contrast, one can only score $Y_T = 0$ if that patient reaches day 5+28 = 33 of the study without Toxicity having occurred. For Y_E, one must wait until day 33 to score it for patient 1, to day 48 to score it for patient 2, and to day 68 to score it for patient 3. If patient 4 arrives before day 68 of the study, the question then arises of how to choose a dose adaptively for that patient. If accrual is sufficiently slow, then this sort of logistical problem does not arise, but if it is rapid then the idea "Pick a dose, treat 3 patients, observe their outcomes, pick a new dose adaptively, repeat" breaks down since it does not say how to deal with new patients who arrive before the previous cohort's outcomes are all evaluated. A simple, commonly used approach is to allow cohort size to vary depending on accrual, for example between 2 and 4. Thus, patient 4 would be treated at the starting dose, and if this sort of situation were to arise later in the trial the new patient would be treated at the current optimal dose recommended by the adaptive design. This flexible approach often works well in practice, provided that the accrual rate is not too high.

As a more extreme case to illustrate practical limitations, suppose that a cohort of 3 patients recently were treated after escalating to a new, higher dose d_j, and then 10 new patients were enrolled very quickly, within a week, before any of the outcomes of the most recently treated cohort were evaluated. If all 10 are simply treated at d_j and it turns out that d_j is too toxic, this would be a disaster. This implies that, after escalating to a new dose for the first time, to ensure a safe and ethical trial one must wait for Toxicity to be evaluated for the most recently treated cohort. This is because, regardless of the assumed dose-outcome model, when escalating to an untried dose d_j for the first time, essentially one must rely on predictions of $\pi_E(d_j)$ and $\pi_T(d_j)$. If, instead, to ensure safety all 10 are treated at d_{j-1} but it later turns out that d_j is acceptably safe and has a much larger Efficacy probability, say $\pi_{E,j} = .60$ while $\pi_{E,j-1} = .30$, then those 10 patients have been deprived of the much higher Efficacy probability. Thus, the solution "treat new patients who arrive before the current cohort's outcomes have been evaluated at one dose level below the current recommended dose" does not work. After all, the therapeutic goal is to achieve Efficacy without an unacceptable risk of Toxicity. A different alternative approach is to make new patients wait to be treated. This usually is not feasible, and it may be impossible or ethically undesirable. A fourth alternative is simply to turn away the 10 new patients and not enroll them in the trial. This certainly solves the logistical problem, but the clinical question then becomes what treatment or treatments, if any, exist, should be given to those 10 patients. This problem is quite complex, and is a practical reality in actual trials that use sequentially outcome-adaptive methods. Formal phase I–II methods for dealing with this problem will be discussed in Chapter 5.

A different sort of setting is one where it simply is not feasible to use Efficacy, as it is clinically defined, for dose-finding. This is the case, for example, if Efficacy is characterized in terms of progression free survival (PFS) time, with the idea that the new agent should extend median PFS, for a disease where this median is large enough so that waiting for disease progression or death in order to choose doses adaptively is not feasible. Another common example is a trial where Efficacy is a longitudinal process observed over a lengthy time period, say 6 to 12 months, such as the level of an immunological biomarker in a T-cell therapy trial. In such settings, the best that one can do is use an adaptive "Toxicity only" method, like the CRM, while making the common implicit assumption that Efficacy must improve with increasing dose, and simply estimate Efficacy at the end of the trial.

1.3.6 Expansion Cohorts

The idea of adding so-called "expansion cohorts" to phase I trials began innocently enough, since it is based on what seems to be common sense. The idea is to first conduct a usual phase I trial to determine an MTD using the 3+3 algorithm or some other method, such as the CRM. Then, to obtain a better estimator of Pr(*Toxicity* | MTD), a small number of additional patients are treated at the MTD. When this practice was begun, typical expansion cohorts sizes were 3 to 10 patients. This is based on the fundamental principle of statistics that a larger sample size provides a more reliable estimator. Unfortunately, the practice of including expansion cohorts is based on the fallacious assumption that an MTD obtained in a usual phase I trial is in some sense the "right" dose of the agent. In recent years, the sizes of expansion cohorts actually used in phase I trials have exploded, from about 10 patients to hundreds.

The fallacious assumption that an MTD is either known or very likely to be a safe dose, and the use of expansion cohorts on that basis, have some very undesirable consequences. This practice is very likely to lead to severe, often intractable problems. These problems arise due to the myopic assumption that, once the MTD is chosen, it must be an acceptably safe dose. As more patients are treated at the selected MTD, however, the resulting additional data easily may contradict the earlier conclusion that the chosen dose is the MTD. For example, suppose that a protocol includes the provision that, once an MTD is chosen, an expansion cohort of an additional 10 patients should be treated at the MTD. If this were done starting with the phase I Toxicity data given in Table 1.4, a wide variety of complicated questions very likely will arise for the various numbers of Toxicities that may be observed in the expansion cohort. As shown above, this is due to the fact that typical phase I estimates of $\pi_T(d)$ typically are very unreliable for any d in the trial, including the MTD. For example, what should one do if two Toxicities are observed in the first three patients of the expansion cohort treated at the chosen MTD of $d = 30$? Given the data, this would result in $1/6 + 2/3 = 3/9$ Toxicities. Should one then continue and treat seven more patients at the MTD until the expansion cohort of 10 has been reached, as mandated by the protocol, or violate the protocol by abandoning the MTD and de-escalating? If one adheres to the protocol and continues to treat patients at the MTD, and ends up with $7/10$ Toxicities, for a total of $1/6 + 7/10 = 8/16$ (50%), what would one then conclude? It seems likely that, regardless of what the protocol may mandate, any clinician who actually did this and ended up with these results would be criticized on ethical grounds. The first $2/3$ Toxicities in the expansion cohort show that something likely is wrong with the assumption that the selected MTD is safe. If, instead of completing the expansion cohort, one de-escalates, the question then becomes what sort of rule or algorithm should be applied thereafter. The general point is that the idea of treating a fixed expansion cohort at a chosen MTD may seem sensible, but in practice it is very foolish. A simple, practical alternative solution is available, however. Any reasonable sequentially adaptive design with an explicit optimality criterion that is used throughout to choose doses for successive cohorts gives well-defined, unambiguous decisions and answers.

What nominally is a large "phase I expansion cohort" is actually a phase II trial conducted without any design, other than a possible specification of sample size. Thus, one sensible alternative approach is to proceed from phase I to phase II, but with a design that includes stopping rules for both Toxicity and Efficacy (cf. Bryant and Day, 1995; Thall et al., 1995). However, it should be kept in mind that, if a phase II trial is stopped due to excessive Toxicity at the chosen MTD, then either the agent must be abandoned or, alternatively, a second dose-finding trial may be conducted with the goal to find a lower dose that is acceptable. This, in turn, raises the question of how the data from the previous phase I and phase II trials may or may not be used in the design and conduct of such a third trial. These problems, and all of the problems arising with an expansion cohort, can be avoided entirely if a phase I–II trial is conducted in the first place.

The current, extreme practice of including very large expansion cohorts of 100 patients or more in what are nominally "phase I" trials might be described as follows:

Step 1. Begin by using a standard method based on Toxicity alone to choose a dose, and call it the "MTD."

Step 2. Thereafter, do not bother with an experimental design, and in particular do not specify safety or futility stopping rules. Instead, simply treat a very large number of patients at the chosen MTD. Call these patients the trial's "expansion cohort."

Step 3. Once all patients have been treated, analyze the resulting data. If possible, identify and select a subset of patients in which the empirical Efficacy rate is highest. Use this as a basis for submitting a New Drug Application to the U.S Food and Drug Administration.

This practice magnifies all of the problems described above that occur with small expansion cohorts. It also ignores decades of scientific research to develop clinical trial designs that ethically and reliably determine reasonably safe and effective doses and schedules of experimental agents at the start of their clinical development. Consequently, it does a very poor job of optimizing the new regime's dose or schedule, fails to protect patient safety adequately, fails to reliably discontinue trials of experimental treatments that are ineffective, and leads to numerous logical and clinical problems, of the sort described above, as patients in the expansion cohort are treated. In summary, the use of very large "phase I expansion cohorts" poorly serves the patients in the trial, future patients, and the pharmaceutical company that provided the experimental agent.

1.3.7   Guessing a Schedule

Many agents have effects that are highly schedule-dependent, given a fixed total dose. As a simple example, consider the two dose-schedule regimes ρ_1 in which total dose d is administered as a single bolus infused over 30 minutes on day 1, and ρ_2 in which $d/2$ is administered as a bolus infused over 30 minutes on each of days 1 and 3. These two (dose, schedule) regimes can be represented formally as $\rho_1 = \{d, 1\}$ and $\rho_2 = \{(d/2, d/2), (1, 3)\}$. Since it is quite possible that ρ_2 may have any sort of effect on the distribution of (Y_E, Y_T) compared to ρ_1, no monotonicity assumptions for the probabilities of either Efficacy or Toxicity may be made about $\pi_k(\rho_1)$ versus $\pi_k(\rho_2)$. Consequently, if one wishes to evaluate these two schedules along with, say, five values of d, then there are a total of 10 (dose, schedule) regimes to evaluate. Numerous other schedules that could be considered, such as giving $d/3$ on each of days 1, 3, and 5 or giving $d/4$

weekly for 4 weeks. If one wishes to evaluate all combinations of four schedules and five doses, this would result in 20 dose-schedule regimes. Moreover, the logistics of defining and evaluating Y for a 4-week regime may be very different from what is needed to evaluate a 1-day regime. Consequently, the problem of determining an optimal or nearly optimal (dose, schedule) regime, and avoiding regimes that are greatly inferior, is very difficult. It is extremely important, however. Designs for jointly optimizing dose and schedule will be presented in Chapter 11.

In practice, because the number of possible schedules is impractically large to investigate, most clinical trialists do not evaluate alternative schedules of a new agent at all. Instead, based on *in vivo* animal experiments and possibly past experience with other agents, the most common practice is to guess a schedule and focus attention on finding a dose to give using that schedule. Since schedules of administration, once adopted, often become conventions, this makes investigation of alternative schedules in a clinical trial less likely and more difficult. The point is that the convention is to guess a schedule rather than search for an optimal or even a better schedule empirically, based on observed patient Efficacy and Toxicity outcomes in a clinical trial. Consequently, if an inferior schedule leading to poor clinical outcomes has been guessed in a setting where a substantively better schedule actually exists, this may doom an agent to failure. It is impossible to know how many agents that were very promising based on pre-clinical data have failed in clinical evaluation for this reason.

1.3.8 Patient Heterogeneity

Most of the designs that we will discuss assume that patients are homogenous with regard to the effects of treatment on Y. In general, this assumption is not true. From a purely mathematical viewpoint, any of the models and designs presented in this book may be elaborated to account for patient prognostic covariates. It simply is a matter of including the covariates in the model, which is trivial, and making the decision rules covariate-specific, which also is relatively straightforward. In practice, however, actually implementing a phase I–II trial with this additional structure is extremely difficult. To see why this is so, consider a common setting where patients are classified as having good, intermediate, or poor prognosis, represented respectively by the categorical covariate values $Z_1 = -1$, 0, or $+1$, and a biomarker is targeted by the agent, represented by the covariate $Z_2 = -1$ or 1 for the patient being biomarker negative or positive. For binary outcomes, incorporating $Z = (Z_1, Z_2)$ into the model requires specification of $\pi_k(d, Z, \theta)$ for each $k = E, T$, so it seems like a simple regression problem. For example, one may assume linear terms $\eta_k = g^{-1}(\pi_k)$ for some link function g to account for prognosis and the biologically motivated possibility that the dose effect may differ in biomarker positive and negative patients. Denoting the indicator of the event A by $[A]$, a reasonable linear term might be

$$\eta_k = \beta_{k,0} + \beta_{k,1}[Z_1 = -1] + \beta_{k,2}[Z_1 = 1] + d\{\beta_{k,3}[Z_2 = -1] + \beta_{k,4}[Z_2 = 1]\}.$$

The parameters $\beta_{k,1}$ and $\beta_{k,2}$ quantify the prognostic subgroup effects, while $\beta_{k,3}$ and $\beta_{k,4}$ quantify dose effects within each of the two biomarker subgroups. Under a bivariate model defined using a copula, there would be a total of $5+5+1 = 11$ model parameters. For implementation, since Z_1 is prognostic by definition its effects on Y_E and Y_T should be well understood. In the context of a Bayesian model, this implies that informative priors on the baseline parameters $(\beta_{E,0}, \beta_{E,1}, \beta_{E,2}, \beta_{T,0}, \beta_{T,1}, \beta_{T,2})$ should be available, obtained either from a preliminary fit of historical data or by elicitation from physicians familiar with the disease. In contrast, the priors on the dose effect parameters $(\beta_{E,3}, \beta_{E,4}, \beta_{T,3}, \beta_{T,4})$ should be non-informative, otherwise there would be no need to do the dose-finding study. This model requires the key assumption that the effects of treating the patient with the new agent at a given dose d are additive in the linear terms, that is, that the baseline parameters do not change when the dose effect parameters are included in the model. So, even for this simple setting, establishing a Bayesian model with a reasonable prior is a non-trivial exercise.

For trial conduct, the dose-finding algorithm should allow the possibility that patients with different covariates Z may receive different optimal doses at the same point in the trial. That is, the algorithm should allow the doses to be "personalized" based on the available data. This implies that the optimal decision at each stage of the trial is not simply one dose d^{opt} for all patients, but rather it is a function $d^{opt}(Z)$ that maps Z to the set of doses. In practice, this may be difficult. For example, suppose that there are five dose levels, so since Z has six possible values (three prognostic subgroups × two biomarker values), there would be $6 \times 5 = 30$ combinations of Z and d. Given that the six values of Z typically will be far from equally likely, many combinations of (d, Z) would have no data for much of the trial. For example, suppose that the levels of Z_1 have population proportions $(.20, .50, .30)$ and $\Pr(Z_2 = 1) = .60$. Assuming independence, the six subgroups determined by Z would have probabilities $(.12, .30, .18, .08, .20, .12)$. At the end of a 60-patient trial, the expected sub-sample sizes would be, roughly, $(7, 18, 11, 5, 12, 7)$. With adaptive dose assignment, each of these 6 subsamples would be divided very unevenly among the 5 doses, so the sample sizes in the 30 subgroups determined by d and Z would be very small and very unevenly distributed, with many (d, Z) combinations having no data. Even at the end of a very large phase I–II trial, say with 120 patients, many of the (d, Z) combinations still would have little or no data. Consequently, in any actual phase I–II trial, the function $d^{opt}(Z)$ that chooses personalized doses would, unavoidably, rely heavily on the underlying model and prior to borrow strength from (d, Z) combinations for which data are available. Given the additional requirements that the trial must be conducted in an ethically acceptable manner, it is not obvious how to make sequentially adaptive decisions with such sparse data based on (Y, Z, d).

Another important practical issue is that the biomarker Z_2 must be evaluated quickly enough so that it may be used to compute the adaptive rule $d^{opt}(Z)$. If, for example, the laboratory procedure for evaluating Z_2 requires one or two weeks, then this would delay each patient's therapy. If the procedure for evaluating Z_2 is imperfect, as often is the case, then some patients will have their biomarker status misclassified. This in turn may invalidate the adaptive procedure by leading to some patients being given the wrong dose. Finally, suppose that several genomic or proteomic biomarkers are involved, rather than only one. Generalizing the model given above to accommodate this very likely would lead to an intractably complex parameterization, so some alternative modeling approach would be needed. Thus, while giving patient-specific, "personalized" treatment regimes during sequentially adaptive clinical trials is a very appealing idea, actually implementing this is extremely challenging. Phase I–II designs for doing this will be presented in Chapter 7.

2

The Phase I–II Paradigm

CONTENTS

2.1 Efficacy and Toxicity 29
2.2 Elements of Phase I–II Designs 30
2.3 Treatment Regimes and Clinical Outcomes 31
2.4 Sequentially Adaptive Decision Making 33
2.5 Risk–Benefit Trade-Offs 35
2.6 Stickiness and Adaptive Randomization 37
2.7 Simulation as a Design Tool 41

2.1 Efficacy and Toxicity

Because most medical treatments have multiple effects, physicians routinely must consider risk–benefit trade-offs between possible good and bad clinical outcomes when deciding how to treat their patients. Depending on the disease being treated, desired treatment effects may be reducing pain, curing an infection, shrinking a solid tumor, bringing acute leukemia into remission, reducing abnormally high blood pressure, or dissolving a blood clot in the brain that caused a stroke. Adverse events may be a heart attack or stroke, infection, liver or kidney dysfunction, or low white blood cell count, or nausea/vomiting from chemotherapy for cancer, depression or insomnia from beta-blockers given to treat high blood pressure, bleeding in the brain from a drug given to dissolve a blood clot, or regimen-related death. We will refer to desirable treatment effects as Efficacy, and undesirable effects as Toxicity. Motivated by the idea that a clinical trial design should reflect the way that physicians think and behave, we will use the (Efficacy, Toxicity) pair as practical basis for constructing the statistical models and trial designs that we will discuss. The designs deal with early phase trials in settings where the effects of the treatment regime on Efficacy and Toxicity in humans are not yet understood.

The problem that treatments may have both desirable and undesirable effects on the patient is especially true in oncology, where virtually all treatment regimes have substantial risks of harming the patient. Consequently, practicing oncologists routinely select each patient's treatment by considering how much risk of adverse outcomes is acceptable as a trade-off for a desired level of therapeutic benefit. Phase I–II clinical trials, which evaluate new treatment regimes being given to humans for the first time, are designed to reflect how physicians actually behave. To do this, phase I–II designs are based on an undesirable clinical outcome, Toxicity, and a desirable outcome, Efficacy, both thought to be related to the treatment regime. These outcomes are defined so that they can be observed soon enough after the start of therapy to facilitate sequential, outcome adaptive decision making during the trial. Often, Toxicity is a composite event defined in terms of several qualitatively different adverse outcomes. It is important to keep in mind that the definitions of these primary outcomes will be used by the trial design to choose treatment regimes for successive cohorts of patients. Consequently, these definitions must be determined very carefully during the collaborative discussion between the statistician and physician, since they must satisfy therapeutic, ethical, and logistical requirements.

2.2   Elements of Phase I–II Designs

One may consider a phase I–II design to be like a Labradoodle, which is obtained by cross-breeding a Labrador Retriever with a Poodle. Labradoodles enjoy the desirable quality of heterosis, or hybrid vigor, since they have greater genetic diversity and hence better overall health than either of their parents. Hybrid clinical trial designs, if carefully constructed, enjoy similar advantages over the simpler designs that motivated them. The analogy is not strict, however, since both Labradors and Poodles both are fine canine breeds, whereas the most commonly used phase I or phase II clinical trial designs suffer from logical and ethical flaws, as we demonstrated in Chapter 1.

    Each of the phase I–II designs reviewed in this book was motivated by the desire to address one or more of the flaws in the conventional paradigm. Denote the set of treatment regimes to be evaluated in a given trial by $\mathcal{R}$ = $\{\rho_0, \rho_1, \cdots, \rho_k\}$. We denote the action "Do not treat" by ρ_0, which corresponds to the belief that none of the regimes $\rho_1, \cdots, \rho_k$ is acceptably safe and efficacious. Phase I–II designs all include the following elements:

1. Effects of each treatment regime on a multivariate outcome, Y, characterizing both Efficacy and Toxicity are evaluated. The goal is to select a best regime based on these estimated effects.

2. Patients are enrolled and treated in successive cohorts, with ρ chosen adaptively for each cohort from $\mathcal{R}$ using the (ρ, Y) data from previous patients.

3. The adaptive decisions are based on an explicit criterion function, $\phi(\rho, \mathcal{D}_n)$, that characterizes and quantifies the risk–benefit trade-off of each ρ being considered.

4. In addition to the criterion function, admissibility rules often are imposed to protect the patients enrolled in the trial from unacceptably toxic or inefficacious regimes.

5. The underlying probability model is Bayesian, and decision criteria are posterior or predictive quantities.

6. Non-model-based safety rules, such as "Do not skip an untried dose when escalating" often are imposed, because the underlying model may not be correct.

7. Computer simulation is used to establish the design's properties, and to calibrate priors and design parameters on that basis.

2.3   Treatment Regimes and Clinical Outcomes

A given treatment regime may be complex, possibly including multiple components. While this depends on the disease and treatment modality, in oncology multi-component regimes are commonplace. In many medical settings, this leads to consideration of multi-stage or multi-cycle dynamic treatment regimes (DTRs) that have within-patient adaptive rules. All but one of the designs that we will discuss consider only one cycle, or stage, of treatment and use only between-patient adaptive decision rules, wherein data from previous patients are used by the rules to choose regimes for new patients.

For most phase I–II trials, the regime is simply the dose of a new agent, and doses for successive cohorts of one, two, or three patients are chosen based on the (dose, Efficacy, Toxicity) data from previous patients. Toxicity typically is a composite outcome defined in terms of several qualitatively different adverse events at specified grades of severity. Efficacy, often called "response," is a desirable outcome thought to characterize an early anti-disease effect. Toxicity and Efficacy most often are defined as binary events, although more elaborate phase I–II designs may define them as ordinal categorical or event time variables. As the case study given in Chapter 14 will show, a phase I–II design may even have three outcomes.

Each design will consider regimes that take one of the following forms:

1. the dose d of a single agent administered either alone or in combination with other agents or treatments that are not varied;

2. the doses (d_1, d_2) of two agents given in combination;

3. the doses (d_1, d_2) of a single agent given to a patient in two successive cycles;

4. a combination (d, s) where d is the per-administration dose and $s = (s_1, \cdots, s_m)$ is the schedule of administration times.

The effects of each regime ρ on patients who receive it are evaluated in terms of a clinical outcome, Y. For most of the phase I–II designs that we will discuss, Y is a pair (Y_E, Y_T) of binary indicators of Efficacy and Toxicity. More generally, Y_E and Y_T may be ordinal categorical variables with three or more levels. For example, if Efficacy has possible values Progressive Disease (PD), Stable Disease (SD), Partial Response (PR), and Complete Response (CR), then Y_E has possible values {PD, SD, PR, CR}. These ordinal events may be represented nominally by the integers {0, 1, 2, 3}. Similarly, if Toxicity is ordinal with possible severity levels None (N), Moderate (M), High (H), Severe (S), then the possible values of Y_T are {N, M, H, S}, which may be represented nominally by the integers {0, 1, 2, 3}.

The simplest phase I–II case is that where Efficacy and Toxicity are disjoint, and Y has the three possible values {N, E, T}, where E and T represent Efficacy and Toxicity, these events are disjoint, and N is the third event that neither Efficacy nor Toxicity occurs. This case arises, for example, if Toxicity is regimen-related death or is an adverse event so severe that it renders Efficacy impossible. This case was dealt with by Thall and Russell (1998) and Mandrekar et al. (2007). For trinary outcomes, a common assumption is that $\pi_E(d) + \pi_T(d)$ and $\pi_T(d)$ both increase with d, that is, the three events are ordered as $N < E < T$. The underlying idea is that there may be an intermediate dose that achieves Efficacy, but if the dose is increased too much then Toxicity occurs.

For event time outcomes subject to right-censoring at follow up time V, the time to event $k = E, T$ is represented by X_k. The observed time is $X_k^o = X_k \wedge V$, the minimum of X_k and V, and $\epsilon_k = I(X_k < V)$ is the indicator that the observed time is the time of the event, i.e., that X_k is not right-censored. In this setting, $Y = (Y_E, Y_T)$ with each $Y_k = (X_k^o, \epsilon_k)$. A possible complication with event time outcomes is that Toxicity may censor Efficacy, but not conversely, if follow up ends at X_T. In this case, $X_E < X_T$ and a semi-competing risks model is required.

There are additional data structures for Y that arise in other settings. The design discussed in Chapter 10 deals with the problem of dose-finding in two cycles of therapy. For this design, the outcome always includes a bivariate binary Y_1 for (Toxicity, Efficacy) in cycle 1, with the possibilities that a second cycle of treatment may or may not be given, depending on the cycle 1 dose and outcome. If a second cycle is given, then the cycle 2 outcome Y_2 also is bivariate binary. Thus, the entire observed outcome is either Y_1 or (Y_1, Y_2), and which it will be for a given patient cannot be known at the start of treatment. Formally, denote the set of possible treatment actions by $\mathcal{R} = \{0, 1, \cdots, m\}$, where the indices $1, ..., m$ represent doses and the decision "Do not treat" is represented by the index 0. A two-stage dynamic treatment regime (DTR) consists of a pair of actions (d_1, d_2), where d_1 chooses an element of $\mathcal{R}$ and $d_2 = d_2(d_1, Y_1)$ chooses an element of $\mathcal{R}$ based on (d_1, Y_1). As the development in Chapter 10 will show, optimizing a two-stage DTR is quite challenging.

In the application discussed in Chapter 14, the outcome is the trivariate binary vector $Y = (Y_G, Y_E, Y_H)$, where both Y_G and Y_E are Efficacy events and Y_H is a Toxicity event. Hybrid outcomes also arise, where Y_T is binary and $Y_E = (X_E^o, \epsilon_E)$ has the event time structure described above.

2.4 Sequentially Adaptive Decision Making

It might seem that determining the best regime from $\mathcal{R}$ based on a sample of N patients may be done simply by randomizing the patients fairly among the regimes. This is because fair randomization ensures that estimators of treatment effects will be unbiased, and thus any comparisons of effects between regimes will be fair. In most early phase trials this would be unethical, since some regimes may be unacceptably toxic. The simplest example is that where the regimes are doses and $\pi_T(d_j)$ increases with d_j. The simplest and most common phase I problem is to choose a dose that has acceptable $\pi_T(d_j)$. The rationale, as explained in Chapter 1, is that $\pi_E(d_j)$ also increases in d_j. Phase I–II dose-finding designs assume explicit models for both $\pi_T(d_j)$ and $\pi_E(d_j)$, and they seek a dose that has both acceptably low $\pi_T(d_j)$ and acceptably high $\pi_E(d_j)$. Since some doses may be either too toxic or unacceptably inefficacious, randomizing patients among the doses is not ethical. This motivates the use of sequentially adaptive designs.

Each design assumes a Bayesian probability model consisting of a distribution $p(Y|\rho, \theta)$ of Y for a patient who receives regime ρ, and a prior $p(\theta|\tilde{\theta})$, where θ is the model parameter vector and $\tilde{\theta}$ is a vector of fixed hyperparameters. One exception is the more general model used for the 2-cycle case in Chapter 10, where some elements of $\tilde{\theta}$ are assumed to follow hyperpriors, also called "Level 2 priors." The data observed from the first n patients in the trial may be represented by

$$\mathcal{D}_n = \{(\rho_{[1]}, Y_1), \cdots, (\rho_{[n]}, Y_n))\},$$

where $\rho_{[i]}$ denotes the regime in $\mathcal{R}$ used to treat the ith patient. The corresponding likelihood for n patients is

$$\mathcal{L}_n(\mathcal{D}_n|\theta) = \prod_{i=1}^{n} p(Y_i|\rho_{[i]}, \theta)$$

and the posterior is

$$p_n(\theta|\mathcal{D}_n, \tilde{\theta}) \propto \mathcal{L}_n(\mathcal{D}_n|\theta)\, p(\theta|\tilde{\theta}). \tag{2.1}$$

For implementing each method, since the models are Bayesian a great deal of attention is paid to establishing the fixed hyperparameters $\tilde{\theta}$ that determine the prior. This is because each design must make decisions affecting patient welfare and possibly survival based on very small amounts of data, especially early in the trial. Because decision criteria are computed from the posterior, the quantitative effect of the prior on the posterior is extremely important. The fact that the posterior depends on $\tilde{\theta}$ is reflected in the notation in (2.1), although we will suppress this hereafter for brevity. Methods for establishing priors will be discussed in Chapter 3.

A design consists of the trial's entry criteria, the set $\mathcal{R}$ of possible treatment regimes or actions, the domain of possible patient outcomes Y, the assumed probability model, trial decision rules, cohort size, maximum sample size N or maximum trial duration. The designs use Bayesian sequential decision rules to choose ρ from $\mathcal{R}$, based on the posterior $p_n(\theta|\mathcal{D}_n)$ computed from the most recent data when a new patient is enrolled. Such a sequentially adaptive decision rule may be expressed as a sequence of functions that use the model and decision regimes to map $\mathcal{D}_n$ to $\mathcal{R}$. In general, each mapping may include several adaptive decision rules used together, such as rules for choosing a dose or a dose pair, deciding what regimes are acceptably safe, or temporarily suspending accrual to wait for outcome data on previously treated patients to be observed. In designs that use patient covariates, Z, the decision regimes map $(Z, \mathcal{D}_n)$ to $\mathcal{R}$.

For cohorts of size 1, the $n \rightarrow n + 1$ iteration of the Bayesian medical decision-making process is given by the sequence of mappings

$$\mathcal{D}_n \longrightarrow p_n(\theta|\mathcal{D}_n, \tilde{\theta}) \longrightarrow \rho_{[n+1]} \longrightarrow Y_{n+1} \longrightarrow \mathcal{D}_{n+1}. \qquad (2.2)$$

In this sequence, under the assumed probability model, Bayes' Theorem is applied to map the current observed data $\mathcal{D}_n$ into a posterior. The decision rules then map this posterior to an action, $\rho_{[n+1]}$, which possibly may be to shut the trial down early if it is decided that no regime is acceptable. If the trial is not shut down early, then ρ_{n+1} is the next patient's regime, the patient is treated, and the patient's outcome Y_{n+1} is observed. The new data $(\rho_{[n+1]}, Y_{n+1})$ are then incorporated into $\mathcal{D}_n$ to give the updated dataset $\mathcal{D}_{n+1}$. This process is repeated until the end of the trial, which may be when a maximum sample size N or maximum trial duration is reached, or because the trial is stopped early.

The process whereby the expanding dataset is used by applying Bayes' Theorem repeatedly to turn $p_n(\theta|\mathcal{D}_n, \tilde{\theta})$ into $p_{n+1}(\theta|\mathcal{D}_{n+1}, \tilde{\theta})$ is an example of "sequential Bayesian learning." It is a formalism for learning about the model parameter vector θ and making decisions on that basis repeatedly as additional data are observed during the trial. It relies on the fact that, if at each stage the posterior $p_n(\theta|\mathcal{D}_n, \tilde{\theta})$ is used as the prior for the next stage with the new likelihood $\mathcal{L}(Y_{n+1}|\rho_{[n+1]}, \theta)$, these $n+1$ iterations of Bayes' Law give the same posterior as if it was applied once with likelihood $\mathcal{L}(\mathcal{D}_{n+1}|\theta)$ and prior $p(\theta|\tilde{\theta})$. This can be seen by expanding the nth posterior and using the fact that the successive observations are independent :

$$p_n(\theta|\mathcal{D}_n,\tilde{\theta})\,\mathcal{L}(Y_{n+1}|\rho_{[n+1]},\theta) \quad \propto \quad \left\{p(\theta|\tilde{\theta})\prod_{i=1}^{n}\mathcal{L}(Y_i|\rho_{[i]},\theta)\right\}\mathcal{L}(Y_{n+1}|\rho_{[n+1]},\theta)$$

$$= \quad p(\theta|\tilde{\theta})\prod_{i=1}^{n+1}\mathcal{L}(Y_i|\rho_{[i]},\theta)$$

There possibly also may be a cohort size, $c > 1$, which is the number of patients treated with each newly chosen regime. Usually, $c = 2$ or 3, with $c = 1$ corresponding to continuous adaptive decision making. For $c > 1$, the mapping in (2.2) jumps from n to $n+c$ at each step. For example, if the cohort size $c = 3$ is used then $\rho_{[n+1]} = \rho_{[n+2]} = \rho_{[n+3]}$ and, formally, Y_{n+1}, Y_{n+2} and Y_{n+3} all must be observed before updating the data and making the next decision. As discussed earlier, in Chapter 1, if Y_{n+1} has not been evaluated fully when patient $n+2$ is accrued then how to decide the next action for the new patient is not so straightforward. A methodology for dealing with this problem is presented in Chapter 5.

2.5 Risk–Benefit Trade-Offs

One may identify three general strategies for defining optimization criteria in phase I–II trials. Each strategy takes a particular approach to quantifying the trade-off between Toxicity and Efficacy, either in terms of their probabilities or the events themselves. The first strategy is to set an upper limit on $\pi_T(\rho_1,\theta),\cdots,\pi_T(\rho_J,\theta)$ and choose the strategy that maximizes $\pi_E(\rho_j,\theta)$ over the set of doses that satisfy the Toxicity limit. For example, if 40% Toxicity is considered to be an upper limit, then a posterior probability criterion such as

$$Pr\{\pi_T(\rho,\theta) > .40 \mid \mathcal{D}_n\} > .90$$

may be used to declare a regime ρ unacceptably toxic. This strategy is asymmetric in π_T and π_E. A similar, alternative approach would be to switch the roles of the two outcomes. If a 20% response rate is considered the lowest acceptable level, then one might set a lower limit on $\pi_E(\rho_1,\theta),\cdots,\pi_E(\rho_J,\theta)$, by using the rule that declares a regime ρ unacceptably inefficacious if

$$Pr\{\pi_E(\rho,\theta) < .20 \mid \mathcal{D}_n\} > .90.$$

One then would choose ρ_j to minimize the mean of $\pi_T(\rho_j,\theta)$ over the set of doses that satisfy this Efficacy limit. The set of regimes having both acceptable Toxicity and acceptable efficacy based on $\mathcal{D}_n$ is denoted by $\mathcal{A}_n$.

A second strategy where the regimes are doses, which is symmetric in

Efficacy and Toxicity, is used in settings where the strategies are doses. This relies on a function $\phi(\pi_E, \pi_T)$ that maps the set of possible (π_E, π_T) pairs to a real number quantifying the pair's desirability, or "trade-off." This is used as a criterion to choose d_j to maximize an estimate of $\phi(\pi_E(d_j), \pi_T(d_j))$. For example, it might be that $\phi(.20, .30) = 1$, $\phi(.40, .30) = 1.5$, and $\phi(.40, .40) = 1$. This says that, compared to $(\pi_E, \pi_T) = (.20, .30)$, increasing π_E from .20 to .40 while keeping the toxicity probability constant at $\pi_T = .30$ increases the desirability from 1 to 1.5, but increasing π_E from .20 to .40 while also increasing π_T from .30 to .40 gives the same desirability. In other words, since $\phi(.20, .30) = \phi(.40, .40) = 1$, starting with $(\pi_E, \pi_T) = (.20, .30)$, a .10 increase in π_T is considered to be a fair trade-off for a .20 increase in π_E. The EffTox method (Thall and Cook, 2004), which will be covered in detail in Chapter 4, takes this approach by defining a trade-off function, $\phi(\pi_E, \pi_T)$, so that it increases in π_E and decreases in π_T. The numerical values of the function ϕ are obtained by a process of elicitation and curve fitting. At each decision, the posterior means $\mu_{E,j,n} = E\{\pi_E(d_j, \theta) \mid \mathcal{D}_n\}$ and $\mu_{T,j,n} = E\{\pi_T(d_j, \theta) \mid \mathcal{D}_n\}$ are evaluated for each d_j, and the dose maximizing $\phi(\mu_{E,j,n}, \mu_{T,j,n})$ is chosen. Since this would choose an optimal d_j in any case, including cases where all doses are unsafe or inefficacious, additional dose admissibility rules are required. These take the same form as the Efficacy and Toxicity acceptability criteria given above in terms of regimes. They ensure that only doses d_j for which $\pi_E(d_j)$ is acceptably high and $\pi_T(d_j)$ is acceptably low are considered before computing $\phi(\mu_{E,j,n}, \mu_{T,j,n})$ to find a nominally "optimal" dose.

A third strategy, which also is symmetric in Efficacy and Toxicity, starts by assigning numerical utilities $U(y)$ to all possible outcomes y of Y, and then chooses ρ_j during the trial to maximize the estimated mean utility $\bar{U}(\rho_j, \theta)$ $= E\{U(Y) \mid \rho_j, \theta\}$. Table 2.1 gives examples of three possible utilities that may be assigned to the elementary outcomes in a setting with two binary outcomes, using the convention that the best possible outcome is assigned utility 100 and the worst outcome is assigned utility 0. Utility 1 reflects the viewpoint that, if Efficacy is achieved, $Y_E = 1$, then there is a small loss in utility for Toxicity, from 100 to 80. Assignment of utility 40 to the event $\{Y_E = 0, Y_T = 0\}$ says that it is much better to have neither event than Toxicity without Efficacy, $\{Y_E = 0, Y_T = 1\}$, which has utility 0. Utility 2 reflects the different viewpoint that Toxicity is much worse, since there is a much larger drop for $Y_E = 1$ if Toxicity occurs, from 100 to 50. Utility 3 reflects the viewpoint that, while there is a price for Toxicity, the most important thing is achieve Efficacy. If the true probabilities were known, and equal to the values for d_1 given in Table 1.5, then the mean utilities for these three numerical utility assignments would be 38, 50, and 54, respectively. In practice, since the outcome probabilities are not known, one must assume a model and estimate its parameter vector, θ, from the trial data. A frequentist version of this approach would compute an estimator $\hat{\theta}_n$ based on $\mathcal{D}_n$ and use $\bar{U}(\rho_j, \hat{\theta}_n)$ to estimate the mean utility for each ρ_j. A Bayesian version computes the posterior mean $u(\rho_j \mid \mathcal{D}_n) = E[\bar{U}(\rho_j, \theta) \mid \mathcal{D}_n]$ for each ρ_j. Like

TABLE 2.1: Some utilities for bivariate binary Efficacy and Toxicity

Utility 1	$Y_E = 0$	$Y_E = 1$
$Y_T = 0$	20	100
$Y_T = 1$	0	80

Utility 2		
$Y_T = 0$	50	100
$Y_T = 1$	0	50

Utility 3		
$Y_T = 0$	60	100
$Y_T = 1$	0	40

the trade-off-based method, since there always exists a ρ_j that maximizes this mean utility criterion, additional dose admissibility rules are required. A major advantage of the utility-based approach is that it can be applied in settings where Efficacy and Toxicity are more complex than binary indicator variables, including ordinal or event times outcomes. Utility-based designs will be discussed generally in Chapter 7.

2.6 Stickiness and Adaptive Randomization

Intuitively, it may seem that it is best at each interim decision to treat the next cohort with the regime that maximizes the optimality criterion, such as a posterior mean utility or Efficacy–Toxicity trade-off function, based on the current data, $\mathcal{D}_n$. Of course, this should be done while also enforcing additional regime acceptability criteria. However, in sequential decision making there is a well-known problem with any "greedy" or "myopic" algorithm that always chooses each successive action by optimizing a given criterion. Any greedy algorithm carries the risk of getting stuck at a suboptimal action. This is because, due to the play of chance, if a greedy algorithm happens to choose a suboptimal action, it may continue to take that suboptimal action and thus fail to explore other possibilities, including a different action that is truly optimal. By repeatedly taking a suboptimal action, a greedy algorithm may fail to take an optimal action often enough, or at all, and thus fail to obtain the necessary data to learn, statistically, which action is truly optimal. This problem is well known in sequential analysis, where it sometimes is called the "optimization versus exploration" dilemma (cf. Robbins, 1952; Gittins, 1979;

Sutton and Barto, 1998). This problem has been recognized only recently in the context of dose-finding trials (Bartroff and Lai, 2010; Azriel et al., 2011; Braun et al., 2012; Thall and Nguyen, 2012; Oron and Hoff, 2013; Thall et al., 2014b; Cai et al., 2014b; Riviere et al., 2015). For phase I trials conducted using the CRM with a one-parameter dose-toxicity model, Carlin et al. (2013) proposed dealing with stickiness by discarding early trial data and limiting the memory of the method to a set of recent cohorts.

A simple example to illustrate what can go wrong with a greedy decision algorithm is as follows. Suppose that two regimes are available, ρ_1 and ρ_2, the outcome is "Response," and the true response probabilities are .50 for ρ_1 and .30 for ρ_2, so in fact ρ_1 is superior. Suppose that one starts by treating two patients with each regime, and thereafter uses the greedy algorithm that simply chooses each successive patient's regime as that having the larger current empirical response rate. Intuitively, this may seem to make perfect sense. After all, why would one want to treat a patient with the regime having the lower empirical response rate? It turns out that this rationale is flawed because it ignores random variation, and it is very short sighted in that it does not take into account what actually may happen with future patients. Suppose that, due to the play of chance, the initial data are 0/2 responses for ρ_1, giving an empirical response rate of 0, and 1/2 responses for ρ_2, giving an empirical response rate of .50. Since the empirical response rate is 0 for ρ_1 and is positive for ρ_2, the greedy rule will assign all remaining patients to the inferior regime, ρ_2. That is, the greedy rule causes one to get stuck at the inferior regime. The problem arises because the interim empirical response rates are only statistical estimates, and are not the actual true rates, but the greedy rule behaves as if the estimates actually equal the true rates. This example can be elaborated so that one gets stuck at some interim point in a clinical trial, or to include more than two regimes. A greedy algorithm is sensible only if the only thing that matters is optimizing the payoff for the next decision and the payoffs for all decisions made after that, including what happens to any future patients, do not matter.

Obviously, any statistical estimator for a response probability based on a sample of size 2 is very unreliable. Perhaps not so obviously, statistical estimators of decision criterion functions $\phi(\rho_1, \mathcal{D}_n), \cdots, \phi(\rho_k, \mathcal{D}_n)$ have very limited reliability for small to moderate maximum sample size N. As an example, ignoring Toxicity and focusing on Efficacy for simplicity, suppose that after $N = 48$ patients have been treated at five dose levels the data in the upper portion of Table 2.2 have been obtained, with each dose's posterior quantities computed assuming a beta(.5,.5) prior. A greedy algorithm based on the posterior mean, and ignoring variability, would simply choose dose level 3 as "best" since its posterior mean is largest. Accounting for uncertainty in terms of independent posterior 95% credible intervals shows that very little actually is known about the five response probabilities, since the subsample sizes are small. The point is that, if one makes a decision based on the fact that .38 is the largest of the posterior means, it must be kept in mind that there is

TABLE 2.2: Response data after a hypothetical phase I–II trial with either $N = 48$ or $N = 480$ patients. Posterior quantities are based on independent beta(.5, .5) priors

	N=48	Posterior Quantities	
Dose	# Responses/# Pats	Mean	95% CI
1	1 / 6	.21	.02 − .56
2	3 / 12	.27	.08 − .53
3	6 / 16	.38	.17 − .62
4	1 / 6	.21	.02 − .56
5	2 / 8	.28	.06 − .59

	N = 480	Posterior Quantities	
Dose	# Responses/# Pats	Mean	95% CI
1	10 / 60	.17	.09 − .28
2	30 / 120	.20	.14 − .27
3	60 / 160	.38	.30 − .45
4	10 / 60	.17	.09 − .28
5	20 /80	.25	.16 − .35

great posterior uncertainty about the five response probabilities. That is, ignoring uncertainty always is a mistake. If the probabilities of response at the two dose levels are denoted by θ_3 and θ_5, then $\Pr(\theta_3 < \theta_5 \mid data_{48}) = .724$, slightly larger than what would be obtained by flipping a coin. One cannot reliably declare any dose to be "best" in terms of response probabilities based on this dataset of 48 patients. Unfortunately, aside from the fact that Toxicity has not been included in order to simplify the illustration, this is a typical sample size encountered in a phase I–II trial.

To illustrate the effect of larger sample size, suppose that all five empirical proportions were exactly the same but obtained from a sample of size $N = 480$ instead of $N = 48$. The data then would be as given in the lower portion of Table 2.2. The posterior 95% credible intervals of dose levels 3 and 5 still would overlap, but the evidence in favor dose level 3 would be far more convincing. For this much larger sample, $\Pr(\theta_3 < \theta_5 \mid data_{480}) = .975$.

An effective way to deal with the problem of stickiness with greedy decision rules is to add some randomness to the decision rule. While this may seem counterintuitive, doing this ensures that there is a non-zero probability of exploring regimes other than the one that currently is empirically optimal. As a simple toy example, if $\hat{\pi}_{n,1}$ and $\hat{\pi}_{n,2}$ are the empirical response rates of two regimes after n patients, then an adaptive randomization (AR) rule is to choose ρ_1 with probability $p_{n,1} = \hat{\pi}_{n,1}/(\hat{\pi}_{n,1} + \hat{\pi}_{n,2})$, and choose ρ_2 with probability $1 - p_{n,1} = p_{n,2} = \hat{\pi}_{n,2}/(\hat{\pi}_{n,1} + \hat{\pi}_{n,2})$. For example, if $\hat{\pi}_{n,1} = .20$ and $\hat{\pi}_{n,2} = .30$ then $p_{n,1} = .40$ and $p_{n,2} = .60$, while if $\hat{\pi}_{n,1} = .20$ and $\hat{\pi}_{n,2} = .40$ then $p_{n,1} = .33$ and $p_{n,2} = .67$.

In a phase I–II trial based on utilities, always choosing an "optimal" regime ρ by maximizing $u(\rho \mid \mathcal{D}_n)$ is an example of a greedy algorithm, even if ρ is restricted to the set of regimes with acceptable Efficacy and Toxicity. A key aspect of this problem is that the posterior mean utilities $u(\rho_1 \mid \mathcal{D}_n), \cdots, u(\rho_J \mid \mathcal{D}_n)$ are statistics, and often are quite variable for most values of n during the trial. Simply choosing ρ_j to maximize among these ignores this variability. It is a mistake to treat the J posterior mean utilities based on an interim sample of size n as if they were the true mean utilities $\bar{U}(\rho_1, \theta), \cdots, \bar{U}(\rho_J, \theta)$ that one could compute if θ were known. This is analogous to the fact that, in the toy example with binary response given above, the empirical response rates $\hat{\pi}_{n,1}$ and $\hat{\pi}_{n,2}$ are statistics and are not the true response probabilities.

The problem of stickiness has both ethical and practical consequences. Because being greedy by maximizing $u(\rho_j \mid data_n)$ for each cohort may cause one to get stuck at a suboptimal regime, a substantial number of patients in the trial could be treated at that regime. It also increases the risk of recommending a suboptimal regime at the end of the trial, which diminishes benefit to future patients. To deal with this problem, AR may be used to improve this greedy algorithm and thus the reliability of the trial design. For ethical reasons, AR must be applied carefully. It is essential to restrict the regimes used to compute the AR probabilities to $\mathcal{A}_n$. Including AR gives a design that, on average, treats more patients at regimes with higher actual utilities and is more likely to choose a regime with maximum true utility, or at least with a high true utility, at the end of the trial. At the same time, it must not allow an unacceptable risk for the patients in each cohort. AR may be implemented in numerous ways, but one practical way with utilities is as follows. Given current data $\mathcal{D}_n$, the next cohort is randomized to regime ρ_j with probability

$$p_{n,j} = \frac{u(\rho_j \mid \mathcal{D}_n)I(\rho_j \in \mathcal{A}_n)}{\sum_{r=1}^{J} u(\rho_r \mid \mathcal{D}_n)\, I(\rho_r \in \mathcal{A}_n)}. \tag{2.3}$$

Similarly, if AR were applied in a phase I–II dose-finding trial using the EffTox method, in the above formula the posterior mean utility $u(\rho_j \mid \mathcal{D}_n)$ of regime j could be replaced by $\phi(\mu_{E,j,n}, \mu_{T,j,n})$ for dose j, to give AR probabilities

$$p_{n,j} = \frac{\phi(\mu_{E,j,n}, \mu_{T,j,n})I(\rho_j \in \mathcal{A}_n))}{\sum_{r=1}^{J} \phi(\mu_{E,r,n}, \mu_{T,r,n}\, I(\rho_r \in \mathcal{A}_n)}. \tag{2.4}$$

In practice, empirical AR probabilities such as $p_{n,1}, \cdots, p_{n,J}$ may be extremely variable for small n at the start of a trial, hence the AR probabilities may not be reliable. This may be dealt with by requiring an initial "burn-in" of some number of patients using the greedy algorithm, e.g., based on posterior values of a trade-off function or mean utility, until enough data have been obtained so that the AR probabilities are sufficiently reliable.

2.7 Simulation as a Design Tool

The following paradigm will be applied repeatedly throughout this book. Bayesian machinery is used to construct a model and design, and then the trial is simulated on the computer using that design, under each of a set of assumed regime-outcome scenarios, to evaluate the design's frequentist operating characteristics (OCs). Preliminary simulation results are used during the process of developing the design as a basis to calibrate numerical design parameters or prior parameters, and this process is iterated until a design with good OCs is obtained. Computer simulation thus is an essential tool in the process of constructing a design. This approach is motivated by the complexity of the model and sequential decision process, which make analytic derivation of a given design's properties infeasible in nearly all practical settings. This general simulation-based approach to Bayesian clinical trial design was used in the context of various early phase trials described by O'Quigley et al. (1990); Thall and Simon (1990, 1994); Gooley et al. (1994); Thall et al. (1995). Computer simulation now is widely accepted, and often required, as the standard approach for establishing the OCs of both Bayesian and frequentist clinical trial designs. More generally, computer simulation now typically is required to establish the properties of any statistical method, such as a new test or estimation procedure. This has supplanted the use of analytic results, often relying on asymptotic theory, that served as the only way to establish the properties of statistical methods prior to the advent of modern computing.

Each simulation scenario usually is characterized by fixed, assumed true values of the probabilities $p(y|\rho_1), \cdots, p(y|\rho_J)$, and possibly other parameters affecting design behavior, such as accrual rate or maximum sample size. In phase I–II designs, the OCs include the selection probability and distribution of sample size for each regime, the probability of stopping the trial early, and distribution of overall sample size. Under a given scenario, it is desirable to have high probabilities of selecting regimes or doses that are truly optimal or nearly optimal. It also is desirable to have a high probability of terminating a trial early under a scenario where, for example, all regimes are unacceptably toxic. One may think of the OCs of a design as generalizations of the size, power, and sample size distribution of a conventional randomized hypothesis-test-based group sequential trial.

The prior always has important consequences in an early phase trial, regardless of how "uninformative" it may appear to be. Simulating a trial based on a Bayesian model also provides a basis for the physician to better understand the consequences of particular numerical prior values or decision criteria. If desired, the physician may use what has been learned from the simulation results to modify his/her prior or decision parameters so that they more accurately reflect what the physician actually believes or intends. In this simulation process, it is important to examine the prior's properties in the natural parameter domain, such as $\pi_T(d, \theta)$, $\pi_E(d, \theta)$, rather than in terms of elements of θ that may have no intuitive meaning to a physician.

In addition to evaluating average design behavior by simulation, it also is useful to examine the first few decisions in the trial. This provides a basis for avoiding a prior or decision rules leading to early decisions that do not make sense. This is especially important because decisions made early in the trial are based on very little data. A simple example is examining how the design chooses the second cohort's dose adaptively based on different possible configurations of data from an initial cohort of three patients.

3

Establishing Priors

CONTENTS

3.1   Pathological Priors 43
3.2   Prior Effective Sample Size 46
3.3   Computing Priors from Elicited Values 50
    3.3.1   Least Squares Algorithm 54
    3.3.2   Pseudo Sampling Algorithm 55

"Bayesian methods . . . involve the serious difficulty of the choice of the prior distribution."

Dennis Lindley

3.1   Pathological Priors

Given a Bayesian model to be used as the basis for a clinical trial design, it might seem that one may deal with the problem of specifying the prior hyper-parameters simply by assuming convenient values for the prior hyper-mean vector $\tilde{\mu}$ and very large prior hyper-variances $\tilde{\sigma}^2$. For example, one might specify $\tilde{\mu}_j = \mathrm{E}(\theta_j) = 0$ and $\tilde{\sigma}_j^2 = \mathrm{var}(\theta_j) = 100^2$ for each parameter in $\theta = (\theta_1, \cdots, \theta_p)$, to ensure that the prior is "uninformative." While this sort of approach is used quite commonly in Bayesian data analysis, it may have very undesirable consequences when the model is used as the basis for an early phase trial design. This is because, early in the trial, adaptive decisions must be made based on posteriors computed from very small amounts of data. For example, the data $(x, Y_T, Y_E) = $ (dose, Toxicity, Efficacy) from each patient in an initial cohort of three patients often must be used to choose a dose adaptively for the second cohort. In this case, a putatively "uninformative" prior may have a non-trivial effect on the posterior and hence the design's adaptive decisions.

To see what can go wrong with prior specification for a Bayesian regression model used in an early phase trial, consider the following example. Suppose that a binary Toxicity indicator Y_T is used in a phase I CRM design to optimize dose, among the 5 standardized values $x = -2, -1, 0, 1, 2$, with target $\pi_T^* = .30$, maximum sample size $N = 45$ and cohort size 3, under the logistic model

$$\pi_T(x, \alpha, \beta \mid \tilde{\theta}) = \frac{e^{\alpha+\beta x}}{1 + e^{\alpha+\beta x}} \tag{3.1}$$

with $\beta > 0$ to ensure that π_T increases with x, where $\tilde{\theta} = (\tilde{\mu}_\alpha, \tilde{\mu}_\beta, \tilde{\sigma}_\alpha^2, \tilde{\sigma}_\beta^2)$ is the vector of prior hyper-parameters. The usual safety rule is imposed to terminate the trial if the lowest dose is too toxic compared to $\pi_T^* = .30$, with the trial stopped early if

$$Pr\{\pi_T(-2, \alpha, \beta \mid \tilde{\theta}) > .30 \mid \mathcal{D}_n\} > .90.$$

Suppose that one assumes the supposedly "uninformative" prior

$$\alpha, \ \log(\beta) \ \sim \ iid \ N(0, 100^2).$$

This prior gives a design with the pathological property that, if the true Toxicity probabilities are $(.25, .30, .35, .40, .45)$, so that dose $x = -1$ is optimal, then the trial is stopped early and no dose is selected with probability .32. If the true Toxicity probabilities are $(.30, .35, .40, .45, .50)$, so that dose $x = -2$ is optimal, then the trial is stopped early and no dose is selected with probability .50. The reason for this pathological behavior is that the seemingly "uninformative" prior actually is far too disperse, and the prior mean 0 for α and $\log(\beta)$, together with $\tilde{\sigma}_\alpha^2 = \tilde{\sigma}_\beta^2 = 100^2$, force the induced prior of the Toxicity probability $\pi_T(-2, \alpha, \beta \mid \tilde{\theta})$ to have far too much probability mass near 1. Because the data early in the trial cannot reliably overcome this, the prior causes the early stopping rule to shut down the trial far too often.

This example illustrates the important point that numerical values of prior hyper-parameters of a given real-valued model parameter θ_j often have no intuitive meaning, whereas the induced priors on outcome probabilities are easy to understand and interpret. This general idea was first presented by Tsutakawa (1975) and Tsutakawa and Lin (1986), and discussed further by Grieve (1988). They recommended that, for Bayesian regression with binary outcomes, priors should be elicited on the domain of the outcome probabilities, rather than in terms of real-valued parameters appearing in their linear components. A discussion of this issue is given by Christensen et al. (2011, Section 8.4). In the example given above, the particular numerical hyper-parameter values have no intuitive meaning, since α and β are essentially statistical objects. While it is clear that larger β corresponds to larger π_T, the numerical values $\beta = .2, 2$, or 20 have no intuitive meaning. In contrast, numerical values of the outcome probabilities are intuitively meaningful, and the behavior of their priors is easy to understand, especially once the induced priors of the $\pi_T(x, \alpha, \beta \mid \tilde{\theta})$'s are plotted and prior values of $Pr\{\pi_T(-2, \alpha, \beta \mid \tilde{\theta}) > .30\}$ are computed. In practice, values of stopping criteria such as $Pr\{\pi_T(-2, \alpha, \beta \mid \tilde{\theta}) > .30 \mid \mathcal{D}_n\}$ should be computed for small

n corresponding to early decisions in the trial. The practical point is that these posterior probabilities are statistics, hence they are variable, and they are highly variable for small n.

At the other extreme, it is important to avoid priors that are overly informative due to $\tilde{\sigma}^2$ being too small, since one's prior assumptions may be wrong. This may cause the design to be unsafe because it does not stop the trial early with sufficiently high probability if the agent actually is too toxic. For example, suppose that an investigator believes, *a priori*, that a new agent is very safe for all x_j. This might motivate constructing a prior to reflect this belief. One method for computing prior means is the pseudo-sampling algorithm described later in this chapter. Given elicited prior mean Toxicity probabilities (.02, .04, .06, .08, .10), reflecting the strong belief that the agent is safe, one may apply the pseudo-sampling algorithm to compute the hyper-means $\tilde{\mu}_\alpha = -2.90$ of α and $\tilde{\mu}_\beta = -3.64$ of β. One then might set the prior hyper-variances to be very small values, say $\tilde{\sigma}_\alpha^2 = \tilde{\sigma}_\beta^2 = \tilde{\sigma}^2 = .25$ to reflect the strength of the investigator's prior belief. The resulting prior is $\alpha \sim N(-2.90, .25)$, $log(\beta) \sim N(-3.64, .25)$. This prior leads to the following decisions. Suppose that .10 has been chosen as an upper limit on $\pi_T(-2, \alpha, \beta \mid \tilde{\theta})$ and the safety rule is to stop the trial if $\Pr\{\pi_T(-2, \alpha, \beta \mid \tilde{\theta}) > .10 \mid \mathcal{D}_n\} > .90$. If 3/3 Toxicities are observed in the first cohort of 3 patients then, based on a simple beta(.10,.90) prior, one would obtain the posterior beta probabilities

$$\Pr\{\pi_T(-2 \mid \tilde{\theta} = (.10, .90)) > .10 \mid \mathcal{D}_3\} = .999$$
$$\Pr\{\pi_T(-2 \mid \tilde{\theta} = (.10, .90)) > .20 \mid \mathcal{D}_3\} = .994$$
$$\Pr\{\pi_T(-2 \mid \tilde{\theta} = (.10, .90)) > .30 \mid \mathcal{D}_3\} = .98.$$

In contrast, under the model with the above informative prior reflecting the strong belief that the agent is safe, these posterior probabilities would be

$$\Pr\{\pi_T(-2, \alpha, \beta \mid \tilde{\theta}) > .10 \mid \mathcal{D}_3\} = .56$$
$$\Pr\{\pi_T(-2, \alpha, \beta \mid \tilde{\theta}) > .20 \mid \mathcal{D}_3\} = .06$$
$$\Pr\{\pi_T(-2, \alpha, \beta \mid \tilde{\theta}) > .30 \mid \mathcal{D}_3\} = .00.$$

The informative prior obviously is pathological. Observation of 3/3 Toxicities at the lowest dose $x = -2$ gives a posterior that quantifies the probability of Toxicity at that dose, $\pi_T(-2, \alpha, \beta \mid \tilde{\theta})$, as being acceptable, which strongly disagrees with the observed data and common sense. The resulting design is unsafe. One could address this problem by choosing larger numerical values for $\tilde{\sigma}_\alpha^2$ and $\tilde{\sigma}_\beta^2$, but the question is precisely what values should be chosen. Recall that if they are too large, then the induced priors on $\pi_T(x, \alpha, \beta \mid \tilde{\theta})$ for $x = -2, ..., +2$ also become pathological, since most of their probability mass is either above .99 or below .01, and the design stops too often.

In the next section, we will discuss prior effective sample size (ESS), which provides a simple, quantitative tool to evaluate how informative a prior actual is before using it. The following example illustrates how ESS can be used to avoid pathological priors like those above and obtain a "Three Bears" prior

TABLE 3.1: Comparison of dose selection percentages and early stopping probabilities of the CRM design with target $\pi_T^* = .30$, maximum sample size 45 and cohort size 3, for each of three priors. The priors with $\tilde{\sigma}^2 = \tilde{\sigma}_\alpha^2 = \tilde{\sigma}_\beta^2 = 10,000$, .25, and 9 are, respectively, uninformative, overly informative, and derived using pseudo-sampling to have effective sample size .7.

		Standardized Dose					
		-2	-1	0	1	2	Stop
				Scenario 1			
$\tilde{\sigma}^2$	π_T^{true}	0.25	0.30	0.35	0.40	0.45	
10,000		29	16	6	4	14	32
.25		5	2	2	4	87	0
9		25	37	20	6	2	11
				Scenario 2			
	π_T^{true}	0.30	0.35	0.40	0.45	0.50	
10,000		31	8	3	1	6	50
.25		12	5	5	6	72	0
9		35	27	8	2	1	28
				Scenario 3			
	π_T^{true}	0.45	0.50	0.55	0.60	0.65	
10,000		4	0	0	0	0	95
.25		53	5	5	4	12	21
9		11	1	0	0	0	88

between the two extremes that is "just right." Consider the trial design discussed above with prior Toxicity probabilities (.05, .10, .20, .30, .45). Applying the pseudo-sampling method and calibrating the hyper-variance to have ESS 0.7, gives the prior $\alpha \sim N(-1.51, 9)$, $log(\beta_T) \sim N(-0.44, 9)$. Table 3.1 summarizes the dose selection percentages and early stopping probabilities for the three priors. The uninformative prior with $\tilde{\sigma}^2 = 10,000$ stops too often in Scenarios 1 and 2. The overly informative prior with $\tilde{\sigma}^2 = .25$ stops far too infrequently in Scenario 3, where all doses are too toxic. The Three Bears prior with $\tilde{\sigma}^2 = 9$ has good operating characteristics for all three scenarios.

3.2   Prior Effective Sample Size

The above examples illustrate the general point that quantifying the amount of information in the prior is a fundamental issue in Bayesian inference. One of the most common criticisms of Bayesian statistics is that inferences depend on the assumed prior, and that this prior is subjective. Criticizing Bayesian statistics on the grounds that priors are subjective is silly, simply because all statistical models and methods rely on subjective assumptions. Still, in Bayesian statistics it is very important to avoid making posterior inferences based on a prior that is inappropriately informative. This is both a scientific and a practical issue. As shown in the above examples, a prior that might be considered "uninformative" also can produce undesirable posterior inferences and actions. Prior variances can be too big, or be they can too small. Like Goldilocks in her adventure with The Three Bears, a practicing Bayesian should establish a prior that is not too informative, not too uninformative, but is just right. Effective sample size (ESS) is a tool that helps one to determine such a prior.

While the problem of quantifying the information in a prior $p(\theta \mid \tilde{\theta})$ is straightforward for some commonly used models, for most models the answer is not obvious. The logistic regression model is an example, as shown by the numerical illustration given above. Another common example is a Bayesian linear regression model for data $(Y_1, X_1), \cdots (Y_n, X_n)$ where it is assumed that $E(Y_i|X_i) = \beta_0 + \beta_1 X_i$ and $\text{var}(Y_i|X_i) = \sigma^2$ for $i = 1, \cdots, n$, with priors

$$\beta_j \sim N(\tilde{\mu}_j, \tilde{\sigma}_j^2), \quad j = 0, 1 \quad \text{and} \quad \sigma^2 \sim IG(\tilde{\alpha}_1, \tilde{\alpha}_2).$$

on the three model parameters $(\beta_0, \beta_1, \sigma^2)$. Under these assumptions, the informativeness of the prior is determined by the numerical values of the six hyper-parameters $\tilde{\theta} = (\tilde{\mu}_0, \tilde{\sigma}_0, \tilde{\mu}_1, \tilde{\sigma}_1, \tilde{\alpha}_1, \tilde{\alpha}_2)$. However, it is not at all clear how much information is provided by, say, $\tilde{\theta} = (0, 1, 0, 1, 10, 5)$.

Morita et al. (2008) provide a general constructive definition of prior ESS, which is an easily interpretable number for quantifying the informativeness of a prior. The basic idea is motivated by the following heuristic example, which serves as a prototype for more complex models. It is widely agreed that a $beta(\tilde{a}, \tilde{b})$ distribution has ESS $= \tilde{a} + \tilde{b}$. This may be argued using the well-known fact that, due to conjugacy, given a binomial random variable Y from a sample of size n with success probability π following a $beta(\tilde{a}, \tilde{b})$ prior, the posterior is $[\pi \mid Y, n] \sim beta(\tilde{a} + Y, \tilde{b} + n - Y)$. This implies that, given a binomial sample of size n, the prior sum $\tilde{a} + \tilde{b}$ becomes the posterior sum $\tilde{a} + \tilde{b} + n$, so the difference (posterior sum - prior sum) $= (\tilde{a} + \tilde{b} + n) - (\tilde{a} + \tilde{b}) = n$ is the sample size. Saying that a $beta(\tilde{a}, \tilde{b})$ distribution has ESS $= \tilde{a} + \tilde{b}$ may be explained by repeating this prior-to-posterior computation, but this time thinking of the $beta(\tilde{a}, \tilde{b})$ distribution as a posterior obtained after starting out with a very non-informative prior. That is, suppose that the $beta(\tilde{a}, \tilde{b})$ distribution is the posterior arising from a sample of size $\tilde{a} + \tilde{b}$ starting with a previous $beta(\tilde{c}, \tilde{d})$ prior having a very small amount of information. This may be formalized by setting $\tilde{c} + \tilde{d} = \epsilon$ for an arbitrarily small $\epsilon > 0$ and solving ESS $=$ (posterior sum - prior sum) $= (\tilde{a} + \tilde{b}) - (\tilde{c} + \tilde{d}) = \tilde{a} + \tilde{b} - \epsilon$. Since ϵ is arbitrarily small, this says that the ESS of a $beta(\tilde{a}, \tilde{b})$ is $\tilde{a} + \tilde{b}$.

The general constructive definition of ESS given by Morita et al. (2008, 2012) is as follows. Let $f(Y \mid \theta)$ be a parametric probability distribution function (pdf) or probability mass function (pmf) for a random vector Y with parameter vector $\theta = (\theta_1, \cdots, \theta_d)$, and let $p(\theta \mid \tilde{\theta})$ be the prior. The first step of the construction is to define an ϵ-*information prior* $q_0(\theta \mid \tilde{\theta}_0)$ that has the same mean vector and correlations as $p(\theta \mid \tilde{\theta})$ but has suitably large variances. How to construct an ϵ-information prior will be explained below. Denote $\mathcal{Y}_m = (Y_1, \cdots, Y_m)$, with $Y_i \sim f(Y_i \mid \theta)$ an i.i.d. sample, so the likelihood is

$$f_m(\mathcal{Y}_m \mid \theta) = \prod_{i=1}^{m} f(Y_i \mid \theta).$$

Given a sample $\mathcal{Y}_m$, with possibly vector-valued predictors $\mathcal{X}_m = (X_1, \cdots, X_m)$, and an ε-information prior $q_0(\theta \mid \tilde{\theta}_0)$, the posterior is

$$q_m(\theta \mid \tilde{\theta}_0, \mathcal{Y}_m, \mathcal{X}_m) \propto q_0(\theta \mid \tilde{\theta}_0) f_m(\mathcal{Y}_m \mid \mathcal{X}_m, \theta).$$

The ESS is the interpolated value of m minimizing the distance between $q_m(\theta \mid \tilde{\theta}_0, \mathcal{Y}_m)$ and $p(\theta \mid \tilde{\theta})$. Morita et al. (2008, 2012) define this distance in several ways, using either the trace or the determinant of the second derivative matrices of $\log\{p(\theta|\tilde{\theta})\}$ and $\log\{q_m(\theta|\tilde{\theta}_0)\}$. They also provide detailed computational algorithms for various cases.

An ε-information prior may be constructed as follows. Suppose that $\theta = (\theta_1, \cdots, \theta_d)$. Denote the prior variances $\tilde{\sigma}_{p,j}^2 = var(\theta_j)$ under $p(\theta \mid \tilde{\theta})$ and $\tilde{\sigma}_{q_0,j}^2 = var(\theta_j)$ under $q_0(\theta \mid \tilde{\theta}_0)$, for $j = 1, \cdots, d$. The first requirement is that $\tilde{\sigma}_{p,j}^2 < \bar{V}_j(\tilde{\theta})$ for a fixed upper bound $\bar{V}_j(\tilde{\theta})$ that may be finite or, if $\tilde{\sigma}_{p,j}^2$ is unbounded, $\bar{V}_j(\tilde{\theta}) = \infty$. For any $\epsilon > 0$, $q_0(\theta \mid \tilde{\theta}_0)$, is an ϵ-*information prior* if it satisfies the inequality

$$\left\{ \frac{\bar{V}_j(\tilde{\theta}) - \sigma_{q_0,j}^2}{\bar{V}_j(\tilde{\theta}) - \tilde{\sigma}_{p,j}^2} \right\} \frac{\tilde{\sigma}_{p,j}^2}{\tilde{\sigma}_{q_0,j}^2} < \varepsilon \qquad \text{for } j = 1, ..., d. \qquad (3.2)$$

If $\bar{V}_j(\tilde{\theta}) = \infty$, then the above inequality is simply $\tilde{\sigma}_{p,j}^2/\tilde{\sigma}_{q_0,j}^2 < \varepsilon$, so one may just choose the fixed prior hyper-variance $\tilde{\sigma}_{q_0,j}^2$ to be sufficiently large to ensure this bound. For cases where the upper bound on the variance is finite, $\bar{V}_j(\tilde{\theta}) < \infty$, the inequality can be written in the form

$$\frac{\bar{V}_j(\tilde{\theta})}{\tilde{\sigma}_{q_0,j}^2} - 1 < \varepsilon \left\{ \frac{\bar{V}_j(\tilde{\theta})}{\tilde{\sigma}_{p,j}^2} - 1 \right\}.$$

In this case, one can specify $\tilde{\theta}_0$ to ensure that $\tilde{\sigma}_{q_0,j}^2$ is close enough to $\bar{V}_j(\tilde{\theta})$ from below so that the inequality holds. The $beta(\tilde{a}, \tilde{b})$ is an example of the latter case, since, denoting $\tilde{\mu} = \tilde{a}/(\tilde{a} + \tilde{b})$, it has variance

$$\tilde{\sigma}_p^2 = \tilde{\mu}(1 - \tilde{\mu})/(\tilde{a} + \tilde{b} + 1)$$

that is bounded above by $\tilde{\mu}(1 - \tilde{\mu})$, which is $< 1/2$ since $0 < \tilde{\mu} < 1$. The ϵ-information prior may be specified as a $beta(\tilde{a}/c, \tilde{b}/c)$, simply by choosing $c > 0$ large enough so that $1/c < \epsilon$.

A key point is that ESS is not a property of a prior alone, but rather it is a property of the prior $p(\theta \mid \tilde{\theta})$, the distribution $f(Y \mid \theta)$ of the observed outcome, and possibly the adaptive experiment that will be conducted using posteriors computed from this model. This is because, when computing prior ESS in the context of an adaptive clinical trial, since the computational algorithm involves the distribution of outcomes that are used by the design's adaptive rules, the ESS also may depend on the design.

In some simple settings, the ESS can be determined analytically from the prior and likelihood, so no computational algorithm is needed. For example, generalizing the beta to k elementary outcomes, a Dirichlet prior $Dir(\tilde{a}_1, \cdots, \tilde{a}_k)$ for parameters $(\theta_1, \cdots, \theta_k)$ of a multinomial likelihood has ESS $= \tilde{a}_1 + \cdots + \tilde{a}_k$. Another example is a gamma$(\tilde{a}, \tilde{b})$ prior for the mean θ of an exponential distribution, which has ESS $= \tilde{a}$. A third example is a $N(0, \sigma^2)$ distribution with σ^2 following an inverse χ^2 prior with parameters $(\tilde{a}, \tilde{b})$, which has ESS $= \tilde{a}$.

A simple way to compute an approximate ESS of a prior $p(\theta \mid \tilde{\theta})$ is to define one or more probabilities $\pi_1(\theta), \cdots \pi_k(\theta)$ and match the prior mean and variance of each probability with those of a $beta(\tilde{a}, \tilde{b})$, which has mean $\tilde{\mu}$ $= \tilde{a}/(\tilde{a} + \tilde{b})$ and variance $\tilde{\sigma}^2 = \tilde{\mu}(1 - \tilde{\mu})/(\tilde{a} + \tilde{b} + 1)$. Denoting the prior mean and variance of the probability $\pi_j(\theta)$ by $\tilde{\mu}_j$ and $\tilde{\sigma}_j^2$, solving the equations

$$\tilde{\mu}_j = \frac{\tilde{a}}{(\tilde{a} + \tilde{b})} \quad \text{and} \quad \tilde{\sigma}_j^2 = \frac{\tilde{\mu}(1 - \tilde{\mu})}{(\tilde{a} + \tilde{b} + 1)}$$

gives the approximate value

$$ESS_j \cong \frac{\tilde{\mu}_j(1 - \tilde{\mu}_j)}{\tilde{\sigma}_j^2} - 1.$$

One may use the arithmetic mean $\sum_{j=1}^k ESS_j/k$ to approximate the ESS of $p(\theta \mid \tilde{\theta})$.

An illustrative example of ESS computation for a logistic regression is given in Section 6 of Morita et al. (2008). For a phase I dose-finding trial with doses $d_1 = 100$, ..., $d_6 = 600$, using the standardized doses $x_j = \log(d_j) - \sum_{r=1}^6 \log(d_j)$, for the model $\pi_T(x_j, \alpha_T, \beta_T) = \exp(\alpha_T + x_j\beta_T)/\{1 + \exp(\alpha_T + x_j\beta_T)\}$. Assuming independent normal priors for α_T and β_T and solving for the two prior means from the equations based on $E\{\pi_T(x_2, \theta)\} = .25$ at $d = 200$ and $E\{\pi_T(x_5, \theta)\} = .75$ at $d = 500$ gives means $\tilde{\mu}_{\alpha_T} = -0.1313$ and $\tilde{\mu}_{\beta_T} = 2.3890$. Assuming variances $\tilde{\sigma}_{\alpha_T}^2 = \tilde{\sigma}_{\beta_T}^2 = 4$ gives ESS $= 2.3$, which is reasonable for a dose-finding trial with cohorts of size 3. An important property of ESS is that it is not additive, in that if θ can be partitioned into subvectors (θ_1, θ_2), the ESS values of the marginals $p(\theta_1|\tilde{\theta}_1)$ and $p(\theta_2|\tilde{\theta}_2)$ do not sum to the ESS of $p(\theta|\tilde{\theta})$. In this example, the prior of α_T has ESS $= 1.4$ and the prior of β_T has ESS $= 6.3$.

3.3   Computing Priors from Elicited Values

Computing prior hyperparameters $\tilde{\theta}$ from elicited values may be done in a straightforward way if the number of elicited values equals the number of parameters in $\tilde{\theta}$. To compute prior means, $\tilde{\mu}$, this often is done by matching each elicited value with its corresponding prior expected value and solving the resulting set of equations for $\tilde{\mu}$. If desired, one also may include prior variances, and possibly other shape or scale parameters in the system of equations. We will not include hyper-variances, since these will be calibrated to control the level of prior informativeness, in order to use the prior as the basis for a trial design. The following is a more detailed account of the type of computation given earlier in Section 3.1.

Consider a simple setting involving only an indicator Y_T of Toxicity and standardized dose $x = 1, 2, 3, 4, 5$, or 6. Suppose that the probability of Toxicity at x follows the logistic regression model

$$\pi_T(x, \theta_T) = \frac{\exp(\alpha_T + \beta_T x)}{1 + \exp(\alpha_T + \beta_T x)},$$

denoting $\theta_T = (\alpha_T, \beta_T)$. For the prior, suppose that α_T and β_T are independent with $\alpha_T \sim N(\tilde{\mu}_{\alpha_T}, \tilde{\sigma}^2_{\alpha_T})$ and $\beta_T \sim N(\tilde{\mu}_{\beta_T}, \tilde{\sigma}^2_{\beta_T})$, so that there are four hyperparameters, $\tilde{\theta}_T = (\tilde{\mu}_{\alpha_T}, \tilde{\mu}_{\beta_T}, \tilde{\sigma}^2_{\alpha_T}, \tilde{\sigma}^2_{\beta_T})$. We focus on the problem of deriving numerical values of the two hyper-means, $(\tilde{\mu}_{\alpha_T}, \tilde{\mu}_{\beta_T})$, from two elicited values, with the plan to then calibrate the numerical values of the two hyper-variances.

The prior mean probability of Toxicity at dose x is

$$\tilde{\mu}_{\pi_T}(x) = E\{\pi_T(x, \theta_T)\} = \int \pi_T(x, \theta_T) p(\theta_T \mid \tilde{\theta}_T) d\theta_T.$$

The notation $\tilde{\mu}_{\pi_T}(x)$ is used to remind us of the fact that the prior mean for each dose x depends on the fixed values $\tilde{\theta}_T$ that determine the prior $p(\theta_T \mid \tilde{\theta}_T)$. If the two elicited means for Toxicity are $\mu_{\pi_T}(2)^{(e)} = .25$ and $\mu_{\pi_T}(5)^{(e)} = .75$, then substituting the prior means $\tilde{\mu}_{\alpha_T}$ for μ_{α_T} and $\tilde{\mu}_{\beta_T}$ for μ_{β_T} in the formula for $\pi_T(x, \theta_T)$ gives the two equations

$$.25 = \tilde{\mu}_{\pi_T}(2) \simeq \frac{\exp\{\tilde{\mu}_{\alpha_T} + \tilde{\mu}_{\beta_T} \, 2\}}{1 + \exp\{\tilde{\mu}_{\alpha_T} + \tilde{\mu}_{\beta_T} \, 2\}}$$

and

$$.75 = \tilde{\mu}_{\pi_T}(5) \simeq \frac{\exp\{\tilde{\mu}_{\alpha_T} + \tilde{\mu}_{\beta_T} \, 5\}}{1 + \exp\{\tilde{\mu}_{\alpha_T} + \tilde{\mu}_{\beta_T} \, 5\}},$$

which may be solved for the two unknown means. The solution in this case is $\tilde{\mu}_{\alpha_T} = 2.56234$ and $\tilde{\mu}_{\beta_T} = 0.7324$. Note that the right-hand sides of the equations are approximations of $\tilde{\mu}_{\pi_T}(2)$ and $\tilde{\mu}_{\pi_T}(5)$ obtained by plugging in the prior means of α_T and β_T. This ignores the nonlinearity of the function $\eta \to e^\eta/(1 + e^\eta)$, but it certainly is a reasonable approximate approach.

For the model of a phase I–II trial, assuming for simplicity that Y_T and Y_E are independent, suppose that we also have the efficacy probability

$$\pi_E(x, \theta_E) = \frac{\exp(\alpha_E + \beta_E x)}{1 + \exp(\alpha_E + \beta_E x)}$$

for each x, and that the four parameters $\alpha_T, \beta_T, \alpha_T, \beta_T$ are independent with $\alpha_k \sim N(\tilde{\mu}_{\alpha_k}, \tilde{\sigma}^2_{\alpha_k})$, and $\beta_k \sim N(\tilde{\mu}_{\beta_k}, \tilde{\sigma}^2_{\beta_k})$ for each $k = E, T$. If the elicited prior mean efficacy probabilities are $\mu_{\pi_E}(2)^{(e)} = .10$ and $\mu_{\pi_E}(5)^{(e)} = .40$, then solving two equations similarly to those given above for Toxicity gives $\tilde{\mu}_{\alpha_E} = \text{-}3.3917$ and $\tilde{\mu}_{\beta_E} = 0.5972$. Given these four hyper-means, one may calibrate the numerical values of the four hyper-variances $\tilde{\sigma}^2_{\alpha_T}, \tilde{\sigma}^2_{\beta_T}, \tilde{\sigma}^2_{\alpha_E}, \tilde{\sigma}^2_{\beta_E}$ to obtain a desired level of informativeness. This could be done using the mean approximate prior effective sample size,

$$\overline{ESS} = \sum_{x=1}^{6} \sum_{k=E,T} ESS[p\{\pi_k(x, \theta_k) \mid \tilde{\theta}_k\}],$$

where $p\{\pi(x|\theta_k) \mid \tilde{\theta}_k\}$ denotes the prior of $\pi_k(x, \theta_k)$. For example, setting all prior variances equal to 3 gives $\overline{ESS} = 0.72$.

This approach may be carried out more generally to solve for $p > 2$ hyperparameters $\tilde{\theta}^{p \times 1}$. Given a regime ρ, parametric functions $\xi_j(\rho, \theta)$ and their corresponding elicited mean values $\xi_j(\rho, \theta)^{(e)}$, for $j = 1, ..., p$, one may formulate a system of p equations

$$\xi_j(\rho, \theta)^{(e)} = \xi_j(\rho, \theta)|_{\theta = \tilde{\theta}}, \qquad j = 1, \cdots, p$$

and solve for p-dimensional hyper-parameter vector $\tilde{\theta}$. The functions $\xi_j(\rho, \theta)$'s may be marginal probabilities, as in the above example, or other quantities, such as interval probabilities of the form $\Pr\{L < \pi_E(\rho, \theta) < U\}$ for given lower and upper limits L and U. For real-valued outcomes, such as an event time T, $\xi_j(\rho, \theta)$ may be a cumulative probability $\Pr(T \le t \mid \rho, \theta)$, or possibly median$(T \mid \rho, \theta)$ or some other percentile. This leads naturally to the question of whether prior variances, and possibly covariances, should be established by the elicitation process, as well. While in theory this certainly can be carried out, as explained above it may lead to pathological or overly informative priors that are inappropriate for use in a Bayesian model that will be the basis for a clinical trial.

A different version of the general approach of matching the number of elicited values with the number of parameters to be determined was given by Bedrick et al. (1996) in the context of generalized linear models. Rather than eliciting only prior means, their method begins by eliciting entire priors on the domain of the observable outcomes, and then transforms these to obtain

priors on the real parameter domain. This follows the general recommendation of Tsutakawa (1975), Tsutakawa and Lin (1986), and Grieve (1988), that
it is much more appropriate, and more realistic, to elicit information on the
observable outcome domain, especially outcome probabilities, rather than to
attempt eliciting information about real-valued model parameters that may
be difficult for a non-statistician to interpret. The formulation used by Bedrick
et al. (1996) assumes that each outcome Y has corresponding covariate vector
x and p-dimensional regression parameter vector $\beta = (\beta_1, \cdots, \beta_p)$ under a
generalized linear model. Each mean $\mu(x) = \mathrm{E}(Y \mid x, \beta)$ is related to a linear
term by the equation $g\{\mu(x)\} = x'\beta$ by a monotone link function g. They
define a conditional mean prior (CMP) obtained by first evaluating prior information at p locations $\tilde{x}_1, \cdots, \tilde{x}_p$ in the covariate space. For each location
$j = 1, \cdots, p$, a prior distribution is specified for the mean of Y at that location, denoted by $\tilde{\mu}_j = E(Y \mid \tilde{x}_j, \beta)$. Thus, each mean is defined conditional
on the covariate vector at its location. The prior on β is then obtained as
that which is induced by the CMP on $\tilde{\mu} = (\tilde{\mu}_1, \cdots \tilde{\mu}_p)$ by applying the usual
transformation theorem for probability distributions. Denoting the $p \times p$ non-
singular matrix $\tilde{X}$ having $\tilde{x}_j$ as its jth row, and G as the vector of mappings
that apply the link g to each $\tilde{\mu}_j$, one may write the one-to-one transformation
from the p means to the parameter vector as $G(\tilde{\mu}) = \tilde{X}\beta$. This implies that β
$= \tilde{X}^{-1}G(\tilde{\mu})$, which yields the induced prior on β from the prior on $\tilde{\mu}$ by the
transformation theorem.

For example, in the binomial case each Y_j is the proportion of successes in
N_j observations at $\tilde{x}_j$, so that $E(Y_j \mid \tilde{x}_j) = \tilde{\mu}_j = F(\tilde{x}_j'\beta)$, where $F = g^{-1}$ is
a continuous cdf such as $F(\eta) = \Phi(\eta)$ or $\exp(\eta)/\{1 + \exp(\eta)\}$ for real-valued
η. Suppose that the elicited priors on the means are independent betas, with
$\tilde{\mu}_j \sim beta(a_{1,j}, a_{2,j})$, for $j = 1, \cdots, p$, so the prior on the vector of p means is

$$p(\tilde{\mu}) \propto \prod_{j=1}^{p} \tilde{\mu}_j^{a_{1,j}-1}(1 - \tilde{\mu}_j)^{a_{2,j}-1}.$$

Denoting $f = F'$, by the transformation theorem the induced prior on β is

$$p(\beta) \propto \prod_{j=1}^{p} F(\tilde{x}_j'\beta)^{a_{1,j}-1} \left[1 - F(\tilde{x}_j'\beta)\right]^{a_{2,j}-1} f(\tilde{x}_j'\beta)$$

An illustration of this methodology for analyzing binomial data is given in
Bedrick et al. (1996).

For application to clinical trial design, the above binomial example might
be made more concrete by considering a two-agent trial with dose x_1 of agent
1 and dose x_2 of agent 2. Suppose that a single binary outcome $Y = 0$ or
1 is observed for each patient, so all $N_i = 1$. Then $x = (1, x_1, x_2)$ and $\beta =$
$(\beta_0, \beta_1, \beta_2)$ with $x'\beta = \beta_0 + \beta_1 x_1 + \beta_2 x_2$, and $\mu(x) = \Pr(Y = 1|x, \beta)$. If
one elicits a $Beta(a_{1,j}, a_{2,j})$ prior at each of three particular dose pairs, $\tilde{x}_j =$
$(1, \tilde{x}_{1,j}, \tilde{x}_{2,j})$, for $j = 1, 2, 3$, and assumes a probit link $F(x'\beta) = \Phi(x'\beta)$ for

any x, then, by the transformation theorem, the induced prior on β is

$$p(\beta) \propto \prod_{j=1}^{3} \Phi(\tilde{x}'_j \beta)^{a_{1,j}-1} \left[1 - \Phi(\tilde{x}'_j \beta)\right]^{a_{2,j}-1} \phi(\tilde{x}'_j \beta),$$

where ϕ denotes the standard normal pdf.

Thinking about how one actually would elicit a prior in a phase I–II setting, however, shows that there is an obvious problem with any method for establishing priors that requires one to match dimensions. The first algorithm matches p elicited prior means values with p corresponding theoretical model-based quantities, substitutes plug-in values of the p prior hyper-parameters $\tilde{\theta}$, and then solves the p equations for $\tilde{\theta}$. This requires the number of elicited values to equal the number of hyperparameters $\tilde{\theta}$ to be determined. So one would need to elicit the means of exactly $\dim(\tilde{\theta})$ values of $\xi_j(\rho, \theta)$'s, but no more since otherwise the set of equations would be overdetermined. Similarly, the method of BCJ, which uses elicited priors rather than single numbers, requires the number of elicited priors to equal the dimension of the regression parameter vector, β, in order to apply the transformation theorem.

To see how trying to apply either method may be problematic in the above two-agent combination trial example, suppose that the dose x_1 of agent 1 has three levels and the dose x_2 of agent 2 has four levels, for a total of 12 dose pairs $x = (x_1, x_2)$. Suppose that one wishes to establish a prior on $\beta = (\beta_E, \beta_T)$ $= (\beta_{E,0}, \beta_{E,1}, \beta_{E,2}, \beta_{T,0}, \beta_{T,1}, \beta_{T,2})$ for the simple model where $g\{\pi_k(x, \theta)\} = \beta_{k,0} + \beta_{k,1} x_1 + \beta_{k,2} x_2$ for $k = E, T$, where Y_E and Y_T are independent, so there are $p = 6$ parameters. Using either method described above, one would need to elicit prior information for β_E at exactly three of the 12 dose pairs, and, similarly, for β_T at exactly three dose pairs. This may not make sense, since in practice one almost certainly would want to elicit priors at more than only three of the 12 dose pairs for each outcome. The question, then, is how one should proceed if either priors or prior means are elicited at more than three dose pairs, so that there are more than six pieces of information. One very simple solution, using either method, is to discard some of the prior information in order to make the dimensions match. Of course, this is very unappealing since it wastes information, and it also leads to the question of which prior information should be discarded.

The following algorithms provide practical approaches for dealing with this problem without throwing away any elicited prior information. For many of the designs that we will discuss, we will establish the hyper-parameters of the prior by applying some version of the following general prior computation algorithm. Assume, for simplicity, that each $\theta_j \sim N(\tilde{\mu}_j, \tilde{\sigma}_j^2)$, for $j = 1, \cdots, p$, and that these are independent, so that $\tilde{\theta} = (\tilde{\mu}, \tilde{\sigma}) = (\tilde{\mu}_1, \cdots, \tilde{\mu}_p, \tilde{\sigma}_1, \cdots, \tilde{\sigma}_p)$, i.e., $\tilde{\theta}$ has $2p$ elements consisting of a p-vector of hyper-means and a p-vector of hyper-variances. This formulation works quite well in many trial design settings, although the algorithm can be generalized easily to accommodate more complex set-ups. Let a given vector $\{x_r, r = 1, \cdots, m\}$ denote possible combinations of doses or schedules in the regime ρ, and in general each x_r also may include patient covariates.

3.3.1   Least Squares Algorithm

Step 1: Identify a set of vectors $x = \{x_1, \cdots, x_m\}$, each consisting of some combination treatment regime and possibly patient characteristics, and k outcome probabilities $\pi(\theta, x) = (\pi_1(\theta \mid x), \cdots, \pi_k(\theta \mid x)))$, that are meaningful to the physicians planning the trial, where $k \geq m$.

Step 2: Elicit the physicians' prior expected values $\pi^{(e)}(x) = (\pi_1^{(e)}(\theta, x), \cdots, \pi_k^{(e)}(\theta, x)$ of $\pi(\theta, x)$.

Step 3: Treat the elicited values $\pi^{(e)}(x)$ like observed outcome variables and the hyper-parameters $\tilde{\theta}$ like usual parameters in a conventional statistical regression setting where each $\pi_j^{(e)}(\theta, x)$ has prior conditional mean $m_j(\tilde{\theta}, x) = \mathrm{E}[\pi_j(\theta, x) \mid \tilde{\theta}]$, and apply nonlinear least squares to estimate $\tilde{\theta}$.

Step 4: Use ESS and possibly simulated design performance to calibrate $\tilde{\sigma}$.

This algorithm regresses the k-dimensional vector $\pi^{(e)}$ of elicited values on the p-dimensional vector $\tilde{\theta}$ of hyper-parameters to obtain numerical estimates, for $k \geq p$. The prior means are given by

$$m_j(\tilde{\theta}, x) = \int_\theta \pi_j(\theta, x) \, p(\theta | \tilde{\theta}) \, d\theta, \quad j = 1, \cdots, k,$$

and we denote the vector $m(\tilde{\theta}, x) = (m_1(\tilde{\theta}, x), \cdots, m_k(\tilde{\theta}, x))$. For example, it might be the case that the prior means of both $\pi_E(\theta \mid x_r)$ and $\pi_T(\theta \mid x_r)$ are elicited for each of five doses, i.e., $r = 1, \cdots, 5$, so $k = 10$. For a binary Y_E with $\pi_j(\theta, x) = \Pr(Y_E = 1 \mid \theta, x)$, the prior means can be written as prior predictive probabilities, $m_j(\tilde{\theta}, x) = \Pr(Y_E = 1 \mid \tilde{\theta}, x_j)$.

Given the above formulation, the main requirement is that $k \geq \dim(\tilde{\theta})$, in order to use nonlinear least squares to solve for $\tilde{\theta}$. This turns the problem that $k > p$, i.e., there are more elicited values than hyperparameters, into a requirement in order to perform a regression analysis. For example, possibly using some appropriately chosen weights $w_1, \cdots, w_k$, one may solve for $\tilde{\mu}$ to minimize

$$\sum_{j=1}^{k} w_j \{\pi_j^{(e)} - m_j(\tilde{\theta}, x_j)\}^2.$$

Regression analysis is an immense field, and there are many ways to do this minimization in a given setting, depending on the forms of the model for $\pi(\theta, x)$ and the prior $p(\theta \mid \tilde{\theta})$. We will not explore such nonlinear regression methods here, since this book is about clinical trial design. However, a very common practical difficulty with nonlinear regression is that, for given data, it may be numerically unstable. Various fix-ups can be used to deal with this, such as including a penalty term, or exploring various starting values. The following sampling-based alternative approach avoids such problems.

3.3.2 Pseudo Sampling Algorithm

Our experiences with a wide variety of Bayesian models and trial designs show that the least squares prior computation algorithm is adequate for small models with relatively few parameters. However, as the model grows more complex with larger numbers of parameters and elicited values, the nonlinear least squares problem can quickly become ill-conditioned and the optimization algorithm may not converge to a solution. Typically, there exist large regions of parameter space where the objective function stays virtually constant even as the parameters vary substantially. As a result, small changes to the elicited values can lead to large changes in the computed parameters.

The pseudo sampling algorithm is an alternative approach to computing the prior model parameters without relying on numerical optimization. It requires that enough prior information be elicited to specify a consistent state of nature, which is called the prior scenario. For example, each dose in a dose-finding trial should have a prior probability for each level of each outcome, with appropriate constraints on these values for the selected model. Once this has been specified, a conceptually appealing but impractical Bayesian approach would be to start with a non-informative prior on the model parameters and compute its posterior mean using a very large dataset simulated from the prior scenario. Unfortunately, this one-step approach requires a huge number of observations to give reliable parameter estimates for nontrivial models, most likely well beyond the capability of MCMC methods. The pseudo sampling algorithm solves this problem by dividing the huge computation into many smaller subproblems, with each being a posterior computation on a large but manageable set of data simulated from the same prior scenario.

To implement the pseudo sampling method, we assume the prior $p(\theta \mid \tilde{\theta})$ follows a multivariate normal distribution $N(\tilde{\mu}, \tilde{\sigma}^2)$, with individual real-valued parameters marginally distributed as $\theta_j \sim N(\tilde{\mu}_j, \tilde{\sigma}_j^2)$, $j = 1, \cdots, p$. For positive-valued parameter θ_j, we may let $\theta_j \sim N_0(\tilde{\mu}_j, \tilde{\sigma}_j^2)$, where N_0 denotes the normal distribution truncated below at 0. Alternatively, one may assume $log(\theta_j) \sim N(\tilde{\mu}_j, \tilde{\sigma}_j^2)$. Parameters with compact support are given independent beta prior distributions over appropriate domains. For example, the association between Efficacy and Toxicity is usually modeled by a parameter with uniform prior distribution on $(-1, +1)$. A priori, we assume there is no correlation between the parameters, and typically also assume that they share the same hyper variance $\tilde{\sigma}_j^2$.

The numerical values of the hyperparameters $\tilde{\theta}$ may be established from the elicited probabilities $\pi^{(e)}$ using the following pseudo-sampling algorithm, similar to that given in Thall and Nguyen (2012). The method requires that the vectors $\{x_1, \cdots, x_m\}$ for which prior mean probabilities are elicited include all regimes that will be considered in the planned trial. For each regime, it requires a prior mean probability for each outcome level of each outcome type. Naturally, these probability values must be coherent and must satisfy all monotonicity constraints, such as higher Toxicity for higher dose. For example, in a single-agent binary-outcome trial with doses $\{x_1, \cdots, x_m\}$, the method would require that the means of both $\pi_E(x_j, \theta)$ and $\pi_T(x_j, \theta)$ be elicited for each $j = 1, \cdots, m,$ for a total of $2m$ values.

Step 1. Assume a non-informative pseudo-prior $p_o(\theta)$ on θ with all entries $\theta_j \sim$ $N(0, \sigma_o^2)$ for large σ_o^2.

Step 2. Use the elicited prior probabilities $\pi^{(e)}(x)$ to simulate a large pseudo-sample of size N balanced equally among the regimes.

Step 3. Compute the pseudo-posterior from the pseudo-prior and pseudo-sample, and record the pseudo-posterior mean.

Step 4. Repeat steps 2 and 3 M times, and set the prior mean of θ equal to the mean of the M pseudo-posterior means.

Step 5. Using ESS as a criterion, calibrate the values of $(\tilde{\sigma}_1^2, \cdots, \tilde{\sigma}_p^2)$ to obtain ESS values of the θ_j's in the range 0.1 to 1.0.

As a practical guideline, this algorithm may be applied effectively with N = 100×[number of regimes], M = 1000 pseudo-samples, and pseudo-prior variances σ_o^2 in the range 100 to 10,000. The particular value of σ_o^2 may be chosen to ensure that the pseudo-posteriors are insensitive to the pseudo-prior. In practice, often one or two unique numerical values may be used for the entries of $(\tilde{\sigma}_1^2, \cdots, \tilde{\sigma}_p^2)$. If desired, an elaboration of Step 5 is to simulate the trial for each of several values of the hypervariances to ensure that the trial will have good operating characteristics across a diverse set of scenarios, as well as the prior being non-informative in terms of ESS. The overall ESS of $p(\theta \mid \tilde{\theta})$ may be computed using the formal method of Morita et al. (2008, 2012) or, alternatively, one may approximate the prior of each $\pi(x, \theta)$ using the beta moment matching method as described earlier.

   In addition to the much easier computation, the pseudo sampling approach has other advantages over optimization-based methods for computing priors. Specifying and sampling a prior scenario is a natural and flexible way to incorporate many types of prior information about the state of nature. For some clinical trial designs, the types of information that can be elicited easily from the physician are actually difficult to integrate effectively into the objective function of an optimization algorithm. As an example, consider the 39 elicited cumulative probabilities of Toxicity and response for three doses at multiple times given in Table 2 of Thall et al. (2013). Another example of this sort of complexity is the variety of probabilities that were elicited in Table 2 of Thall et al. (2014b). It would be practically impossible to achieve least squares convergence for either example while using all of the elicited values. Also, when different elicited data types are combined, there is the additional complication in choosing the relative weights for different types of residuals within an objective function. On the other hand, the pseudo sampling method takes all of the prior information into account naturally, with the relative importance of different data types implicitly handled through a fair sampling of the prior scenario.

4

Efficacy–Toxicity Trade-Off-Based Designs

CONTENTS

4.1	General Structure	59
4.2	Probability Model	60
4.3	Dose Admissibility Criteria	62
4.4	Trade-Off Contours	63
4.5	Establishing a Prior	64
4.6	Steps for Constructing a Design	67
4.7	Illustration	69
4.8	Sensitivity to Target Contours	71
4.9	Sensitivity to Prior ESS	71
4.10	Trinary Outcomes	74
4.11	Time-to-Event Outcomes	79

"Life is a series of trade-offs."

Jennifer Kunst

4.1 General Structure

The Efficacy–Toxicity (EffTox) trade-off-based design, introduced by Thall and Cook (2004) has three basic components. The first component is a Bayesian model for the probabilities of Efficacy (also referred to as "response") and Toxicity, each an explicit function of dose. The second component consists of two posterior probability criteria for deciding which doses are acceptable. Suppressing notation for dose and denoting the outcome probabilities by $\pi = (\pi_E, \pi_T)$, one acceptability criterion is based on a fixed lower limit $\underline{\pi}_E$ on π_E, and the other criterion is based on a fixed upper limit $\overline{\pi}_T$ on π_T. The third design component is a family of Efficacy–Toxicity trade-off contours that partition the two-dimensional domain $[0, 1]^2$ for all possible π pairs and are used to quantify the desirability of each dose. The contours are obtained by first constructing a target trade-off contour, which is defined using several π pairs considered to be equally desirable. The set of all trade-off contours are then obtained as transformed versions of the target contour. During the trial, based on posterior mean probabilities of Efficacy and Toxicity for each dose, computed from the current data, each successive cohort is treated with the most desirable acceptable dose.

The trade-off contours are an explicit structure that reflects subjective risk–benefit considerations weighing the hope of Efficacy against the fear of Toxicity. This sort of thinking is central to most medical decision making when treatments may have good or bad outcomes, and sometimes both may occur. The EffTox design is based on the general idea that a clinical trial design should reflect the way that the physicians who will treat the patients in the trial actually will behave. Practical refinements have been given by Thall et al. (2008) to include patient covariates, and by Jin et al. (2014) to accommodate late-onset outcomes. These extensions will be discussed in Chapters 5 and 7. Thall et al. (2014a) provided extremely important refinements and guidelines for how the numerical parameters that determine the prior and the target trade-off contour should be established when implementing EffTox. Because these two refinements substantially improve the EffTox design's performance, the account given here will include them.

4.2   Probability Model

The bivariate binary outcome, $Y = (Y_E, Y_T)$, takes on the four possible values (1,1), (1,0), (0,1), and (0,0.) The central problem is that Y is a stochastic function of dose, so while knowing what dose a patient received helps to predict which of these four elementary outcomes will occur, there is always uncertainty. This is why we do clinical trials. It is useful to think of these outcomes in terms of what the patient experiences. The best possible outcome is (1,0), Efficacy without Toxicity, which may be described as a therapeutic "win-win." The worst possible outcome is (0,1), Toxicity without Efficacy, a "lose-lose" outcome that, therapeutically, is a complete disaster. The physician and patient naturally hope for (1,0), but must acknowledge the possibility of (0,1). The outcome (0,0) is that neither event occurs. This outcome can be achieved by not treating the patient, and can be made likely by giving a very low dose of the agent. The outcome (1,1), that both Efficacy and Toxicity occur, has the important property that it is both good and bad. Therapeutic success has been achieved, but with a price.

Given a set of doses, $d_1 < d_2 < \cdots < d_k$, to stabilize numerical computations the standardized doses

$$x_j = \log(d_j) - J^{-1} \sum_{r=1}^{J} \log(d_r), \quad j = 1, \cdots, J.$$

will be used. The EffTox model's linear terms are defined to be

$$\eta_{E,j}(\theta_E) = \mu_E + \beta_{E,1}x_j + \beta_{E,2}x_j^2,$$

which is reasonably flexible and allows non-monotone dose-response, and

$$\eta_{T,j}(\theta_T) = \mu_T + \beta_T x_j,$$

where the parameter subvectors are $\theta_E = (\mu_E, \beta_{E,1}, \beta_{E,2})$ and $\theta_T = (\mu_T, \beta_T)$. Using a logit link, the marginal probabilities are

$$\pi_{k,j}(\theta_k) = \text{logit}^{-1}\{\eta_{k,j}(\theta_j)\} \quad \text{for } k = E, T.$$

Requiring $\beta_{T,1} > 0$ ensures that $\pi_{T,j}(\theta_T)$ increases with dose, which is the case with cytotoxic agents. Other forms of $\eta_{E,j}(\theta_E)$ and $\eta_{T,j}(\theta_T)$ may be used. One may ensure that $\pi_E(x, \theta)$ is increasing in x by setting $\beta_{E,2} = 0$ and requiring $\beta_{E,1} > 0$. To allow the possibility that there is an unknown upper bound below 1 on the probability of outcome k, one may multiply $\pi_{k,j}(\theta_j)$ by a parameter $0 < \alpha_k < 1$. Bretz et al. (2005) give a variety of functional forms for $\pi_T(x)$ and $\pi_E(x)$ that may be used in various phase I–II settings.

Given the marginals, a bivariate distribution for $[Y_E, Y_T|x_j]$ may be defined using a copula (Nelsen, 2006). Denote the joint probabilities

$$\pi(a, b \mid x_j, \theta) = \Pr(Y_E = a, Y_T = b \mid x_j, \theta).$$

Suppressing x_j and θ for brevity, the Fairlie–Gumbel–Morgenstern (FGM) copula is quite tractable, and is given by

$$\pi(a, b) = \pi_E^a \, (1 - \pi_E)^{1-a} \, \pi_T^b \, (1 - \pi_T)^{1-b}$$

$$+ (-1)^{a+b} \left(\frac{e^\psi - 1}{e^\psi + 1} \right) \pi_E \, (1 - \pi_E) \, \pi_T \, (1 - \pi_T),$$

for $(a, b) = (1,1)$, $(1,0)$, $(0,1)$, or $(0,0)$, and real-valued association parameter ψ. The overall model parameter vector $\theta = (\theta_T, \theta_E, \psi)$ has six entries.

Denoting $Y_i = (Y_{i,E}, Y_{i,T})$ the observed data from n patients are $\mathcal{D}_n = \{(Y_i, x_{[i]}), i = 1, \cdots, n\}$, the likelihood is the product

$$\mathcal{L}(\mathcal{D}_n \mid \theta) = \prod_{i=1}^{n} \pi(Y_i | x_{[i]}, \theta).$$

and the posterior is

$$p(\theta \mid \mathcal{D}_n, \tilde{\theta}) \propto \mathcal{L}(\mathcal{D}_n \mid \theta) \times p(\theta \mid \tilde{\theta}).$$

4.3   Dose Admissibility Criteria

Since it is possible that no dose is both acceptably safe and acceptably effica-cious, the following two dose acceptability criteria are imposed. Let $\underline{\pi}_E$ be a fixed lower limit on $\pi_{E,j}(\theta_E)$ and $\overline{\pi}_T$ a fixed upper limit on $\pi_{T,j}(\theta_T)$. Both of these fixed limits must be elicited from the physician, and they depend on the definitions of Efficacy and Toxicity and what is considered acceptable in the particular clinical setting. Let p_E and p_T be fixed lower probability cut-offs, usually in the range .05 to .20. Given the current data, a dose x_j has *acceptable Efficacy* if it satisfies the Efficacy admissibility criterion

$$\Pr\{\pi_{E,j}(\theta_E) > \underline{\pi}_E | \mathcal{D}_n, \tilde{\theta}\} > p_E,$$

and has *acceptable Toxicity* if it satisfies the Toxicity admissibility criterion

$$\Pr\{\pi_{T,j}(\theta_T) < \overline{\pi}_T | \mathcal{D}_n, \tilde{\theta}\} > p_T.$$

These criteria say that, given the current data, it is not unlikely that the probability of Efficacy at x_j is at least the lower limit $\underline{\pi}_E$, and it is not unlikely that the probability of Toxicity at x_j is below the upper limit $\overline{\pi}_T$. A dose x_j is *acceptable* if it has both acceptable Toxicity and acceptable Efficacy.

Only acceptable doses are given to patients during the trial, and if all doses are unacceptable the trial is stopped with no dose selected. These two admissibility rules may be thought of as gatekeepers that decide which doses may be included in the pool of doses that may be used to treat patients. It is very important to bear in mind that the posterior probabilities used to define the admissibility criteria are statistics that may be quite variable, but they become more reliable as patients are treated and their data are acquired throughout the trial. For example, due to the fact that the dataset used to compute the posteriors is expanding, a dose that is declared unacceptable at some point in the trial may later be declared acceptable, and conversely. In practice, $\overline{\pi}_T = .10$ is roughly the smallest Toxicity limit that may be used to obtain a design with reasonable properties. If $\overline{\pi}_T = .01$ were used, then the design would be very likely to stop the trial if even one Toxicity were observed. That is, using the upper limit .01 essentially says that no Toxicity will be acceptable. Similarly, using $\underline{\pi}_E = .90$ or .95 essentially requires that nearly every patient must have a response in order for the trial to continue.

The two admissibility criteria may not seem to make sense, intuitively, since in practice the small probability cut-offs $p_E = p_T = .10$ typically are used. It might seem more sensible to use large cut-offs, such as .90. If this is done, however, then in almost every case the design is very likely to stop the trial early with all doses declared inadmissible. It thus is useful to state the two rules in the following equivalent forms. Using $p_E = p_T = .10$, *a dose x_j is unacceptable* if, given the current data and the two numerical limits $\underline{\pi}_E$ and $\overline{\pi}_T$, either

$$\Pr\{\pi_{E,j}(\theta_E) < \underline{\pi}_E \mid \mathcal{D}_n, \tilde{\theta}\} > 1 - p_E = .90$$

or

$$\Pr\{\pi_{T,j}(\theta_T) > \bar{\pi}_T \mid \mathcal{D}_n, \tilde{\theta}\} > 1 - p_T = .90.$$

This says x_j is unacceptable if it is either likely to be inefficacious or likely to be too toxic. Although these two rules are equivalent to the previous forms, when described in this alternative way they may seem to make more sense.

4.4 Trade-Off Contours

The target Efficacy–Toxicity probability trade-off contour, $\mathcal{C}$, and corresponding family of contours partitioning $[0, 1]^2$ may be defined in various ways. The basic idea motivating trade-off contours is that they should be constructed so that all π pairs on each contour are equally desirable. Each time a decision must be made in the trial, this structure is used to compute the desirabilities of all the doses in order to choose a best dose for treating the next cohort.

The EffTox program constructs contours as follows. The target contour is determined by three user-specified, equally desirable outcome probability pairs $\pi_1^* = (\pi_{1,E}^*, 0)$, $\pi_2^* = (1, \pi_{2,T}^*)$ and $\pi_3^* = (\pi_{3,E}^*, \pi_{3,T}^*)$, subject to the constraints $\pi_{1,E}^* < \pi_{3,E}^*$ and $\pi_{3,T}^* < \pi_{2,T}^*$. Initially, these values are elicited from the physicians. In practice, however, the practical consequences of a particular $\mathcal{C}$ are extremely important and often are not obvious. *A key point is that $\mathcal{C}$ must be calibrated to be sufficiently steep so that a design with good OCs is obtained.* We will explain how to do this below, in terms of an illustrative example.

The following derivation is based on the fact that, in this particular set-up for constructing trade-off contours, $\mathcal{C}$ is determined by the numerical values of the four probabilities $\pi_{1,E}^*, \pi_{2,T}^*, \pi_{E,3}^*, \pi_{T,3}^*$, subject to the above constraints. Given $\mathcal{C}$, the *desirability function* of $(\pi_E, \pi_T) = \pi \in [0, 1]^2$ is defined as

$$
\begin{aligned}
\phi(\pi) &= 1 - \|\pi - (1,0)\|_r \\
&= 1 - \left\{ \left(\frac{\pi_E - 1}{\pi_{1,E}^* - 1} \right)^r + \left(\frac{\pi_T - 0}{\pi_{2,T}^* - 0} \right)^r \right\}^{1/r}
\end{aligned}
\tag{4.1}
$$

where $r > 0$. The EffTox program solves the equation $\phi(\pi_{E,3}^*, \pi_{T,3}^*) = 0$ for r using the bisection method. Once r has been determined, this gives $\phi(\pi) = 0$ for all π on $\mathcal{C}$. A family of contours that partition the unit square $[0, 1]^2$ of all $\pi = (\pi_E, \pi_T)$ pairs is generated from the elicited target contour $\mathcal{C}$ as follows. Given $\mathcal{C}$ and r, for each desirability δ one may define the contour

$$\mathcal{C}_\delta = \{\pi \in [0, 1]^2 : \phi(\pi) = \delta\}.$$

Thus, all π on $\mathcal{C}_\delta$ have desirability δ, and the target contour is $\mathcal{C} = \mathcal{C}_0$.

The desirability function $\phi(\pi)$ increases as π moves along any straight line from a point in $[0, 1]^2$ toward the ideal probability pair (1,0). In this way, $\phi(\pi)$ induces an ordering on all probability pairs π in terms of the values of $\phi(\pi) = \delta$. At each point in the trial when a dose must be chosen, the EffTox method exploits this structure by computing the posterior mean probabilities

$$\mu_{E,j,n} = E\{\pi_{E,j}(\theta_E)|\mathcal{D}_n\} \quad \text{and} \quad \mu_{T,j,n} = E\{\pi_{T,j}(\theta_T)|\mathcal{D}_n\}$$

for each dose $j = 1, ..., J$. The desirability of dose x_j is then defined to be $\phi(\mu_{E,j,n}, \mu_{T,j,n})$. Among the set of acceptable doses, the x_k having largest desirability is selected for treating the next patient cohort.

There are several alternative ways to construct a family of trade-off contours from $\mathcal{C}$. One simple approach is as follows. For given π, let $\pi_{\mathcal{C}}$ denote the point where the straight line from π to (1,0) intersects $\mathcal{C}$. The desirability of π is defined as the Euclidean distance from π to (1,0) divided by the Euclidean distance from $\pi_{\mathcal{C}}$ to (1,0), formally

$$\phi(\pi) = \frac{\|\pi_{\mathcal{C}} - (1,0)\|_2}{\|\pi - (1,0)\|_2}.$$

To avoid infinite values, the function $\phi(\pi)$ may be replaced by $1 - e^{-\phi(\pi)}$, although any monotone transformation will do.

4.5 Establishing a Prior

The following algorithm, given by Thall et al. (2014a), may be used to establish a prior on θ for the EffTox model based on elicited prior means. The algorithm provides a way to specify a prior having a given level of informativeness in terms of ESS. First, the fixed priors $\psi \sim N(0, 1)$ and $\beta_{E,2} \sim N(0, .20)$ are assumed, since they work well in general. For the remaining parameters, we assume that $\mu_k \sim N(\tilde{\mu}_{k,\mu}, \tilde{\sigma}^2_{k,\mu})$ and $\beta_{k,1} \sim N(\tilde{\mu}_{k,\beta}, \tilde{\sigma}^2_{k,\beta})$ for $k = E, T$. It thus remains to determine the priors of $(\mu_E, \beta_{E,1}, \mu_T, \beta_{T,1})$ by specifying numerical values of the four hyper-means and four hyper-standard deviations, denoted respectively by

$$\tilde{\mu} = (\tilde{\mu}_{E,\mu}, \tilde{\mu}_{T,\mu}, \tilde{\mu}_{E,\beta}, \tilde{\mu}_{T,\beta}) \quad \text{and} \quad \tilde{\sigma} = (\tilde{\sigma}_{E,\mu}, \tilde{\sigma}_{E,\beta}, \tilde{\sigma}_{T,\mu}, \tilde{\sigma}_{T,\beta}).$$

It also will be convenient to rearrange these eight hyperparameters and express them as vectors in terms of the two outcomes,

$$\tilde{\theta}_k = (\tilde{\mu}_{k,\mu}, \tilde{\mu}_{k,\beta}, \tilde{\sigma}_{k,\mu}, \tilde{\sigma}_{k,\beta}) \quad \text{for } k = E, T.$$

Given $\tilde{\mu}$, the hyper-standard deviations $\tilde{\sigma}$ determine the informativeness of the prior. In general, the degree of prior informativeness cannot be known from the numerical values of its hyper-parameters. Larger values of $\tilde{\sigma}_{k,\mu}$ and

$\tilde{\sigma}_{k,\beta}$ give more informative priors on μ and β, but, for example, it is not at all clear precisely how informative the priors are using values of $\tilde{\sigma}_{k,\mu}$ or $\tilde{\sigma}_{k,\beta}$ equal to 1, 10, or 100. The practical question is whether, given $\tilde{\mu}$, particular numerical values of $\tilde{\sigma}_{j,\mu}$ and $\tilde{\sigma}_{j,\beta}$ will yield a design with good properties.

The following algorithm provides a practical way to establish a prior having given ESS. To speed up computation, the algorithm relies on the method, given in Chapter 3, of matching the first two moments of each prior with those of a beta distribution to obtain an approximate ESS. For the EffTox model, this is applied to obtain ESS values of the marginal priors of $(\mu_E, \beta_{E,1})$ and $(\mu_T, \beta_{T,1})$, since the priors of $\beta_{E,2}$ and ψ, have been specified. Using the beta-approximated value $ESS_{k,j}$ of the prior of $\pi_{k,j}(\mu_k, \beta_{k,1} \mid \tilde{\theta}_k)$ for each outcome k and dose j, the mean

$$\overline{ESS}_k(\tilde{\theta}_k) = J^{-1} \sum_{j=1}^{J} ESS_{k,j}(\tilde{\theta}_k)$$

over the J doses is an approximate ESS of the marginal prior $p(\mu_k, \beta_{k,1} \mid \tilde{\theta}_k)$ for each $k = E, T$. The mean $\{\overline{ESS}_E(\tilde{\theta}_E) + \overline{ESS}_T(\tilde{\theta}_T)\}/2$ may be considered an approximate average marginal ESS. We avoid the more complex formal derivation of the ESS of the prior based on the entire vector θ to speed up computation and facilitate practical application. Thus, to apply the algorithm, one must specify values of the targeted prior effective sample size $ESS_{target,E}$ for $p(\theta_E \mid \tilde{\theta}_E)$ and $ESS_{target,T}$ for $p(\theta_T \mid \tilde{\theta}_T)$. These targets are used for $\overline{ESS}_E(\tilde{\theta}_E)$ and $\overline{ESS}_T(\tilde{\theta}_T)$ to calibrate $\tilde{\sigma}$.

The algorithm determines $(\tilde{\mu}, \tilde{\sigma})$ from the elicited mean outcome probabilities $(\mu_{E,1}^{(e)}, \mu_{T,1}^{(e)}), \cdots, (\mu_{E,J}^{(e)}, \mu_{T,J}^{(e)})$ by exploiting two key ideas. The first is the fact that the prior means of the $\pi_{k,j}(\theta_k)$'s are functions of $(\tilde{\mu}, \tilde{\sigma})$. The second is that ESS is an intuitively straightforward criterion for calibrating the numerical values of $\tilde{\sigma}$. An important technical point is that, even for $J = 3$ dose levels, there are $2J = 6$ elicited means, a number larger than $\dim(\tilde{\mu}) = 4$, so any set of equations in $\mu^{(e)}$ and $\tilde{\mu}$ would be over-determined. While a simple approach would be to use only 4 of the $2J$ elicited values, as discussed earlier, this would require one to discard elicited information.

An alternative approach to eliciting the prior means is to elicit probability intervals for the $\pi_{k,j}(\theta)$'s, such as prior coverage intervals of the form $\Pr\{L < \pi_{k,j}(\theta) < U\} = .90$, in order to obtain information about $\tilde{\sigma}$. However, with this approach, pairs (L, U) having small $U - L$ might lead to overly informative priors that dominate the data, which could have disastrous consequences during trial conduct if the physician's prior optimism about Toxicity turns out to be wrong.

For $k = E, T$ and $j = 1, \cdots, J$, the prior mean outcome probabilities are

$$\tilde{\mu}_{k,j} = \mu_{k,j}(\tilde{\theta}_k) = E\{\pi_{k,j}(\theta_k) \mid \tilde{\theta}_k\} = \int_{\theta_k} \pi_{k,j}(\theta_k) p(\theta_k \mid \tilde{\theta}_k) d\theta_k.$$

Recall that the corresponding elicited mean is denoted by $\mu_{k,j}^{(e)}$. In practice, ESS values between 0.3 and 1.5 usually work well, with $ESS_{target,E} = ESS_{target,T}$. For $k = E, T$ the objective functions are

$$
\phi_k(\tilde{\theta}_k) = \sum_{j=1}^{J} \left\{ \mu_{k,j}^{(e)} - \mu_{k,j}(\tilde{\theta}_k) \right\}^2
$$
$$
+ \ 0.1 \left\{ \overline{ESS}_k(\tilde{\theta}_k) - ESS_{target,j} \right\}^2 + \ 0.02 \left(\tilde{\sigma}_{k,\mu} - \tilde{\sigma}_{k,\beta} \right)^2. \quad (4.2)
$$

The hyperparameter vector $\tilde{\theta}_k$ that minimizes (4.2) can be found quickly and easily using the Nelder–Mead algorithm (Nelder and Mead, 1965). To initialize the algorithm, values of $\tilde{\mu}$ are obtained by solving the linear equations

$$
\text{logit}\{\mu_{k,j}^{(e)}\} = \tilde{\mu}_{k,\mu} + \tilde{\mu}_{k,\beta} x_j, \quad k = E, T,
$$

using the lowest and highest doses, $x_j = x_1$ and $x_j = x_K$. Using a first-order Taylor expansion approximation, the initial $\tilde{\sigma}$ is obtained by solving the equations

$$
var\{\pi_{k,j}(\theta_k \mid \tilde{\theta}_k)\} \doteq [\{\text{logit}^{-1}(\tilde{\mu}_{k,\mu} + \tilde{\mu}_{k,\beta} x_j)\}']^2 (\tilde{\sigma}_{k,\mu}^2 + \tilde{\sigma}_{k,\beta}^2 x_k^2), \quad k = E, T.
$$

Applying the beta approximation for ESS, the left-hand side of this equation takes the form

$$
var\{\pi_{k,j}(\theta_k \mid \tilde{\theta}_k)\} \doteq \frac{\mu_{k,j}^{(e)}(1 - \mu_{k,j}^{(e)})}{(ESS_{target,k} + 1)}.
$$

This is evaluated for x_1 and x_K, and the geometric mean is then computed. The right-hand side of the equation is obtained evaluating it at x_1 and x_K and taking the arithmetic mean. The final step is to equate the left-hand and right-hand sides and solve for $\tilde{\sigma}$.

The two penalty terms are included to stabilize the Nelder–Mead algorithm. The penalty term $\left\{ \overline{ESS}_k(\tilde{\theta}_k) - ESS_{target,k} \right\}^2$ ensures that the marginal of $(\mu_k, \beta_{k,1})$ will have the desired degree of informativeness in terms of the specified $ESS_{target,k}$. The penalty term $(\tilde{\sigma}_{k,\mu} - \tilde{\sigma}_{k,\beta})^2$ ensures that the prior standard deviations $\tilde{\sigma}_{k,\mu}$ and $\tilde{\sigma}_{k,\beta}$ do not have different orders of magnitude, which can destabilize the Nelder–Mead algorithm and cause it to fail to converge. Both penalty terms converge to 0 as the Nelder–Mead algorithm approaches its minimum. The particular tuning parameters in (4.2) were determined empirically. The value 0.1 that multiplies the penalty term $\left\{ \overline{ESS}_k(\tilde{\theta}_k) - ESS_{target,k} \right\}^2$ was determined by examining a range of values with the two aims to (1) obtain results that are robust to the numerical values of elicited means and starting values of the hyperparameters $\tilde{\theta}_k$ and (2) reduce the number of iterations needed to obtain convergence. Similarly, if for example the value 0.02 that multiplies the penalty term $(\tilde{\sigma}_{k,\mu} - \tilde{\sigma}_{k,\beta})^2$ were replaced by 1, in many cases the Nelder–Mead algorithm would take longer to converge.

The small value 0.02 works well in practice because, when $\phi_k(\tilde{\theta}_k)$ is far from its minimum, this value avoids problems caused by the term $(\tilde{\sigma}_{k,\mu} - \tilde{\sigma}_{k,\beta})^2$ dominating $\phi_k(\tilde{\theta}_k)$, whereas if $\phi_k(\tilde{\theta}_k)$ is near its minimum $(\tilde{\sigma}_{k,\mu} - \tilde{\sigma}_{k,\beta})^2$ then converges to 0 and its tuning parameter no longer matters.

4.6 Steps for Constructing a Design

When constructing any phase I–II design, it is essential that the outcomes be defined collaboratively by the physician and statistician in a manner that is appropriate for the particular trial at hand. The definitions of Efficacy and Toxicity may vary widely depending on the particular clinical setting. The two fixed probability limits used for deciding the acceptability of each dose will depend on the particular disease being treated, the trial's entry criteria, and the probabilities of Efficacy and Toxicity that may be expected with whatever standard therapies may be available. For example, chemotherapy of acute myelogenous leukemia (AML) is very different from chemotherapy of solid tumors, such as lung or breast cancer. AML originates in the bone marrow, whereas solid tumors do not. Since chemotherapy is only marginally more toxic for cancer cells than for similar normal cells, in order to be effective, chemotherapy for AML must be far more aggressive, and thus far more toxic for normal bone marrow cells, than chemotherapy used to treat solid tumors. Consequently, rates of marrow Toxicity, such as infection due to low white blood cell counts, considered unremarkable in AML patients undergoing chemotherapy would be considered unacceptable in solid tumor patients. Additionally, nausea and vomiting are much more likely to limit dose escalation of drugs used for chemotherapy of solid tumors. Thus, the definitions of "Toxicity" in the two settings are usually quite different. "Response" in AML is generally defined as complete remission by 42 days from the start of therapy, which requires recovery of white cells and platelets to specified functional levels and reduction of blasts (undifferentiated blood cells) to < 5%, since leukemia is essentially caused by abnormal proliferation of blastic leukemia cells. In sharp contrast, "Response" in treatment of a solid tumor often is defined as a 50% or greater reduction in the size of the tumor, based on MRI or PET imaging, by a given time from the start of therapy.

The definitions of the outcomes, disease and patient prognosis as determined by the trial's entry criteria, what is achievable with standard therapy, and what may be anticipated with the experimental therapy to be evaluated all help the physician determine the numerical probability limits $\overline{\pi}_T$ and $\underline{\pi}_E$. For example, the upper Toxicity probability limit $\overline{\pi}_T = .45$ may be used in a chemotherapy trial of AML, whereas $\overline{\pi}_T = .20$ may be appropriate for a breast cancer trial. Similarly, the numerical values of $\underline{\pi}_E$ in the EffTox design used for an AML trial and a solid tumor trial likely will be very different.

One may construct a phase I–II trial design applying the EffTox method by taking the following steps. This process must be carried out in collaboration with the physicians planning the trial, since their input is needed to provide essential design features and parameters.

STEP 1. Determine the disease, trial entry criteria, treatment, doses to be studied, definitions of Efficacy and Toxicity, and the numerical limits $\overline{\pi}_T$ and $\underline{\pi}_E$ that will be used in the dose admissibility rules.

STEP 2. Determine N = maximum sample size, and c = cohort size, which in practice is 1, 2, or 3, and the anticipated accrual rate. Initially, each of the design parameters may be a set of several feasible values, and possible combinations of N and c may be studied by simulation. In general, larger K = number of dose levels will require larger N, since the maximum number of cohorts, N/c, should be large enough to explore the J dose levels reliably. Generally, N = 18 to 24 is roughly the smallest trial that can be run feasibly using EffTox, and only with J = 3 or 4 doses. If J = 3, then N = 18 may be feasible, but the trial's overall reliability will be very limited. When choosing N, it is important to keep in mind that the EffTox design completes both phase I and phase II simultaneously.

STEP 3. Elicit prior mean probabilities of Efficacy and Toxicity at each dose. Elicit the three probability pairs used to determine an initial target contour $\mathcal{C}$. Recall that it often is necessary to adjust $\mathcal{C}$ to be sufficiently steep to obtain a design with good properties. This must be explained to the physician.

STEP 4. Specify the ESS target values, usually in the range .4 to 1.5, and derive the prior hyperparameters.

STEP 5. Specify a set of simulation scenarios in terms of assumed true values of $(\pi_{E,j}, \pi_{T,j})$, $j = 1, \cdots, J$.

STEP 6. Conduct preliminary simulations to calibrate the design parameters, with particular attention initially to $\mathcal{C}$. This may be done using 100 to 400 replications per scenario to save time. Iteratively adjust $\mathcal{C}$ to be sufficiently steep so that the design performs well in a scenario where all $\pi_{T,j}$ are low and $\pi_{E,j}$ increases substantially with j. Since the EffTox program interface gives a picture of $\mathcal{C}$ that can easily be modified interactively, this tool should be used during this process.

STEP 7. Iterate Steps 1–6, if necessary, until a design with good OCs is obtained.

STEP 8. Conduct a final set of simulations, with 1000 to 4000 replications per scenario, to establish the design's final operating characteristics (OCs). Include a table of these OCs in the trial protocol as part of the design specification. Including four to 12 scenarios is generally appropriate.

The design may be implemented using the computer program EffTox freely

available from the website
https://biostatistics.mdanderson.org/SoftwareDownload/.
Figure 4.1 illustrates the graphical user interface of the EffTox program.

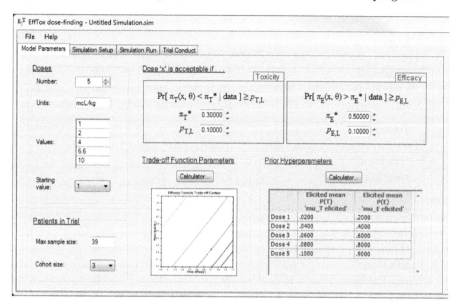

FIGURE 4.1: Graphical user interface of the EffTox program.

4.7   Illustration

The EffTox method is illustrated by a phase I–II of valproic acid (VA) + idarubicin (IDA) in patients with AML or myelodysplastic syndrome (MDS) who have poor prognosis. A fixed dose of 12 mg/m^2 idarubicin is given as a bolus intravenously daily for 3 days, and VA is given orally as a pill daily for 21 days at a dose of 20, 30, 40, or 50 mg/m^2. Toxicity was defined as death or severe infection within 42 days from the start of therapy, and Efficacy is defined as CR by day 42. The prior means of $\pi_{E,j}$ and $\pi_{T,j}$ are the values given in Scenario 1 of Table 4.1, and the prior informativeness was set to $E\bar{S}S_{target}$ = .90. The Efficacy lower limit of $\underline{\pi}_E$ = .40 and Toxicity upper limit $\overline{\pi}_T$ = .45, with acceptability cut-offs probability $p_{L,T} = p_{L,T}$ = .10. The target contour was determined by the three equally desirable probability pairs $\pi_1^* = (.40,0)$, $\pi_2^* = (.60,.30)$, $\pi_3^* = (1,.75)$. The maximum sample size was 60 with cohort size of 3, and the first cohort treated at the lowest VA dose $d_1 = 20$ mg/m^2.

Table 4.1 gives OCs of the design under each of four simulation dose-outcome scenarios. In general, a well-behaved design has dose selection prob-

TABLE 4.1: Operating characteristics for the AML/MDS trial EffTox design with maximum $N = 60$ patients

	Dose (mg/m^2)				
	20	40	60	80	None
Scenario 1					
True (π_T, π_E)	(.20, .25)	(.25, .35)	(.35, .55)	(.60, .60)	
Trade-off	63	71	87	69	
Selection %	3	20	50	14	13
Num. Patients	7	15	21	11	
Scenario 2					
True (π_T, π_E)	(.10, .30)	(.15, .45)	(.20, .60)	(.25, .80)	
Trade-off	77	93	113	146	
Selection %	4	22	21	53	0
Num. Patients	6	16	14	24	
Scenario 3					
True (π_T, π_E)	(.30, .60)	(.55, .65)	(.70, .70)	(.80, .75)	
Trade-off	100	78	68	64	
Selection %	83	8	0	0	9
Num. Patients	46	9	1	0	
Scenario 4					
True (π_T, π_E)	(.65, .50)	(.70, .60)	(.75, .65)	(.80, .70)	
Trade-off	55	59	59	60	
Selection %	5	0	0	0	95
Num. Patients	13	2	0	0	

abilities that follow the distribution of the numerical dose trade-off (desirability) values. A design also must have high probabilities of stopping the trial early in scenarios where no dose has both acceptable Efficacy and acceptable Toxicity, as in Scenario 4 of Table 4.1. To see the effect of maximum sample size, Table 4.2 gives the probability of making the best possible decision under each of the four scenarios, as functions of N varying from 24 to 84. These results show that, for this particular trial, the design performs reasonably well for $N \geq 48$, with a steady loss of reliability as N declines, but reliability, safety, or both drop substantially for $N = 36$ or 24.

TABLE 4.2: Probability of making the best possible decision under each scenario, as a function of N = maximum sample size

	N					
Decision	24	36	48	60	72	84
Select d_3 in S_1	35	38	47	50	52	56
Select d_4 in S_2	45	47	47	50	52	53
Select d_1 in S_3	78	80	81	83	86	86
Stop Early in S_4	78	88	92	95	95	96

4.8 Sensitivity to Target Contours

The EffTox design's behavior is very sensitive to how the target contours are specified. Most importantly, the target C must be sufficiently steep so that the algorithm reliably escalates to higher doses that are safe and have larger values of $\pi_{E,j}$, especially when the dose-Efficacy curve is steep. Figure 4.2 shows four different families of contours that may be specified. Starting with the design contour denoted by C_1 in the upper left corner, the target contours C_2, C_3, and C_4 are successively less steep. The consequence is that, moving from C_1 to C_4, the trade-off values change dramatically and the design's operating characteristics become more degraded and the design has successively smaller probabilities of correctly choosing the best dose level, as summarized in Table 4.3. The contour C_2 is not sufficiently steep since it reduces the probability of choosing the highest dose level from .53 to .33, and the target contours C_3, and C_4 may be considered pathological, since they lead to designs with very poor properties. The problem is that these contours do not provide a sufficiently large reward for escalating to dose levels d_3 or d_4, so the method gets stuck at levels d_2 or d_3.

4.9 Sensitivity to Prior ESS

The EffTox design's behavior is also very sensitive to the informativeness of its prior. Table 4.4 show how the design's dose selection percentages vary with $\overline{ESS}_{target}$ set equal to 10, .90, or .30. Recall that $\overline{ESS}_{target}$ = .90 is the recommended value. Setting $\overline{ESS}_{target}$ = 10 causes the design to choose suboptimal d_2 = 40 far too often in Scenario 1, choose suboptimal d_2 = 40 and d_3 = 60 far too often in Scenario 2, and degrades the safety in Scenario 4 by not stopping often enough. Setting $\overline{ESS}_{target}$ = .3 causes the design to

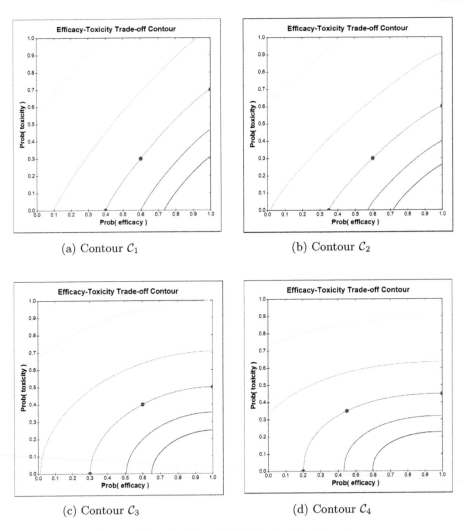

FIGURE 4.2: Four families of Eff-Tox trade-off contours.

TABLE 4.3: Sensitivity to the target contour in scenario 2

	Dose (mg/m^2)			
	20	30	40	50
True (π_T, π_E)	(.10, .30)	(.15, .45)	(.20, .60)	(.25, .80)

C_1 Target $(\pi_E, \pi_T)^*$ Pairs: (.40, 0), (.60, .30), (1, .75)

Trade-off	77	93	113	146
Selection %	4	22	21	53
Num. Patients	6	16	14	24

C_2 Target $(\pi_E, \pi_T)^*$ Pairs: (.35, 0), (.60, .30), (1, .60)

Trade-off	84	99	115	142
Selection %	5	34	28	33
Num. Patients	9	21	16	14

C_3 Target $(\pi_E, \pi_T)^*$ Pairs: (.30, 0), (.60, .40), (1, .50)

Trade-off	98	116	134	157
Selection %	4	36	39	20
Num. Patients	8	22	20	9

C_4 Target $(\pi_E, \pi_T)^*$ Pairs: (.20, 0), (.45, .35), (1, .45)

Trade-off	112	130	143	149
Selection %	6	47	38	9
Num. Patients	9	27	18	4

choose suboptimal $d_2 = 40$ far too often in Scenario 1, and choose suboptimal $d_2 = 40$ and $d_3 = 60$ far too often in Scenario 2.

It is interesting to note that $\overline{ESS}_{target} = 10$ gives hyper standard deviations in the range $\tilde{\sigma} = .65$ to .70, $\overline{ESS}_{target} = .90$ gives $\tilde{\sigma} = 2.8$ to 2.9, and $\overline{ESS}_{target} = .30$ gives $\tilde{\sigma}$ in the range 6.5 to 6.9. These numerical values have no intrinsic meaning with regard to whether they are uninformative or not, aside from their comparative magnitudes. It also should be kept in mind that these numerical values of $\tilde{\sigma}$ would change if different prior means were assumed. This numerical example shows why one cannot just choose a very large hyper standard deviation, like $\tilde{\sigma} = 10$, since this would lead to a design with even worse properties than that obtained with $\tilde{\sigma} = 6$ or 7. While these numerical hyper parameter values have no intuitive meaning, recommending that one use a prior ESS close to 1 is simple to understand. The prior with ESS $= .9$ satisfies the Three Bears Criterion. It is not too large, like ESS $= 10$, and not too small, like ESS $= .3$. It is just right.

4.10   Trinary Outcomes

The first phase I–II design for settings with acceptability criteria for $\pi_E(d, \theta)$ and $\pi_T(d, \theta)$ was proposed by Thall and Russell (1998), for the case where E and T are disjoint The three elementary outcomes are E, T, and $N =$ [Neither E nor T]. A prototype example is a chemotherapy dose-finding trial for a rapidly fatal disease, such as salvage therapy for relapsed or treatment-resistant (refractory) acute leukemia, where E is the event that the patient is alive and in complete remission (CR) at day 42 from the start of therapy and T is death within 42 days. The third event, N, occurs if the patient is alive but not in CR at day 42. In this case, $Y = (Y_E, Y_T)$ takes on the three possible values (1,0), (0,0), (0,1) corresponding to E, N, T, respectively. The set of possible (π_E, π_T) pairs is the triangular subset $\{\pi = (\pi_E, \pi_T) : \pi_E + \pi_T \leq 1\}$ of $[0, 1]^2$, and $\pi_N = 1 - \pi_E - \pi_T$.

There are two simple alternative dose-response models that may be assumed. The first is the four-parameter continuation ratio (CR) model. It may be motivated by thinking of the three events as being ordered as $N < E < T$, with a higher dose producing an outcome higher on the ordinal scale. The idea is that one would like a dose high enough to make $\pi_E(x)$ large but not so high that $\pi_T(x)$ becomes unacceptably high. The CR model may be characterized by the linear terms

$$\eta_T(x, \theta) = \text{logit}^{-1}\{\pi_T(x, \theta)\}$$
$$\eta_E(x, \theta) = \text{logit}^{-1}\{P(Y_E = 1 \mid Y_E = 1 \text{ or } Y_N = 1, x, \theta)\}, \quad (4.3)$$

where $\eta_k(x, \theta) = \beta_{k,0} + \beta_{k,1}x$ for $k = E, T$ and standardized dose x, subject

TABLE 4.4: Selection percentages of the AML/MDS trial EffTox design using different $\overline{ESS}_{target}$ values to determine the prior

	Dose (mg/m^2)				
	20	40	60	80	None
Scenario 1					
True (π_T, π_E)	(.20, .25)	(.25, .35)	(.35, .55)	(.60, .60)	
Trade-off	63	71	87	69	
$\overline{ESS}_{target}$					
10	1	69	30	0	1
.9	3	20	50	14	13
.3	5	37	37	2	19
Scenario 2					
True (π_T, π_E)	(.10, .30)	(.15, .45)	(.20, .60)	(.25, .80)	
Trade-off	77	93	113	146	
$\overline{ESS}_{target}$					
10	0	46	50	4	0
.9	4	22	21	53	0
.3	8	43	32	15	3
Scenario 3					
True (π_T, π_E)	(.30, .60)	(.55, .65)	(.70, .70)	(.80, .75)	
Trade-off	100	78	68	64	
$\overline{ESS}_{target}$					
10	99	0	0	0	1
.9	83	8	0	0	9
.3	88	2	0	0	10
Scenario 4					
True (π_T, π_E)	(.65, .50)	(.70, .60)	(.75, .65)	(.80, .70)	
Trade-off	55	59	59	60	
$\overline{ESS}_{target}$					
10	15	1	0	0	84
.9	5	0	0	0	95
.3	6	0	0	0	94

to the constraints $\beta_{T,1} > 0$ and $\beta_{E,1} > 0$. The parameter vector is $\theta = (\beta_{T,0}, \beta_{T,1}, \beta_{E,0}, \beta_{E,1})$, and the three outcome probabilities are

$$\pi_T(x, \theta) = \frac{e^{\eta_T(x,\theta)}}{1 + e^{\eta_T(x,\theta)}}$$

$$\pi_E(x, \theta) = \frac{e^{\eta_E(x,\theta)}}{(1 + e^{\eta_T(x,\theta)})(1 + e^{\eta_E(x,\theta)})}$$

$$\pi_N(x, \theta) = \frac{1}{\{1 + e^{\eta_T(x,\theta)}\}\{1 + e^{\eta_E(x,\theta)}\}}. \tag{4.4}$$

The requirement $\beta_{T,1} > 0$ guarantees that $\pi_T(x, \theta)$ must increase in x, but in general $\pi_E(x, \theta)$ is not monotone in dose.

A second dose-response model is the three-parameter proportional odds (PO) model with the same form for $\pi_T(x, \theta)$ as the CR model but

$$\text{logit}^{-1}\{\pi_E(x, \theta) + \pi_T(x, \theta)\} = \beta_{T,0} + \beta_E + \beta_{T,1}x,$$

with the additional constraint $\beta_E > 0$ to ensure that $\pi_E(x, \theta) > 0$. For this model, $\theta = (\beta_{T,0}, \beta_{T,1}, \beta_E)$. Mandrekar et al. (2007) argue that the three-parameter PO model is inadequate, and that the four-parameter model is preferable. However, this is not true in all cases. An illustration comparing the CR and PO models is given by Scenario 3 of the simulation study presented by Thall and Cook (2004, Section 6). In this case, perhaps counter-intuitively, the three-parameter PO model produces better design performance than the four-parameter CR model. This is essentially because the PO model happens to be closer to the actual dose-response functions in Scenario 3 than the CR model, so the CR model is over-parameterized in this case.

The design proposed by Thall and Russell (1998) did not involve an Efficacy–Toxicity trade-off. For this design, the best acceptable dose is defined as that having largest $\Pr\{\theta_E(x, \theta) \geq \overline{\pi}_E | \mathcal{D}_n\}$. Its rules for trial conduct are as follows:

1. Treat the first cohort at the lowest dose.

2. Do not skip an untried dose when escalating.

3. Never treat a cohort at a dose with either unacceptable Efficacy or unacceptable Toxicity.

4. If all doses are unacceptable, stop the trial and do not select any dose.

5. Among the current acceptable doses, treat the next cohort at the best acceptable dose.

6. At the end of the trial, choose the best acceptable dose.

Rather than using $\Pr\{\theta_E(x, \theta) \geq \overline{\pi}_E | \mathcal{D}_n\}$ as the criterion for quantifying dose desirability in the trinary outcome setting, one may define a trade-off contour and proceed as in the EffTox design for bivariate binary outcomes. This was proposed by Thall and Cook (2004). To implement the trade-off-based EffTox design for trinary outcomes using the four-parameter CR model, one may proceed as follows. For priors, assume that $\beta_{k,r} \sim N(\tilde{\mu}_{k,r}, \tilde{\sigma}_{k,r}^2)$, for $k = E, T$ and $r = 0, 1$. Further assuming that $\tilde{\sigma}_{k,0} = \tilde{\sigma}_{k,1} = \tilde{\sigma}_k$ for each k, the hyper-parameter vector is $\tilde{\theta} = (\tilde{\mu}_{E,0}, \tilde{\mu}_{E,1}, \tilde{\mu}_{T,0}, \tilde{\mu}_{T,1}, \tilde{\sigma}_E, \tilde{\sigma}_T)$. These six hyperparameters may be computed by applying the same algorithm as that used for the bivariate binary outcome model. One may use the command line driven program EffToxTrinaryPriorSolver.txt to compute the prior hyperparameters. This program requires one to input the three vectors of standardized doses $(x_1, \cdots, x_J)$, prior means $(\mu_T(x_1), \cdots, \mu_T(x_J))$ and $(\mu_E(x_1), \cdots, \mu_E(x_J))$, and the target prior ESS. Simulations and trial conduct may be implemented by specifying the "Trinary" outcome type in EffTox version v2.1. Both programs are freely available at the website https://biostatistics.mdanderson.org/SoftwareDownload/. An important point with regard to using this software for trial simulation is that, under the above CR model parameterization,

$$P(Y_E = 1 \mid Y_E = 1 \text{ or } Y_N = 1, x, \theta) = \frac{\pi_E(x, \theta)}{1 - \pi_T(x, \theta)},$$

and this conditional probability increases with dose. Thus, when specifying simulation scenarios it is important to check that the numerical values of the specified pairs $(\pi_E(x)^{true}, \pi_T(x)^{true})$ satisfy this constraint. If this is not done, then the simulations may show that the method behaves pathologically. If one does not believe that $P(Y_E = 1 \mid Y_E = 1 \text{ or } Y_N = 1, x, \theta)$ increases with dose for their application, then this CR model and software should not be used, and a different model, method, and software should be applied.

The design is illustrated by a trial of allogeneic human mesenchymal stem cells (MSCs) for patients with acute respiratory distress syndrome (ARDS). The MSC doses were 10^6, 5×10^6, and 10^7 cells per kg body weight, administered intravenously weekly for four weeks, with standardized values $x = 1, 2, 3$. Efficacy was defined as $E = $ [Alive at day 30 post initial MSC infusion without grade 3,4 (severe) infusional toxicity], and Toxicity was defined as $T = $ [Death within 30 days post initial MSC infusion or severe infusional toxicity]. Thus, $N = $ [Alive at day 30 post initial MSC infusion with severe infusional toxicity]. ARDS is rapidly fatal, with historical 30-day death rate 64% with standard care, which relies on steroids. The design was implemented with $\overline{\pi}_T = .50$ and $\underline{\pi}_E = .25$, and prior hyperparameters computed from elicited means $\mu_T(= (.10, .15, .20)$ and $\mu_E(= (.20, .25, .30)$, with prior ESS = 1. Thus, an acceptable dose had to have Toxicity probability well below the historical value of .64. The trade-off contour was generated from the three equally desirable pairs $(\pi_E, \pi_T) = (.50, 0), (.53, .25), (.39, .61)$, illustrated by Figure 4.3. A maximum of 60 patients were treated in cohorts of size 3, starting at the lowest dose. The operating characteristics of the design are given in Table 4.5

TABLE 4.5: Operating characteristics of the trinary outcome EffTox design for the trial of MSCs for ARDS

	Dose (cells/kg/week)			
	10^6	5×10^6	10^7	None
Scenario 1				
True (π_T, π_E)	(.30, .40)	(.50, .30)	(.70, .20)	
Trade-off	.70	.54	.38	
Selection %	88	2	0	1
Num. Patients	47.2	6.3	1.4	
Scenario 2				
True (π_T, π_E)	(.10, .20)	(.15, .50)	(.40, .40)	
Trade-off	.66	1.04	.70	
Selection %	0	76	21	3
Num. Patients	4.2	34.1	20.2	
Scenario 3				
True (π_T, π_E)	(.10, .10)	(.15, .45)	(.20, .75)	
Trade-off	.56	.96	1.50	
Selection %	0	18	81	1
Num. Patients	3.0	10.0	46.5	
Scenario 4				
True (π_T, π_E)	(.70, .10)	(.75, .15)	(.80, .20)	
Trade-off	.33	.34	.35	
Selection %	1	2	0	97
Num. Patients	11.4	3.4	0.5	

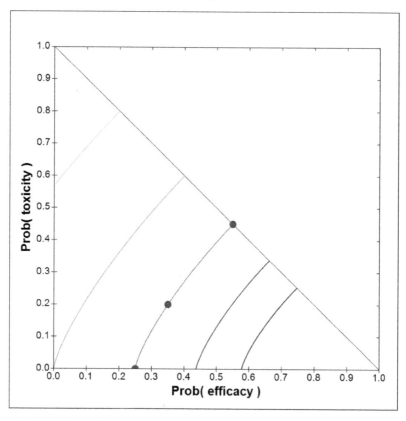

FIGURE 4.3: Trade-off contours for the MSC EffTox trial design.

4.11   Time-to-Event Outcomes

The EffTox design treats Toxicity and Efficacy as bivariate binary outcomes. This makes the design straightforward to implement, but it has some drawbacks. One limitation is that using binary outcomes ignores the information of when each of the two outcomes occurs, which may be important clinically, and also may help to characterize the drug effect (Estey, Shen, and Thall, 2000). For example, in addition to maintaining a low Toxicity probability, delaying the onset of Toxicity can be another goal of a trial design. Patients may hope to delay drug-related adverse events in order to improve their quality of life. At the extreme, considering death as the most severe adverse event, the longer the patient's survival time, the better.

A logistical limitation of using discrete outcomes is that they must be observed soon enough, relative to accrual rate, to make adaptive decisions for each new cohort. This is a general problem with any sequentially outcome-adaptive clinical trial design that assumes discrete outcomes, which requires that the outcomes of previous patients must be fully observed in order to make the adaptive decision for new patients. If accrual is fast, the design may require suspending patient accrual to wait for the Toxicity and Efficacy events to occur, or be scored as not occurring, among patients already treated before enrolling the next new patient. Repeatedly suspending patient accrual typically is not feasible in practice, and may result in an undesirably long study. An alternative approach is to only count previously treated patients whose outcomes have been fully evaluated, which wastes information. These issues, which may be referred to collectively as the problem of "late-onset" outcomes, will be addressed generally in Chapter 5.

A natural way to overcome these difficulties is to model Toxicity and Efficacy as time-to-event (TTE) outcomes (Yuan and Yin, 2009). For all patients who have been treated but for whom one or both events have not been observed, the occurrence times are censored at the current time of decision making. For convenience, we refer to the resulting design as the TTE EffTox design.

The following probability model describes the times to Efficacy and Toxicity as functions of dose. Let x denote dose standardized to have mean of 0 and variance of 1. For a patient treated at x, let $h_T(t_T|x, \beta_T)$ denote the hazard function for the time to Toxicity, assumed to follow the proportional hazards model,

$$h_T(t_T|x, \beta_T) = h_{0T}(t_T)\exp(\beta_T x).$$

Because the sample sizes of phase I–II trials typically are small, the baseline hazard $h_{0T}(t)$ is modeled parametrically using a Weibull distribution, with survival function given by

$$S_T(t_T|x, \theta_T) = \exp\{-\lambda_T t_T^{\alpha_T}\exp(\beta_T x)\}, \tag{4.5}$$

where λ_T and α_T are the scale and shape parameters of the Weibull distribution, respectively, and $\theta_T = (\beta_T, \lambda_T, \alpha_T)$.

Efficacy is a qualitatively different endpoint from Toxicity. Unlike Toxicity, a significant number of patients in the trial may not respond to the treatment and never achieve Efficacy. To model this, the patient population is considered to consist of two subpopulations: a susceptible subpopulation who possibly may respond to the treatment, and a non-susceptible subpopulation who will never respond to the treatment. This type of patient heterogeneity can be accommodated using a mixture cure rate model (Yuan and Yin, 2009). Let $S_E(t_E|x, \theta_E)$ denote the survival function for the time to Efficacy for susceptible patients, and let ω denote the proportion of susceptible patients in the target population. The survival function of the mixture cure rate model (Berkson and Gage, 1952) is given by

$$S_E^*(t_E|x, \theta_E) = 1 - \omega + \omega S_E(t_E|x, \theta_E), \tag{4.6}$$

where $S_E(t_E|x, \theta_E)$ follows the Weibull baseline hazard

$$S_E(t_E|x, \theta_E) = \exp\{-\lambda_E t_E^{\alpha_E}\exp(\beta_E x)\}. \tag{4.7}$$

The function $S_E^*(t_E|x,\theta_E)$ is an improper population survival distribution because $\lim_{t\to\infty} S_E^*(t_E|x,\theta_E) = 1 - \omega > 0$. One may think of the distribution of time-to-Efficacy as having probability mass ω distributed on the positive reals for susceptible patients and mass $1-\omega$ at ∞ for non-susceptible patients. Mixture cure rate models are discussed by Kuk and Chen (1992); Maller and Zhou (1996); Chatterjee and Shih (2001), among others.

Given the marginal distributions $S_T(t_T|x,\theta_T)$ and $S_E(t_E|x,\theta_E)$, the joint distribution of (t_T, t_E) may be modeled using the Clayton (1978) copula,

$$S(t_T, t_E|x,\theta) = \{S_T(t_T|x,\theta_T)^{-1/\phi} + S_E(t_E|x,\theta_E)^{-1/\phi} - 1\}^{-\phi}, \qquad (4.8)$$

where $\phi > 0$ characterizes association and the model parameter vector is $\theta = (\beta_T, \alpha_T, \lambda_T, \beta_E, \alpha_E, \lambda_E, \pi, \phi)$. The relationship between Kendall's τ and ϕ is $\tau = 1/(2\phi+1)$. A small value of ϕ represents high correlation. When $\phi \to 0$, the correlation approaches 1, and when $\phi \to \infty$, the correlation converges to 0.

With a slight abuse of notation, for $k = E$ or T, we use Y_k to denote the observed times of the events or right-censoring, define ϵ_k as the indicator that the event time is not right-censored. The observed data from the ith patient are thus $\mathcal{D}_{[i]} = (Y_{i,T}, Y_{i,E}, \epsilon_{i,T}, \epsilon_{i,E}, x_{[i]})$. The likelihood for the ith patient is given by

$$\mathcal{L}_{[i]}(\mathcal{D}_{[i]}|\theta) = L_1^{\epsilon_T \epsilon_E} L_2^{\epsilon_T(1-\epsilon_E)} L_3^{(1-\epsilon_T)\epsilon_E} L_4^{(1-\epsilon_T)(1-\epsilon_E)},$$

where

$$L_1 = \omega\frac{\partial^2 S(Y_T, Y_E|x)}{\partial Y_T \partial Y_E}$$

$$L_2 = -(1-\omega)\frac{\partial S_T(Y_T|x)}{\partial Y_T} - \omega\frac{\partial S(Y_T, Y_E|x)}{\partial Y_T}$$

$$L_3 = -\omega\frac{\partial S(Y_T, Y_E|x)}{\partial t_E}$$

$$L_4 = (1-\omega)S_T(Y_T|x) + \omega S(Y_T, Y_E|x).$$

For a given patient, L_1, L_2, L_3 and L_4 correspond, respectively, to the likelihood components that (1) both Toxicity and Efficacy are observed, (2) Toxicity is observed but Efficacy is censored, (3) Toxicity is censored but Efficacy is observed, and (4) both Toxicity and Efficacy are censored. Note that Efficacy could be censored either due to non-susceptibility or because the event has not occurred yet. Therefore, for a subject with a censored Efficacy outcome, the likelihood contributions L_2 and L_4 each consist of two parts: the first part corresponds to a patient who is non-susceptible to Efficacy, and the second part for a patient who is susceptible to Efficacy but censored.

We assume that λ_k, α_k and β_k follow independent gamma priors, $k = E, T$. Prior hyper-parameters may be established using the methods described in Chapter 3 or Section 4.5. For the correlation parameter ϕ and the susceptibility probability ω, uniform priors work well. The posterior full conditional distributions do not have closed forms, but can be computed by a Gibbs sampler using the adaptive rejection Metropolis sampling method (Gilks, Best, and Tan, 1995).

The Efficacy–Toxicity trade-off described in Section 4.4 is not used here because Y_T and Y_E are now time-to-event outcomes. In this case, a desirable dose is one that reaches a high response rate in a relatively short time while inducing a low Toxicity probability, with the event occurring as slowly as possible. This corresponds to a sharply dropping survival curve for the time to Efficacy and to a slowly decaying survival curve for the time to Toxicity. This consideration motivates the use of the ratio of the areas under the survival curves (AUSC) of Toxicity and Efficacy (see Figure 4.4) as the trade-off, with a higher value of the AUSC corresponding to a more desirable dose.

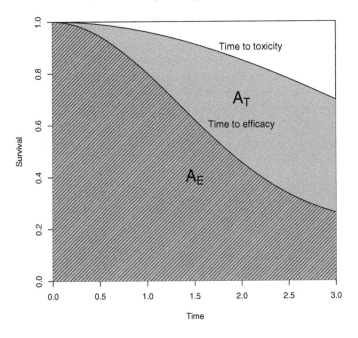

FIGURE 4.4: Illustration of the areas under the survival curves corresponding to Toxicity and Efficacy, the AUSC ratio=A_T/A_E.

Let A_T and A_E denote the AUSCs of Toxicity and Efficacy up to a pre-specified follow-up time τ. The AUSC ratio is given by

$$\frac{A_T}{A_E} = \frac{\alpha_T^{-1}\{\lambda_T\exp(\beta_T x)\}^{-1/\alpha_T}\Gamma(\alpha_T^{-1}, \lambda_T\exp(\beta_T x)\tau^{\alpha_T})}{(1-\omega)\tau + \omega\alpha_E^{-1}\{\lambda_E\exp(\beta_E x)\}^{-1/\alpha_E}\Gamma(\alpha_E^{-1}, \lambda_E\exp(\beta_E x)\tau^{\alpha_E})}, \quad (4.9)$$

where $\Gamma(a, b)$ is the incomplete gamma function $\Gamma(a, b) = \int_0^b e^{-z}z^{a-1}dz$. When

$\pi = 1$ and $\tau \to \infty$, A_T/A_E may be interpreted as the ratio of the mean survival times between Toxicity and Efficacy.

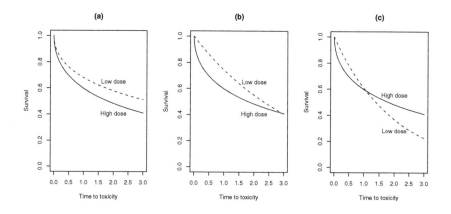

FIGURE 4.5: Survival curves of the time to Toxicity for two different doses. Panel (a) shows a case where the high dose induces a higher Toxicity rate and a shorter time to observe Toxicity, i.e., the survival curve of the high dose is consistently below that of the low dose. Panel (b) displays a case where two doses have the same Toxicity probability, but Toxicity occurs sooner with the higher dose. Panel (c) illustrates a case where the survival curves of two doses cross.

The AUSC ratio simultaneously accounts for two distinct features of drug effects: (1) the Toxicity and Efficacy occurrence rates, evaluated at the end of the follow-up period τ, and (2) how quickly patients experience Toxicity or achieve remission/cure. The TTE EffTox method bases dose selection on these two features, rather than solely on the Toxicity and Efficacy occurrence probabilities. In contrast, the Efficacy–Toxicity trade-off based on binary outcomes completely ignores the path of the survival curve. To illustrate this point, we consider two different doses and focus on time to Toxicity. Figure 4.5 (a) shows typical survival curves for the time to Toxicity under two doses — a high dose and a low dose. The high dose induces a higher Toxicity rate and a shorter event time, i.e., the survival curve (for Toxicity) of the high dose consistently stays below that of the lower dose. Therefore, either the AUSC or the Toxicity rate provides a reasonable criterion to select the low dose as more desirable. However, it may happen that the two doses have similar Toxicity rates at the end of the follow-up, but the survival curve of the high dose declines much faster than that of the low dose because patients experience Toxicity sooner under the high dose, see Figure 4.5 (b). In this case, the low dose is still more desirable because Toxicity is delayed so that the patient's quality of life is improved. The AUSC is able to distinguish between these two doses and tends to choose the low dose with a high probability. In contrast, if we only use the

Toxicity probability as the selection criterion, the EffTox trade-off would regard these two doses as having the same desirability. In practice, it is unlikely that the survival curves for the time to Toxicity at two different doses cross, since this would correspond to a dose that induces Toxicity sooner but results in a lower overall Toxicity probability. See Figure 4.5 (c).

These arguments also apply to the time to Efficacy. Given two doses having the same response rate at the end of the follow-up, the AUSC allows investigators to select the dose that achieves a quicker response. In practice, it may be critical to consider how soon patients achieve response, in addition to the response probability. For example, in cord blood cell transplantation, it is highly desirable to achieve engraftment more quickly, so both the probability of engraftment and mean time-to-engraftment are important (Thall, Wooten, and Shpall, 2006). Thus, for a given Efficacy probability, a dose that helps patients achieve Efficacy more quickly within the follow-up window $[0, \tau)$ more often is more desirable.

Define the Toxicity and Efficacy probabilities of dose x_j to be $\pi_T(x_j|\theta_T) = 1 - S_T(\tau|x_j, \theta_T)$ and $\pi_E(x_j, \theta_E) = 1 - S_E^*(\tau|x_j, \theta_E)$, for $j = 1, \cdots, J$. Because very limited information is available at the beginning of the study, the trial begins with the following start-up rule. Initially, patients are treated in cohorts of 3, and no new patients are assigned until the currently-treated patients have been fully evaluated. The first cohort of 3 patients is treated at the lowest dose x_1. Given the current dose level j, the dose assignment for the next cohort is as follows:

1. If 2 patients experience Toxicity, then switch to the AUSC-ratio based dose-finding procedure starting at dose level $j - 1$. If j is the lowest dose level, then terminate the trial.

2. If 1 patient experiences Toxicity, then switch to the AUSC-ratio based dose-finding procedure, starting at dose level j.

3. If no patients experience Toxicity, then escalate to $j+1$ for the next cohort. If j is the highest dose level, then switch to the AUSC-ratio based dose-finding procedure starting at j.

Although the start-up phase prolongs the trial duration, it is needed to avoid treating patients at excessively toxic doses. As more data accumulate over time, the following AUSC-ratio based dose-finding procedure will seamlessly take effect for the rest of the trial.

Let x_h denote the highest dose tried so far. Assume that n patients have been treated. The dose assigned to the next cohort is chosen as follows. Let $p_T^\dagger$ be a fixed probability limit for escalation, such as $p_T^\dagger = 0.85$ or 0.90.

1. If the posterior probability of observing Toxicity at x_h satisfies

$$\Pr\{\pi_T(x_h) < \bar{\pi}_T | \mathcal{D}_n, \theta\} > p_T^\dagger, \tag{4.10}$$

escalate to dose level $h + 1$. This says that, if x_h is safer than the upper Toxicity limit $\bar{\pi}_T$ with a high probability $p_T^\dagger$, then escalate. If $h = J$, treat the next cohort at dose x_J.

2. If (4.10) is not satisfied, determine the set of admissible doses $\mathcal{A}_n$ that satisfy the usual Toxicity and Efficacy admissibility criteria:

$$\Pr\{\pi_T(x_j) < \bar{\pi}_T | \mathcal{D}_n, \theta\} \quad > \quad p_T \tag{4.11}$$
$$\Pr\{\pi_E(x_j) > \underline{\pi}_E | \mathcal{D}_n, \theta\} \quad > \quad p_E. \tag{4.12}$$

Then,

(i) If $\mathcal{A}_n$ is empty, the trial is terminated and no dose is selected.

(ii) Otherwise, the next cohort is treated at the most desirable dose from $\mathcal{A}_n$, defined as that maximizing A_T/A_E.

3. Once the maximum sample size is reached, the dose from $\mathcal{D}_N$ that maximizes A_T/A_E is recommended.

The values of $p_T^\dagger$, p_T and p_E are determined by using preliminary simulations so that the design has good operating characteristics.

The TTE EffTox design is illustrated by a phase I–II trial of a novel mitotic inhibitor for treating prostate cancer. Five doses of the drug were investigated, $0.1, 0.3, 0.5, 0.7$, and 0.9 g/m^2. The maximum sample size was 48 patients with cohort size 3. The limits $\bar{\pi}_T = 0.3$ and $\underline{\pi}_E = 0.4$ were used, with admissibility cutoffs $p_T = 0.30$, $p_E = 0.25$ and escalation cutoff $p_T^\dagger = 0.8$. The follow-up time for each patient was 3 months, with accrual rate 3 patients per month.

Table 4.6 summarizes the operating characteristics of the design. Under each scenario, the first row is the assumed marginal probability of Toxicity and Efficacy evaluated at τ, i.e., $\pi_T(x)^{true}$ and $\pi_E(x)^{true}$. The second row is the AUSC ratio when the true hazard of Efficacy is decreasing. The third to fifth rows show the results when the true hazard of Efficacy is decreasing, constant, and increasing, respectively. Different shapes of the true hazard of Efficacy are used to evaluate the robustness of the TTE design. Additional details of the simulations are provided in Yuan and Yin (2009).

Scenarios 1 to 3 represent the most common situations in which $\pi_T(x_j)$ and $\pi_E(x_j)$ both increase with the dose. The main difference among the three scenarios is the location of the most desirable dose. This is the middle dose level 3 in Scenario 1, level 2 in Scenario 2, and level 5 in Scenario 3. In all scenarios, the TTE EffTox design selects the most desirable dose with percentage over 67%, and treats a majority of the patients at the target dose.

Figure 4.6 illustrates trial conduct when applying the TTE EffTox design to the prostate cancer trial. In the start-up phase, the first 3 cohorts entered the trial and each was fully followed for 3 months. As the first 2 cohorts did not experience any events, the dose was escalated to level 3 for treating cohort 3. When two toxicities and two efficacies were observed in cohort 3, the trial switched to the AUSC dose-finding algorithm, and chose dose level 2. After one Efficacy event was observed in cohorts 4 and 5, the dose was escalated

TABLE 4.6: Operating characteristics of the TTE EffTox design

			Dose		
	0.1	0.3	0.5	0.7	0.9
			Scenario 1		
(π_T, π_E)	(0.05, 0.22)	(0.11, 0.41)	(0.23, 0.65)	(0.44, 0.82)	(0.72, 0.85)
A_T/A_E	1.11	1.24	1.54	2.06	2.44
$\downarrow \lambda_E$	0.4 (3.7)	13.0 (9.2)	**74.4 (22.4)**	4.2 (9.8)	0.0 (1.0)
const λ_E	0.0 (3.7)	8.8 (8.9)	**67.6 (22.4)**	16.0 (9.8)	1.2 (0.9)
$\uparrow \lambda_E$	0.0 (3.8)	7.2 (9.0)	**67.0 (21.5)**	17.6 (10.0)	0.8 (1.0)
			Scenario 2		
(π_T, π_E)	(0.11, 0.41)	(0.24, 0.53)	(0.45, 0.65)	(0.74, 0.75)	(0.95, 0.82)
A_T/A_E	1.24	1.31	1.34	1.26	1.02
$\downarrow \lambda_E$	10.4 (9.4)	**70.6 (25.1)**	10.6 (9.9)	0.2 (0.7)	0.0 (0.0)
const λ_E	11.6 (9.6)	**71.6 (25.3)**	8.2 (9.6)	0.0 (0.7)	0.0 (0.0)
$\uparrow \lambda_E$	9.8 (9.1)	**68.4 (25.0)**	10.4 (9.5)	0.2 (0.6)	0.0 (0.0)
			Scenario 3		
(π_T, π_E)	(0.07, 0.15)	(0.08, 0.35)	(0.10, 0.65)	(0.12, 0.83)	(0.15, 0.85)
A_T/A_E	1.06	1.20	1.64	2.78	4.36
$\downarrow \lambda_E$	0.0 (3.6)	0.2 (4.9)	0.4 (6.9)	2.6 (7.1)	**92.2 (23.8)**
const λ_E	0.0 (3.7)	0.2 (5.0)	0.4 (7.1)	2.6 (6.9)	**88.8 (22.3)**
$\uparrow \lambda_E$	0.0 (3.6)	0.2 (4.9)	0.4 (6.9)	2.4 (7.1)	**89.0 (22.6)**

*The column of the target dose is in boldface.

to level 3, at which most of the remaining patients were treated. Cohorts 11 and 12 were treated at dose level 4, but an excessive number of toxicities were observed. The trial ended with the conclusion that dose level 3 was the most desirable, satisfying both Toxicity and safety requirements.

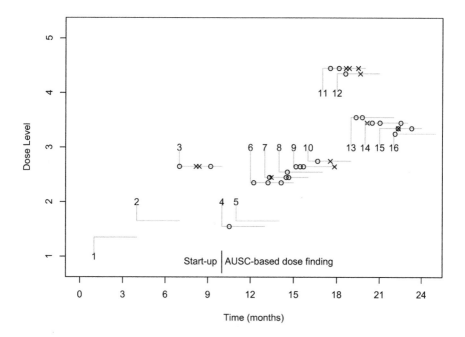

FIGURE 4.6: Dose allocation of the prostate cancer trial using the TTE EffTox design. The number represents the order in which each cohort of 3 patients entered the trial, and the line attached to each number denotes the 3-month follow-up time with the time to Efficacy and Toxicity indicated by circles and crosses, respectively.

5

Designs with Late-Onset Outcomes

CONTENTS

5.1   A Common Logistical Problem 89
5.2   Late-Onset Events as Missing Data 91
5.3   Probability Model 96
5.4   Imputation of Delayed Outcomes 97
5.5   Illustration 99

5.1   A Common Logistical Problem

A common logistical problem with sequentially outcome-adaptive clinical trial designs arises from the fact that the outcomes of previously treated patients must be observed soon enough to apply a design's decision rules to choose treatments for new patients. For example, if outcomes take up to six weeks to evaluate and the accrual rate is one patient per week, then on average three new patients will be accrued while waiting to evaluate the outcomes of the previous three patients. The question is how to treat the new patients. This problem, often known as the late-onset (or delayed) outcome problem, persists throughout the trial. It is not only logistical, but the way that it is handled also affects the design's statistical properties and may have serious ethical implications.

One solution is to turn away new patients and treat them off protocol. This may be less desirable than giving the experimental regimen, or impossible if no alternative treatment exists. Another solution is to give all new patients the dose or treatment that is optimal based on the most recent complete dose-outcome data. This can have disastrous consequences if the most recently chosen dose later turns out to be overly toxic. For example, suppose that a cohort of three patients is treated after an escalation at a new, higher dose d_j, but not yet evaluated for Toxicity and, motivated by the desire to complete the trial quickly, the next two cohorts of patients also are treated at d_j. If it turns out that all three patients in the first cohort experience severe late-onset Toxicities, then the six new patients already have been treated at an excessively toxic dose. Examples of late-onset Toxicities include neurotoxicity with certain chemotherapies, and a variety of Toxicities associated with radiation therapy. This problem is a major reason that dose-finding usually is done sequentially with small cohorts of patients treated at successively chosen doses. Alternatively, suppose that the most recently chosen dose d_j is safe but only marginally effective, say with true probabilities $\pi_T(d_j) = .10$ and $\pi_E(d_j) = .25$, and the next higher dose also is safe but is substantially more efficacious, with $\pi_T(d_{j+1}) = .15$ and $\pi_E(d_{j+1}) = .50$. In this case, treating new patients at d_j because the previous cohort's outcomes have not yet been evaluated deprives the new patients of this greater chance of anti-disease effect, which is the primary motivation for treating them. A third solution, motivated by a very limited focus on safety that ignores Efficacy entirely, is to treat a new cohort at one dose level below the most recent dose. This approach is even more likely to deprive new patients of a higher probability of Efficacy at a higher dose. A fourth solution is to delay new patients' treatments while waiting for previous patients' outcomes to be scored so that an adaptive statistical rule can be applied. This is very undesirable, and often impossible to do. That is, applying outcome-adaptive decision rules may be at odds with clinical practice.

In phase I–II trials, the late-onset outcome problem arises if either Toxicity or Efficacy is not scored sufficiently soon, relative to the accrual rate. To quantify the severity of the problem, we introduce the following indices. Consider phase I–II designs where Efficacy and Toxicity are characterized as binary variables, Y_E and Y_T, evaluated either during or at the end of specified time intervals, $[0, Q_E]$ for Y_E and $[0, Q_T]$ for Y_T. We refer to Y_E and Y_T as "late-onset outcomes" because they are not observed immediately. Denote accrual rate by α. We quantify the severity of the problem defining the *logistical difficulty indexes*,

$$\zeta_k = Q_k \alpha$$

for each outcome $k = E, T$, and overall index $\zeta = \max\{\zeta_E, \zeta_T\}$. When $\zeta \leq 1$, there is no logistic difficulty applying a standard adaptive decision rule. This is because $\zeta \leq 1$ implies that $Q_k \leq \alpha^{-1}$, which is the mean inter-arrival time between two patients. Thus, by the time the next new patient arrives, all enrolled patients have completed their outcome evaluation and their outcomes are available to apply the adaptive design rule.

Logistic difficulties are more likely to arise when $\zeta > 1$ because, in this case, by the time the next new patient arrives, it is more likely that some previously treated patients might not have completed their two outcome evaluations. This problem worsens with larger evaluation windows Q_E, Q_T, i.e., the outcomes require longer amounts of time to be evaluated, or with faster accrual rate, α. For example, if $\alpha = 1$ patient/month and $Q_E = Q_T = 3$ months, then $\zeta = 3$, and on average, there are up to 2 patients whose Y_E or Y_T may not be scored when a new patient arrives. Doubling the accrual rate to $\alpha = 2$ gives the problematic value $\zeta = 6$, under which it is likely that up to 5 patients might not have their Y_E or Y_T scored when a new patient arrives. From the definition of ζ_k, for an adaptive design, whether an outcome should be regarded as late-onset (and causing logistical difficulties for adaptive designs) depends on both the evaluation times Q_E, Q_T and accrual rate α. This is in contrast with the common misconception that a late-onset outcome requires a long time to be evaluated. For example, an outcome that requires 3 months to be scored is not a late-onset outcome if the accrual rate is 1 patient per 3 months, whereas an outcome that takes 1 month to be scored is a late-onset outcome if the accrual rate is 3 patients/month.

We distinguish two cases, based on whether the Efficacy endpoint Y_E can be scored in real time during its evaluation window, or only at the end of the evaluation window, at Q_E. These are illustrated by the following two examples.

Case 1. Consider a phase I–II trial of chemotherapy for acute leukemia, where both the Toxicity and Efficacy events may occur at any time during a common 6-week evaluation period, doses are chosen adaptively for cohorts of size 3, and the accrual rate is 1 patient per 1.5 weeks. On average, the first cohort will be accrued in 4.5 weeks with all of their outcomes scored by week 10.5, when adaptive rules are applied using their data to choose the second cohort's dose. Since one also can expect to accrue 4 new patients between weeks 4.5 and 10.5, the question is how to deal with these new patients therapeutically.

Case 2. A second example is an autologous stem cell transplantation trial for multiple myeloma (MM). Toxicity may occur at any time during the first 30 days, but Efficacy is evaluated only at day 90 post-transplant, and is defined as no detectable MM protein in the urine or blood serum and $< 5\%$ plasma cells in the bone marrow. If the accrual rate is 3 patients per month, one may expect to accrue 9 patients before Efficacy is scored for any patients, so applying an adaptive rule to choose a dose for patients 4, 5, and 6, (cohort 2), using both Y_E and Y_T from patients 1, 2, and 3, (cohort 1), is not possible without delaying the second cohort's therapy. The severity of this problem increases with accrual rate and persists throughout the trial.

In Phase I, the problem of dealing with late-onset Toxicity was addressed by Cheung and Chappell (2000), who introduced the time-to-event continual reassessment method (TiTE-CRM), and later by Braun (2006), Liu et al. (2013), and Yuan and Yin (2011). In this chapter, we describe a general methodology to handle late-onset outcomes that can be applied to any outcome-dependent adaptive design.

5.2   Late-Onset Events as Missing Data

The data structure assumed by most phase I–II dose-finding methods consists of assigned doses and two binary outcomes. We denote this by $\mathcal{D}(Y) = \{(d_{[1]}, Y_{1,E}, Y_{1,T}), \cdots, (d_{[n]}, Y_{n,E}, Y_{n,T})\}$. Suppressing the sample size index n, to account for the fact that, at any interim decision, one or both of Y_E and Y_T may not yet be observed for a given patient, we denote the data including only the observed Y_k's by $\mathcal{D}_{\mathrm{obs}}(Y)$ and the unobserved ("missing") Y_k's by $\mathcal{D}_{\mathrm{mis}}(Y)$. In other words, we will treat the delayed outcome problem as a missing data problem. Our strategy is to use $\mathcal{D}_{\mathrm{obs}}(Y)$ and partial follow up data to impute any missing Y_k's in $\mathcal{D}_{\mathrm{mis}}(Y)$, thereby construct a completed version of $\mathcal{D}_{\mathrm{obs}}(Y)$ that has the form of $\mathcal{D}(Y)$, and then apply the phase I–II methodology based on $\mathcal{D}(Y)$.

Let X_k denote time to outcome $k = E, T$. Corresponding to the acute leukemia trial and the stem cell transplantation trial described previously, we distinguish between two data structures, depending on how the binary variable Y_E is observed. In Case 1, Y_E is observed in real time, and $Y_E = I(X_E \leq Q_E)$. In Case 2, Y_E is evaluated only at follow up time Q_E, and there is no X_E. In both cases, $Y_T = I(X_T \leq Q_T)$. To simplify the exposition, we focus primarily on Case 1 since it is more complex, and later explain how to deal with Case 2. For trials where Efficacy is evaluated periodically, X_E is interval censored. We include this case by smoothing the interval censored data, placing X_E at the midpoint or at a randomly chosen value in the interval where Efficacy was known to occur. We accommodate patient death during therapy by defining X_T as the time to either non-fatal Toxicity or death. For Efficacy, if the patient dies prior to Q_E we define $Y_E = 0$, which is implied by defining $X_E = \infty$ in this case. Denote $Q = \max\{Q_T, Q_E\}$ and $V =$ follow up time, where by design $V \leq Q$.

A central concept for the statistical analysis of missing data is the missing-data mechanism, which determines what type of method is appropriate to use. In general, missing-data mechanisms can be classified into three types: missing completely at random, missing at random, and nonignorable missing data (or not missing at random) (Little and Rubin, 2002). Denote the missingship indicators $M_k = I(Y_k = missing)$ for $k = E, T$, and denote the observed and missing components of Y_k as $Y_{k,\mathrm{obs}}$ and $Y_{k,\mathrm{mis}}$, respectively, with $Y_k = (Y_{k,\mathrm{obs}}, Y_{k,\mathrm{mis}})$. The missing-data mechanism is characterized by the conditional distribution of M_k given Y_k, say $f(M_k|Y_k, \theta)$, where θ is a vector of unknown parameters. The data are called *missing completely random* (MCAR) if

$$f(M_k|Y_k, \theta) = f(M_k|\theta),$$

that is, if missingness does not depend on the value of the observed or missing Y_k. In this case, $Y_{k,\mathrm{obs}}$ is a randomly sampled value of Y_k, and analyses based on $Y_{k,\mathrm{obs}}$ yield valid inferences. The data are called *missing at random* (MAR) if

$$f(M_k|Y_k, \theta) = f(M_k|Y_{k,\mathrm{obs}}, \theta),$$

that is, if missingness depends only on the observed data $Y_{k,\mathrm{obs}}$. In this case, to obtain valid conclusions, statistical inference must be conditional on $Y_{k,\mathrm{obs}}$. The data are called *nonignorable* or *not missing at random* if

$$f(M_k|Y_k, \theta) = f(M_k|Y_{k,\mathrm{mis}}, \theta),$$

that is, if missingness depends on the missing values of Y_k. When the missing data are nonignorable, to obtain valid inference, one must jointly model the missing data mechanism and the observable outcome process. This is because the indicator M_k of whether Y_k is missing contains information about the observable value of Y_k.

We now examine the missing-data mechanism for the missing values of Y_k, $k = E, T$, induced by late-onset Toxicity and Efficacy. Suppose that a decision must be made for a patient enrolled in the trial, with observable time X_k, at $X_k^o = V \wedge X_k$ during the evaluation interval $[0, Q_k]$. We assume that V is independent of X_k. It follows that

$$Y_k = \begin{cases} missing & \text{if } X_k > V \text{ and } V < Q_k & (X_k^o = V), \\ 1 & \text{if } X_k \leq V \leq Q_k & (X_k^o = X_k), \\ 0 & \text{if } X_k > V = Q_k & (X_k^o = Q_k). \end{cases} \tag{5.1}$$

That is, $Y_k = missing$ if the patient has not yet experienced the event and has not been fully followed to Q_k, while Y_k is observed if the patient either has experienced the event ($Y_k = 1$) or has completed the defined follow-up time without the event, formally $V = Q_k$ and $Y_k = 0$. In this case, the following Theorem holds.

Theorem. Under the missing data mechanism (5.1), the missing data induced by late-onset outcomes are nonignorable with $\Pr(M_k = 1 | Y_k = 0) > \Pr(M_k = 1 | Y_k = 1)$ for $k = E, T$.

A proof of the theorem can be found in Liu et al. (2013). In general, missing data are more likely to occur for patients who would not experience the Toxicity/Efficacy event in $[0, Q_k]$. This phenomenon is illustrated in Figure 5.1. Patient 2, who will not experience Toxicity during the assessment period, is more likely to have a missing outcome at the decision-making times (e.g., weeks 2 to 6) than patient 1, who has experienced Toxicity between weeks 1 and 2. As a result, the observed data $\mathcal{D}_{\mathrm{obs}}(Y)$ represent a biased sample of the complete data $\mathcal{D}(Y)$ and contain more events than they should. Thus, the naive approach of simply discarding the missing data and making dose-escalation decisions solely based on $\mathcal{D}_{\mathrm{obs}}(Y)$ is problematic, and leads to biased results.

The fact that patients who would not experience the Toxicity/Efficacy event are more likely to have missing data is formalized by the inequality $\Pr(M_k = 1 | Y_k = 0) > \Pr(M_k = 1 | Y_k = 1)$. By Bayes' Law, this implies that

$$\frac{\pi_k}{1 - \pi_k} > \frac{\Pr(Y_k = 1 | M_k = 1)}{\Pr(Y_k = 0 | M_k = 1)}.$$

This says that the odds of the event $Y_k = 1$ occurring decreases if it is known that Y_k is missing. This illustrates the key point that the missingship indicator M_k contains information about the future value of Y_k. Consequently, to be

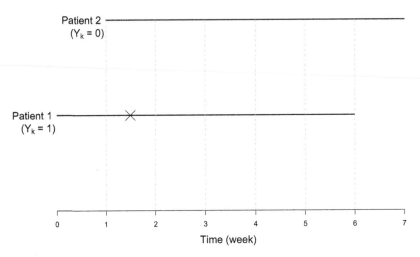

FIGURE 5.1: Illustration of missing outcomes when the evaluation period is 6 weeks and accrual rate is 1 patient per week for the acute leukemia trial. For each patient, the horizontal line segment represents the 6-week evaluation period, during which occurrence of the Toxicity or Efficacy event is indicated by a cross. The outcome of patient 1 is missing at week 1, but observed between weeks 1 and 2. The outcome of patient 2 is missing between weeks 1 and 7.

valid any inference must condition on both $\mathcal{D}_{\mathrm{obs}}(Y)$ and M_k. Because X_k^o determines M_k, as specified by (5.1), a practical approach for incorporating the information provided by M_k is to extend the ith patient's data vector from its standard form $(d_{[i]}, Y_{i,E}, Y_{i,T})$ to $(d_{[i]}, Y_{i,E}, Y_{i,T}, X_{i,E}^o, X_{i,T}^o)$, and base inferences on this extended data vector. Denote the extended interim data for the first n patients by

$$\mathcal{D}_n = \{(d_{[1]}, Y_{1,E}, Y_{1,T}, X_{1,E}^o, X_{1,T}^o), \cdots, (d_{[n]}, Y_{n,E}, Y_{n,T}, X_{n,E}^o . X_{i,T}^o)\},$$

which will be used to impute any missing Y_k's and thereby obtain a completed binary dataset $\mathcal{D}(Y)$ for implementing the phase I–II design.

Statistical analyses involving nonignorable missing data often are plagued by the nonidentifiability problem. This arises when the observed data contain no information about the nonignorable missing data mechanism. However, the missing data that we consider here are a special case of nonignorable missing data, since the missing data mechanism is known, and is defined by (5.1). This feature is essential, because it eliminates the nonidentifiablity problem.

Although we focus on phase I–II trials, the above methodology for treating late-onset outcomes as a missing data problem is very general. It can be applied to handle late-onset outcomes for any existing outcome-dependent designs, e.g., phase I, II, or III trials, or adaptive randomization. This may be done, in general, via the following steps:

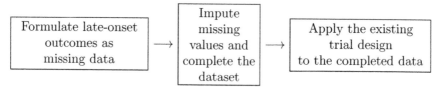

The imputation of the missing data can be explicit, as in using multiple imputation, or implicit, as an iteration step of Markov Chain Monte Carlo. The latter, which we will describe below, is known as Bayesian data augmentation (Tanner and Wong, 1987). One attractive feature of the missing-data approach to late-onset outcomes is that the resulting design always contains the original complete-data design as a special case when outcomes are not late-onset, that is, when there are no missing data.

Compared to other existing methods, such as the weighting method used by the TiTE-CRM, the missing-data approach has several important advantages. First, it is generally applicable to all outcome-dependent adaptive designs. The imputation step for missing data can be viewed as an "add-on" to any existing adaptive designs, and the resulting design always contains the original, complete-data-based design as a special case. This approach has been applied to phase I trials (Liu et al., 2013), drug-combination trials (Liu and Ning, 2013), phase II trials (Cai, Liu and Yuan, 2014, SIM), and phase I–II trials (Jin et al., 2014). Second, because it is fully likelihood-based, it is efficient. In contrast, the weighting method proposed by Cheung and Chappell (2000) for the TiTE-CRM is based on a pseudo likelihood that may not always correspond to the actual data likelihood. Third, the missing-data approach is robust to misspecification of the imputation model, e.g., the time-to-Efficacy and time-to-Toxicity models, because it keeps the observed response data intact. That is, the model misspecification only affects the imputed data. An important point is that such effects attenuate during the trial and eventually disappear because, eventually, all patients' outcomes are observed. In terms of robustness, the missing-data approach is preferable to the alternative approach that directly treats Toxicity/Efficacy as time-to-event outcomes and handles unobserved delayed outcomes as censored observations. The latter approach must assume a particular survival distribution in order to estimate Toxicity and Efficacy probabilities at the end of their assessment periods, and is sensitive to misspecification of the survival model, with such sensitivity persisting throughout the trial.

5.3 Probability Model

The key to the method is that X_k^o provides useful information about Y_k, because

$$\Pr(Y_k = 1 \mid X_k^o = V < X_k) = 1 - \frac{\Pr(Q_k < X_k)}{\Pr(X_k^o = V < X_k)}$$

must decrease as X_k^o increases from 0 to Q_k. This fact also underlies the TiTE-CRM. (Cheung and Chappell, 2000). To construct flexible survival functions, we assume piecewise exponential marginals for $[X_k \mid d, Y_k = 1]$, $k = E, T$, by partitioning $[0, Q_k]$ into L_k intervals, $[0, h_{k,1}), [h_{k,1}, h_{k,2}), \cdots, [h_{k,L_k-1}, h_{k,L_k}]$, and assuming hazard $\lambda_{k,l}$ on $[h_{k,l-1}, h_{k,l})$. The marginal survival function for X_k at time t is

$$S_k(t \mid Y_k = 1, \lambda_k) = \exp\left\{ -\sum_{l=1}^{L_k} w_{k,l}(t) \lambda_{k,l} \right\}, \qquad t > 0,$$

denoting $\lambda_k = (\lambda_{k,1}, \cdots, \lambda_{k,L_k})$, and weights $w_{k,l}(t) = h_{k,l} - h_{k,l-1}$ if $t > h_{k,l}$, $w_{k,l}(t) = t - h_{k,l-1}$ if $t \in [h_{k,l-1}, h_{k,l})$, and $w_{k,l}(t) = 0$ otherwise. In theory, a more elaborate form of S_k can be constructed for more flexibility, for example replacing $\lambda_{k,l}$ by $\lambda_{k,l}\exp(\gamma_k d)$, where $\gamma_k > 0$, to allow the event time distributions varied with dose in a proportional hazard model with piecewise exponential baseline hazard. Numerical studies show that such an elaborated model does not improve the performance of the design, however, due to the fact that there is little or no information to estimate the γ_k's.

The imputation method requires the joint conditional survival probabilities

$$S(t_E, t_T \mid a, b) = \Pr(X_E > t_E, X_T > t_T \mid Y_E = a, Y_T = b)$$

for $(a, b) = (0,1)$, $(1,0)$, and $(1,1)$. We assume conditional independence, $S_k(t_k \mid Y_E, Y_T) = S_k(t_k \mid Y_k)$ for $k = E, T$, which implies that $S(t_E, t_T \mid 1, 0)$ is determined by the marginal of X_E and $S(t_E, t_T \mid 0, 1)$ is determined by the marginal of X_T. Determining $S(t_E, t_T \mid 1, 1)$ requires accounting for association between X_E and X_T. We do this by defining a joint distribution using the Clayton copula, (Clayton, 1978), given for $\phi \geq 0$ by

$$
\begin{aligned}
S(t_E, t_T \mid 1, 1) &= \left\{ S_E(t_E \mid Y_E = 1)^{-1/\phi} + S_T(t_T \mid Y_T = 1)^{-1/\phi} - 1 \right\}^{-\phi} \\
&= \left\{ \exp\left\{ \sum_{l=1}^{L_E} \lambda_{E,l} w_{E,l}/\phi \right\} + \exp\left\{ \sum_{l=1}^{L_T} \lambda_{T,l} w_{T,l}/\phi \right\} - 1 \right\}^{-\phi}.
\end{aligned}
$$

The likelihood of $\mathcal{D}$ depends on Y_E, Y_T, and the censoring patterns of X_E and X_T. Define censoring indicator $\epsilon_k = I(X_k^o = X_k)$, and denote $\lambda = (\lambda_E, \lambda_T)$, $\xi = (\phi + 1)/\phi$, the pdf of X_k by $f_k(\cdot)$, and

$$W(X_E^o, X_T^o) = S_E(X_E^o \mid Y_E = 1)^{-1/\phi} + S_T(X_T^o \mid Y_T = 1)^{-1/\phi} - 1.$$

TABLE 5.1: Possible forms of the likelihood for $\mathcal{D}|(\lambda, \phi)$ as a function of the censoring indicators for Y_E and Y_T

(ϵ_E, ϵ_T)	$\mathcal{L}(\mathcal{D}|\lambda, \phi)$
(0,0)	$W(X_E^o, X_E^o)^{-\phi}$
(0,1)	$W(X_E^o, X_E^o)^{-\phi-1} f_T(X_T^o|Y_T = 1) S_T(X_T^o|Y_T = 1)^\xi$
(1,0)	$W(X_E^o, X_E^o)^{-\phi-1} f_E(X_E^o|Y_E = 1) S_E(X_E^o|Y_E = 1)^\xi$
(1,1)	$\xi W(X_E^o, X_E^o)^{-\phi-2} \prod_{k=E}^{T} f_k(X_k^o|Y_k = 1)\left\{ \prod_{k=E}^{T} S_k(X_k^o|Y_k = 1)\right\}^\xi$

When $(Y_E, Y_T) = (1,1)$, depending on the censoring patterns, there are four possible forms for the likelihood, given in Table 5.1.

When $(Y_E, Y_T) = (1,0)$ or $(0,1)$, the likelihoods are given by

$$\mathcal{L}(\mathcal{D}|\lambda, \phi) = \left[\{f_E(X_E^o|Y_E = 1)\}^{\epsilon_E} \{S_E(X_E^o|Y_E = 1)\}^{1-\epsilon_E} \right]^{Y_E(1-Y_T)}$$

$$\times \left[\{f_T(X_T^o|Y_T = 1)\}^{\epsilon_T} \{S_T(X_T^o|Y_T = 1)\}^{1-\epsilon_T} \right]^{Y_T(1-Y_E)}.$$

5.4 Imputation of Delayed Outcomes

Bayesian data augmentation to impute values of Y_E or Y_T that are not yet known is carried out as follows. Let $\pi_{a,b}(d, \theta) = \Pr(Y_E = a, Y_T = b|d, \theta)$ for $a, b \in \{0,1\}$ denote the joint distribution of (Y_E, Y_T). If no outcomes are missing the likelihood is the usual product

$$\mathcal{L}(\mathcal{D}_n(Y)|\theta) = \prod_{i=1}^{n} \prod_{a=0}^{1} \prod_{b=0}^{1} \{\pi_{a,b}(d_{[i]}, \theta)\}^{I\{(Y_{i,E}, Y_{i,T})=(a,b)\}}, \qquad (5.2)$$

with posterior $f(\theta|\mathcal{D}_n(Y)) \propto \mathcal{L}(\mathcal{D}_n(Y)|\theta) f(\theta)$, for prior $f(\theta)$. To obtain a completed version of the likelihood, of the form (5.2), if some $Y_{i,k}$'s are missing, Bayesian data augmentation is done by iterating between (1) an imputation step sampling missing Y_k's from their full conditionals, and (2) a step computing the posterior using the completed data. A key point is that the imputation depends on the assumed dose-outcome model.

Since there are two binary outcomes, the imputation must account for three possible missingship patterns: (1) $Y_E = missing$ and Y_T is observed,

(2) $Y_T = missing$ and Y_E is observed, and (3) both $Y_E = missing$ and $Y_T = missing$. Since missing values are imputed by sampling from their full conditional posteriors, these distributions must be specified for each missingship pattern. These posteriors are defined in terms of the following conditionals for X_E and X_T, given each of the four possible future outcome pairs. For brevity, we denote these by

$$S_{ab} = \Pr(X_E > V, X_T > V | Y_E = a, Y_T = b), \qquad a, b \in \{0, 1\}. \qquad (5.3)$$

In any case, $S_{00} = 1$ due to the fact that $\Pr(X_k > V | Y_k = 0) = 1$ for $0 \leq V \leq Q_k$, which also implies that $S_{10} = \Pr(X_E > V | Y_E = 1, Y_T = 0)$ and $S_{01} = \Pr(X_T > V | Y_E = 0, Y_T = 1)$. Thus, only S_{11} involves a joint distribution for (X_E, X_T) given $Y_E = Y_T = 1$.

Consistent estimates when imputing the missing Y_k's are obtained by conditioning on the actual data $\mathcal{D}$. The following posterior conditional distributions are derived in Jin et al. (2014). When $Y_E = missing$ and Y_T is observed, Y_E is imputed from its conditional posterior

$$\Pr(Y_E = 1 | \mathcal{D}) = \left\{ \frac{\pi_{1,1} S_{10}}{\pi_{1,1} S_{10} + \pi_{0,1}} \right\}^{Y_T} \left\{ \frac{\pi_{1,0} S_{10}}{\pi_{1,0} S_{10} + \pi_{0,0}} \right\}^{1-Y_T}.$$

When $Y_T = missing$ and Y_E is observed, Y_T is imputed from its conditional posterior

$$\Pr(Y_T = 1 | \mathcal{D}) = \left\{ \frac{\pi_{1,1} S_{01}}{\pi_{1,1} S_{01} + \pi_{1,0}} \right\}^{Y_E} \left\{ \frac{\pi_{0,1} S_{01}}{\pi_{0,1} S_{01} + \pi_{0,0}} \right\}^{1-Y_E}.$$

When both Y_E and Y_T are missing, the pair (Y_E, Y_T) is imputed from the joint conditional posterior

$$\Pr(Y_E = y, Y_T = z | \mathcal{D}) = \frac{\pi_{y,z} S_{yz}}{\sum_{a=0}^{1} \sum_{b=0}^{1} \pi_{a,b} S_{ab}}, \qquad \text{for } y, z = 0, 1.$$

Each of these conditional posteriors is a *predictive probability*, since it is of the general form $\Pr(\text{Future Event} | \text{Observed Data})$.

At the posterior step using the completed data, for this model the parameters are sampled from their full conditional posteriors in two steps: (1) sample θ from $f(\theta | \mathcal{D}(Y))$, and (2) sample ϕ and $\lambda_{k,l}$ for each $l = 1, \cdots, L_k$ and $k = E, T$ from $f(\lambda, \phi | \mathcal{D}, \theta)$. This is iterated until the Markov chain converges, with posteriors computed using adaptive rejection Metropolis sampling (Gilks et al., 1995).

Recall that, in Case 2, Y_E is evaluated at Q_E, and there is no random event time involved in defining Y_E. Analytically, Case 2 is much simpler than Case 1, and Y_E is MCAR at all follow-up times $V < Q_E$. For the same reason, trial conduct in Case 2 is much harder logistically than in Case 1. For example, in the illustrative multiple myeloma trial, for each patient one must wait Q_E

= 90 days to evaluate Y_E, with no earlier information about what its value will be. Inference for π_E relies entirely on observed Y_E values from previously treated patients, while Y_T may be imputed by exploiting the event time data (X_T^o, ϵ_T) using the marginal of X_T.

5.5 Illustration

To make things concrete, we apply the method to the EffTox design described in Chapter 4. We refer to the resulting design as the Late-onset EffTox (LO-EffTox) design. We assume that the marginal probabilities take the quadratic forms $\pi_k = \text{logit}^{-1}\{\mu_k + \beta_{k,1}d + \beta_{k,2}d^2\}$ for $k = E, T$, and use the FGM copula to obtain joint probabilities. For priors, we assume $\mu_T, \mu_E, \beta_{T,1}, \beta_{E,1}, \beta_{T,2}, \beta_{E,2} \sim$ iid Cauchy$(0, 2.5)$, and shift the six Cauchy prior location parameters from 0 to $\tilde{\mu} = (\tilde{\mu}_{\mu_T}, \tilde{\mu}_{\beta_{T,1}}, \tilde{\mu}_{\beta_{T,2}}, \tilde{\mu}_{\mu_E}, \tilde{\mu}_{\beta_{E,1}}, \tilde{\mu}_{\beta_{E,2}})$, to reflect prior opinion. To obtain $\tilde{\mu}$, as before one may first elicit the means $\tilde{m}_{E,d_j}$ and $\tilde{m}_{T,d_j}$ of $\pi_E(d_j, \theta)$ and $\pi_T(d_j, \theta)$ from the physician for each dose $d_j, j = 1, ..., J$, and use least squares to solve for $(\tilde{\mu}_{\mu_k}, \tilde{\mu}_{\beta_{k,1}}, \tilde{\mu}_{\beta_{k,2}})$ by assuming $E\{\text{logit}(\tilde{m}_{k,d_j})\} = \tilde{\mu}_{\mu_k} + \tilde{\mu}_{\beta_{k,1}}d_j + \tilde{\mu}_{\beta_{k,2}}d_j^2$. To obtain a vague prior on λ, we assume $[X_k|Y_k = 1] \sim \text{Unif}(0, Q_k)$, which implies that the hazard at the midpoint of the subinterval $[h_{k,l-1}, h_{k,l}]$ of the partition is

$$\tilde{\lambda}_{k,l} = L_k/\{Q_k(L_k - l + 0.5)\}. \tag{5.4}$$

We assume that

$$\lambda_{k,l} \sim Gam(\tilde{\lambda}_{k,l}/C, 1/C),$$

where $Gam(a, b)$ denotes the gamma distribution with mean a/b and variance a/b^2. Thus, $\lambda_{k,l}$ has prior mean $\tilde{\lambda}_{k,l}$ and variance $C\tilde{\lambda}_{k,l}$, so C is a tuning parameter that determines $\text{var}(\lambda_{k,l})$ and that can be calibrated by simulation. In preliminary simulations, we found that $C = 2$ yields a reasonably vague prior and a design with good operating characteristics. Finally, we assume $\psi \sim \text{Normal}(0, 1)$ and $\phi \sim Gam(0.2, 0.2)$.

The following illustrative cases are constructed to mimic dose-finding trials of either chemotherapy for acute leukemia in Case 1, or of an agent that is part of a preparative regimen in a stem cell transplantation trial for multiple myeloma in Case 2. Recall that, in Case 1, X_E may occur at any time during $[0, Q_E]$, and, in Case 2, Y_E is observed at Q_E. For Case 1, we assumed that $Q_E = Q_T = 6$ weeks with accrual rate $\alpha = 1.5$ patients per week. For Case 2, we assumed $Q_E = 90$ days, (12.85 weeks), Toxicity evaluation interval $Q_T = 30$ days (4.3 weeks), and accrual rate $\alpha = 2.1$ patients per week. The logistical difficulty indices are $\zeta = 1.5 \times 6 = 9$ for Case 1 and $\zeta = \max(12.85, 4.3) \times 2.1 = 27$ for Case 2. We kept all other parameters for Case 2 the same as those in Case 1.

The illustrations consider five standardized doses (-0.75, -0.21, 0.11, 0.34, 0.51), which are centered around 0 and have standard deviation 0.5. Prior means 0.15, 0.20, 0.25, 0.30, 0.35 are assumed for $\pi_E(d_1, \theta)$, ..., $\pi_E(d_5, \theta)$ and 0.15, 0.20, 0.27, 0.35, 0.45 for $\pi_T(d_1, \theta)$, ..., $\pi_T(d_5, \theta)$. Applying the least squares method gives location hyper-parameters $(\tilde{\mu}_{\mu_E}, \tilde{\mu}_{\beta_{E,1}}, \tilde{\mu}_{\beta_{E,2}}) = (-1.21, 0.96, 0.35)$ and $(\tilde{\mu}_{\mu_T}, \tilde{\mu}_{\beta_{T,1}}, \tilde{\mu}_{\beta_{T,2}}) = (-1.16, 1.39, 0.85)$ for the shifted Cauchy priors. For the Gamma piecewise exponential event rate priors, we assumed $K = 6$. The formula (5.4) gives $(\tilde{\lambda}_{E,1}, \cdots, \tilde{\lambda}_{E,6}) = (\tilde{\lambda}_{T,1}, \cdots, \tilde{\lambda}_{T,6}) = (0.182, 0.222, 0.286, 0.400, 0.667, 2.000)$ in Case 1, and $(\tilde{\lambda}_{T,1}, \cdots, \tilde{\lambda}_{T,6}) = (0.364, 0.444, 0.571, 0.800, 1.333, 4.000)$ in Case 2.

The trade-off contour, $\mathcal{C}$, was determined by fitting a quadratic curve to the trade-off target probability pairs $(\pi_E, \pi_T) = (0.15, 0), (0.45, 0.20), (1, 0.60)$, which gives target contour function $\pi_T = -0.0952 + 0.6239\pi_E + 0.0713\pi_E^2$. Figure 5.2 illustrates the target contour by a solid line, with contours on which all (π_E, π_T) have the same desirability $\delta(\pi_E, \pi_T)$ shown as dashed lines. Dose acceptability limits were $\underline{\pi}_E = 0.25$ for Efficacy and $\bar{\pi}_T = 0.35$ for Toxicity, with decision cutoffs $p_E = p_T = 0.10$. The LO-EffTox method was applied for a 48-patient trial with 16 cohorts of size three.

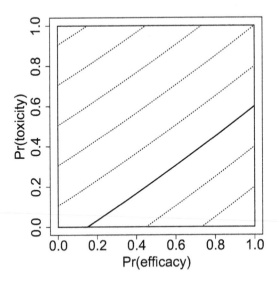

FIGURE 5.2: Trade-off contours. The target contour is represented by a solid line. Other contours on which all (π_E, π_T) have the same desirability are shown as dashed lines.

The LO-EffTox design was compared to three methods that often are used in practice to deal with the late-onset problem. The first method is the "One Level Down" rule. With this method, if some patients treated at the current

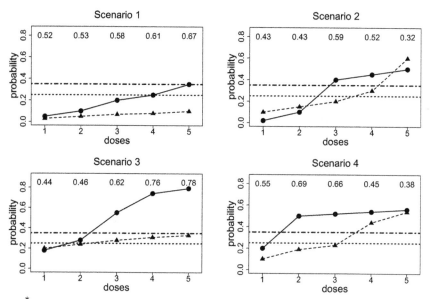

[*] The solid lines with circles represent $\pi_E^{true}(d)$ and the dashed lines with triangles represent $\pi_T^{true}(d)$. The two horizontal lines represent $\bar{\pi}_T$ and $\underline{\pi}_E$.

FIGURE 5.3: Dose-Toxicity and dose-Efficacy curves for the simulation scenarios.

optimal dose $d^{opt} = d_j$ have not yet been evaluated fully, i.e., $Y_{i,E}(d_j) = missing$ or $Y_{i,T}(d_j) = missing$, then any new patient is treated at d_{j-1}. The second method is the "Look Ahead" rule (Thall et al., 1999) which says that, for each possible value $\tilde{\mathcal{D}}_{mis}(Y)$ that $\mathcal{D}_{mis}(Y)$ may take on, use the completed data $\mathcal{D}_{obs}(Y) \cup \tilde{\mathcal{D}}_{mis}(Y)$ to compute d^{opt}. If this dose is the same for all possible $\tilde{\mathcal{D}}_{mis}(Y)$, then use that dose to treat the next patient immediately. Otherwise, the only two options for new patients are to make them wait to be treated, which usually is impossible in practice, or to turn them away and treat them off protocol. The third method uses only complete cases, where both Y_E and Y_T are observed, to compute d^{opt} and treat the next patient immediately, and ignores patients for whom either Y_E or Y_T is missing.

Two summary criteria are used to evaluate each method's performance and compare the three methods. Denote the true desirability of dose d_j by δ_j^{true} and the true set of acceptable doses by $\mathcal{A}^{true}$. The first criterion is the *desirability-weighted selection percentage*,

$$\bar{\delta} = \frac{\sum_{j=1}^{5} \delta_j^{true} \, \Pr(\text{select } d_j) I(d_j \in \mathcal{A}^{true})}{\sum_{j=1}^{5} \delta_j^{true} \, I(d_j \in \mathcal{A}^{true})},$$

which quantifies dose selection reliability and thus the potential benefit for future patients. The second criterion is the ratio N_E/N_T, where N_E and N_T

TABLE 5.2: Simulation scenarios. For each scenario, the first line gives the true probability pair $(\pi_{E,j}^{true}, \pi_{T,j}^{true})$. The second line is the desirability $\delta(\pi_{E,j}^{true}, \pi_{T,j}^{true})$.

			Dose Level		
Scenario	1	2	3	4	5
1	(.05, .03)	(.10, .05)	(.20, .07)	(.25, .08)	(.35, .10)
	.52	.53	.58	.61	.67
2	(.02, .10)	(.10, .15)	(.40, .20)	(.45, .30)	(.50, .60)
	.43	.43	.59	.52	.32
3	(.18, .20)	(.28, .24)	(.55, .28)	(.74, .31)	(.79, .33)
	.44	.46	.62	.76	.78
4	(.20, .10)	(.50, .19)	(.52, .23)	(.54, .44)	(.56, .54)
	.55	.69	.66	.45	.38

denote the numbers of patients who experience Efficacy and Toxicity, respectively. This criterion quantifies benefit to the patients in the trial, hence may be considered an index of ethical desirability.

Figure 5.3 gives the assumed true dose-Toxicity and dose-Efficacy curves that characterize the scenarios used in the simulation study. Figure 5.4 illustrates the results in terms of $\bar{\delta}$ plotted on the horizontal axis and N_E/N_T on the vertical axis under these scenarios. The true Efficacy and Toxicity probabilities at each dose, $\pi_{k,j}^{true}$, for $k = E, T$ and $j = 1, ..., 5$, are given in Table 5.2. In Figure 5.4, values in the upper right portion of the figure are more desirable, while values in the lower left are less desirable. The One Level Down rule produces designs with very poor properties, in terms of both $\bar{\delta}$ and N_E/N_T. These two criteria are roughly equivalent for LO-EffTox and the Look Ahead version of EffTox. However, since the Look Ahead rule turns away many patients, more than 50 patients in each of the four scenarios, and produces a very long trial (see Figure 5.5), the apparent equivalence in terms of the two criteria in Figure 5.4 only tells part of the story. Compared to the Complete Case method, LO-EffTox has either similar or much larger $\bar{\delta}$ values and similar N_E/N_T.

The simulation results for the Case 2 are summarized in Figure 5.6. Again, LO-EffTox generally outperforms the One Level Down, Look Ahead, and Complete Case methods, in terms of both selection percentages and N_E/N_T. In addition, as in Case 1, the Look Ahead rule has selection percentages similar to those of the LO-EffTox design, but the price is a much longer trial with many patients turned away.

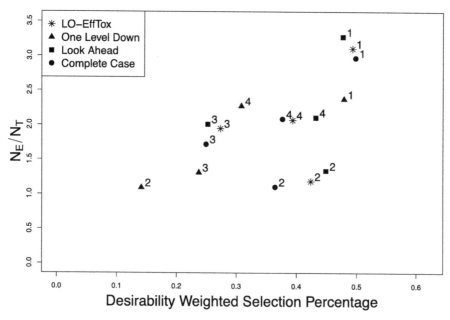

FIGURE 5.4: Simulation results for case 1. Simulation scenarios are identified by integers.

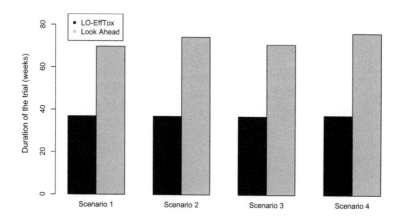

FIGURE 5.5: Trial duration under the LO-EffTox and Look Ahead designs.

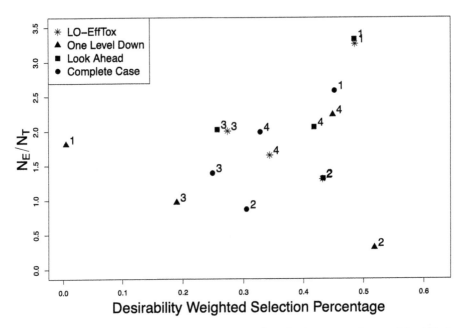

FIGURE 5.6: Simulation results for case 2. Simulation scenarios are identified by integers.

6

Utility-Based Designs

CONTENTS

6.1   Assigning Utilities to Outcomes 105
6.2   Subjectivity of Utilities 111
6.3   Utility-Based Sequential Decision Making 113
     6.3.1   Utility Elicitation 113
     6.3.2   Computing Mean Utilities 114
     6.3.3   Regime Acceptability Criteria 115
     6.3.4   Design Evaluation Criteria 116
     6.3.5   Utility Sensitivity Analyses 117
     6.3.6   More Elaborate Utilities 118
6.4   Optimizing Radiation Dose for Brain Tumors 119

"Nothing can have value without being an object of utility."

Karl Marx

6.1   Assigning Utilities to Outcomes

Many of the designs that we will discuss rely on numerical utilities assigned to the possible elementary clinical outcomes. The motivation for doing this arises from settings where the outcome that is the basis for evaluating the treatment regimes is more complex than a single binary indicator. Recall that, for sequential decision making, the regime-outcome data $(\rho_{[1]}, Y_1), \cdots, (\rho_{[n]}, Y_n)$ on the first n patients are used as a basis for deciding what regime to give patient $n+1$. This requires one to formulate a probability model $p(y \mid \rho, \theta)$ for the relationship between each regimen ρ and the observable outcome Y, and moreover to construct decision rules that quantify the desirability of each possible value y of Y, or of its probability. In the simple case where Y is a binary indicator of a desirable anti-disease effect, such as $\geq 50\%$ tumor shrinkage achieved by a pre-specified time, then $Y = 1$ is better than $Y = 0$, so the probability $\pi(\rho, \theta) = \Pr(Y = 1 \mid \rho, \theta)$ unambiguously quantifies how good ρ is. Regardless of the assumed model, bigger $\pi(\rho, \theta)$ is better and, aside from the usual uncertainty that accompanies any statistical inference, including estimation of each $\pi(\rho, \theta)$, the regime with the largest average $\pi(\rho, \theta)$ is best.

Example 1. Next, suppose that things are slightly more complex, in that Y is a three-level ordinal variable with possible values $[Y = 0] = [\text{No response}]$, $[Y = 1] = [\text{Partial response}]$, and $[Y = 2] = [\text{Complete response}]$, and denote the probabilities $\pi_y(\rho, \theta)$ for $y = 0, 1, 2$. Assume, for the sake of illustration, that there are two treatment regimes, ρ_1 and ρ_2, and that the six probabilities $\{\pi_y(\rho_j, \theta) : y = 0, 1, 2\}$ are known to be (.30, .20, .50) for ρ_1 and (.10, .50, .40) for ρ_2. That is, the model parameter vector θ is known. Even with this knowledge, the question of which regime is better does not have an obvious answer. While ρ_1 has a higher complete response rate, ρ_2 has a much higher partial response rate and lower rate of no response. Thus, the question of how to compare the two regimes based on these two probability vectors, in order to decide which is better, does not have an obvious answer.

This problem can be solved by assigning numerical utilities to the three elementary outcomes that quantify their relative desirability. One then may compute the mean utility for each regime, and declare the one with the larger mean utility to be more desirable. For example, the utility assignment $U(0) = 0$, $U(1) = 60$, $U(2) = 100$ gives mean utility $\bar{U}(\rho_1) = 0 \times .30 + 60 \times .20 + 100 \times .50 = 62$ for ρ_1 and $\bar{U}(\rho_2) = 0 \times .10 + 60 \times .50 + 100 \times .40 = 70$ for ρ_2, so ρ_2 is superior to ρ_1. But the utility assignment $U(0) = 0$, $U(1) = 20$, $U(2) = 100$ gives $\bar{U}(\rho_1) = 54$ for ρ_1 and $\bar{U}(\rho_2) = 50$ for ρ_2, so for this utility ρ_1 is superior to ρ_2, The reason for this reversal is that the second utility places much less value on partial response compared to the first utility. In this illustration, as we will do in all of our other applications, we have taken the general approach of assigning utility 100 to the best possible outcome and 0 to the worst possible outcome. In theory, any other finite interval could be used, but we have found that the domain [0, 100] for utilities of clinical outcomes works quite well in practice when communicating with physicians.

Example 2. Suppose that a phase I–II trial is being planned with Y_E and Y_T both binary indicators, as in the EffTox design, so the regime ρ is a dose, x, and the four possible elementary outcomes are $y = (0,0)$, $(0,1)$, $(1,0)$, or $(1,1)$. Before considering the utility structure in this case, it is worthwhile to re-visit the alternative approach of using only Y_T for dose-finding, rather than (Y_E, Y_T). Since smaller $\pi_T(x)$ is better, this would seem to imply that one simply should not treat the patient at all, which may be denoted by x_0, since this ensures that $\pi(x_0, \theta) \equiv 0$ for any θ, i.e., Toxicity is impossible. Recall that, as explained in Section 1.2, the only logical and ethical rationale for using Toxicity alone for dose-finding is the *implicit* assumption that there also is a desirable Efficacy outcome, Y_E, that is affected by the experimental treatment, and moreover that the distribution of Y_E becomes more favorable as x increases. If, for example, Y_E is progression-free survival (PFS) time, then the implicit assumption is that the mean of Y_E increases with x. When no early Efficacy outcome is available to use in an outcome-adaptive sequential dose-finding design, assuming that mean or median PFS time increases with x may be a reasonable rationale for using a design based on Toxicity alone. If, instead, one may observe a binary indicator Y_E of an early Efficacy event, such as engraftment of a stem cell transplant within 30 days or shrinkage of a solid tumor by at least 50% within the first two cycles of chemotherapy, then the implicit assumption is that $\pi_E(x) = \Pr(Y_E = 1 \mid x)$ increases with dose x. The phase I–II paradigm makes this assumption explicitly by including both Y_E and Y_T as outcomes in the design, and assuming parametric models for $\pi_E(x, \theta)$, $\pi_T(x, \theta)$, and possibly for the joint probabilities $\pi(a, b, \theta) = \Pr(Y_E = a, Y_T = b, \theta)$. Recall that the EffTox method, presented in various versions in Chapters 4, 5, and 6, uses an explicit trade-off function $\phi(\pi_E, \pi_T)$ between the marginal probabilities π_E and π_T as a basis for decision making.

For a utility-based design, numerical utilities first must be assigned to the four elementary outcomes. Following our general approach, we first assign $U(1, 0) = 100$ to the best possible outcome, Efficacy and no Toxicity, and $U(0, 1) = 0$ to the worst possible outcome, No Efficacy and Toxicity. Thus, only the two utilities $U(1, 1)$ and $U(0, 0)$ must be elicited from the physicians. These both must be numbers between 0 and 100, since (1,0) is a more desirable outcome and (0,1) is a less desirable outcome compared to either (1,1) or (0,0). Otherwise, there is no additional constraint, and it may be the case that either $U(1, 1) > U(0, 0)$ or $U(1, 1) < U(0, 0)$.

Denoting the joint probabilities at dose x by $\pi(a, b \mid x, \theta)$ for $a, b = 0, 1$, as before, given x and θ the mean utility is

$$\overline{U}(x, \theta) = \sum_{a=0}^{1} \sum_{b=0}^{1} U(a, b)\, \pi(a, b \mid x, \theta). \tag{6.1}$$

In practice, θ and thus the $\pi(a, b \mid x, \theta)$'s and $\overline{U}(x, \theta)$'s are unknown. For illustration, we temporarily assume that, for a given x, the probabilities are known to be $\pi(0, 0 \mid x) = .40$, $\pi(0, 1 \mid x) = .10$, $\pi(1, 0 \mid x) = .30$, and $\pi(1, 1 \mid x) = .20$. The mean utility of x is then

$$
\begin{aligned}
\overline{U}(x) &= U(0, 0) \times .40 + U(0, 1) \times .10 + U(1, 0) \times .30 + U(1, 1) \times .20 \\
&= U(0, 0) \times .40 + 0 \times .10 + 100 \times .30 + U(1, 1) \times .20 \\
&= 30 + U(0, 0) \times .40 + U(1, 1) \times .20.
\end{aligned}
$$

Thus, given known probabilities, the mean utility $\overline{U}(x)$ of dose x depends on $U(0, 0)$ and $U(1, 1)$. To complete the example, if $U(0, 0) = 40$ and $U(1, 1) = 70$, then $\overline{U}(x) = 60$. One way to think about this utility is in terms of the ratios $U(1, 0)/U(1, 1) = 100/70 = 1.43$, which says that for patients who achieve Efficacy it is 43% better to not have Toxicity, and $U(1, 0)/U(0, 0) = 100/40 = 2.5$, which says that for patients who do not have Toxicity, it is 150% better to achieve Efficacy than not. This sort of comparison can also be done in terms of the differences $U(1, 0) - U(1, 1) = 30$ and $U(1, 0) - U(0, 0) =$

60. Below, we will discuss the problem of estimating $\overline{U}(\rho, \theta)$ for each regime ρ and using the estimates as a basis for making decisions.

In the bivariate binary outcome setting, there is an approximate mapping from any utility function $\{U(a, b) : a, b = 0, 1\}$ to a corresponding EffTox trade-off contour. This mapping may be constructed by first assuming that Y_E and Y_T are independent, so that approximate joint probabilities are $\pi(1, 1)^* = \pi_E \pi_T$, $\pi(1, 0)^* = \pi_E(1 - \pi_T)$, and so on. These may be used to compute the approximate mean utilities

$$\overline{U}^*(\pi_E, \pi_T) = \sum_{a=0}^{1} \sum_{b=0}^{1} U(a, b)\, \pi(a, b)^*.$$

One then may define the approximate trade-off contour $\mathcal{C}_\delta^*$ in $[0, 1]^2$ on which all pairs (π_E, π_T) have desirability δ to be

$$\mathcal{C}_\delta^* = \{(\pi_E, \pi_T) : \overline{U}^*(\pi_E, \pi_T) = \delta\}.$$

Trade-off contours only make sense if π_E increases with π_T, formally $\partial \pi_E / \partial \pi_T > 0$. That is, the rationale underlying the trade-off requires the probability of Efficacy to increase with the probability of Toxicity. To see why this is so on $\mathcal{C}_\delta^*$, we first note that, after some algebra, $\partial \pi_E / \partial \pi_T = (c + d\pi_E)^2/(bc - ad)$ where $a = \overline{U} - U(0, 0)$, $b = U(0, 0) - U(1, 0)$, $c = U(0, 1) - U(0, 0)$, and $d = U(0, 0) - U(0, 1) - U(1, 0) + U(1, 1)$. Since $U(0, 1) = 0$ and $U(1, 0) = 100$, denoting $x = U(0, 0)/100$ and $y = U(1, 1)/100$, we can write $bc - ad = 100\overline{U}(1 - x)(1 - y) + 100(100 - \overline{U})xy$, which must be positive.

Families of approximate contours are illustrated in Figure 6.1, which gives the EffTox trade-off contours obtained, using the above approximation, for four different utility functions on the 2×2 outcome set. All four utilities have $U(0, 0) = 30$, and since $U(1, 0) \equiv 100$ and $U(0, 1) \equiv 0$, the only utility being varied between the four cases is $U(1, 1)$. Given the discussion of trade-off contours in Chapter 4, it should be clear that the upper left contour family is pathological. This family is determined by $U(1, 1) = 10$, which says that, since $U(1, 0) - U(1, 1) = 100\text{-}10 = 90$, for a patient who has the Efficacy event, also having Toxicity decreases the utility by 90%. Another way to look at this utility function is to note that $U(1, 1) - U(0, 1) = 10\text{-}0 = 10$, so for a patient who has Toxicity the increase in utility from achieving Efficacy is only 10, which says that Efficacy has relatively little value. The family of contours in the upper right plot is obtained if $U(1, 1) = 50$, which says that for a patient who has Toxicity, achieving Efficacy increases the utility substantially, by $U(1, 1) - U(0, 1) = 50\text{-}0 = 50$. This is a reasonable utility in many settings. The lower left family is generated from $U(1, 1) = 70$, so the decrease $U(1, 0) - U(1, 1) = 100\text{-}70 = 30$ due to Toxicity among patients with Efficacy is the same as the decrease in utility for patients who do not have Efficacy, $U(0, 0) - U(0, 1) = 30 - 0 = 30$. This is an example of the case where the contours are straight lines, which occurs when $U(0, 0) + U(1, 1) = 100$. The lower right family of contour places very little value on avoiding a Toxicity,

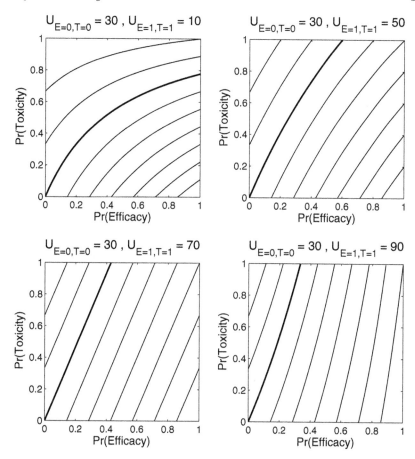

FIGURE 6.1: Approximate trade-off contours for four utility functions.

since $U(1,0) - U(1,1) = 100\text{-}90 = 10$, which would be reasonable only if, from a clinical perspective, Toxicity were an adverse event considered to be of little importance.

Example 3. The third example arises from a phase I–II trial (Thall and Nguyen, 2012) of radiation therapy (RT) for diffuse intrinsic pontine gliomas (DIPGs). These are very aggressive pediatric brain tumors, with median patient age less than one year, and no treatment with substantive antidisease effect currently exists. Thus, the primary therapeutic motivation for RT is palliation, not cure. The scientific goal of the trial is to determine the optimal radiation dose among the three values 40.00, 45.76, and 53.39 in gray units (Gy). Toxicity is defined on a 4-level ordinal scale as {low, moderate, high, severe}, with each of these levels defined in terms of fatigue, nausea/vomiting, headache, skin

TABLE 6.1: Elicited consensus utilities of the 16 elementary outcomes in the trial to optimize radiation therapy dose for brain tumors

	Toxicity Severity			
	Low	Moderate	High	Severe
Efficacy				
0	50	25	10	0
1	85	50	15	5
2	92	60	20	7
3	100	75	25	10

inflammation or desquamation, blindness, and brain edema or necrosis, evaluated during the 42-day period from the start of radiation therapy. Efficacy, scored at day 42, is defined as the sum of three indicators of any improvement, compared to baseline, in (1) clinical symptoms, (2) radiographic appearance of the tumor, or (3) quality of life. Thus, the possible Efficacy scores are $\{0, 1, 2, 3\}$. The elicited consensus utilities of the resulting $4 \times 4 = 16$ elementary outcomes are given in Table 6.1. This table contains many more utilities than in the previous examples, but it was constructed using the same general approach. We first assigned the best possible outcome the utility $U(3, Low) = 100$, assigned the worst possible outcome the utility $U(0, Severe) = 0$, and then elicited the 14 additional intermediate utility values from the radiation oncologists. This was done subject to the obvious constraints that $U(y_E, y_T)$ must decrease moving from left to right in each row of Table 6.1, i.e., as Toxicity gets worse for any given Efficacy level, and it must increase moving from top to bottom in each column, i.e., as Efficacy gets better for any given Toxicity level. The utilities quantify the trade-off between Efficacy and Toxicity in many ways. For example, since $U(1, Moderate) = U(0, Low) = 50$, this says that a *Moderate* Toxicity is a trade-off for obtaining $Y_E = 1$, that is, improvement in one of the three desirable outcomes. Since $U(2, Moderate) = 60$ while $U(2, High) = 20$, this says that, for a patient with improvement in two of the three efficacy events, suffering a *High* Toxicity reduces the patient's utility to 1/3 of its value compared to only a *Moderate* Toxicity occurring.

This example illustrates a very important advantage of assigning utilities to bivariate ordinal outcomes. Since $U(0, Moderate) = U(3, High) = 25$, these two outcomes are considered to be equally desirable. That is, Toxicity severity increasing from *Moderate* to *High* is considered a fair trade-off for achieving all three Efficacy events compared to achieving none. Suppose that, instead, one were to take the commonly used approach of dichotomizing Toxicity by defining $Y_T = 1$ if Toxicity severity $= High$ or *Severe* and $Y_T = 0$ if Toxicity severity $= Low$ or *Moderate*. With this simplification, the event $(0, Moderate)$ would give $Y_T = 0$, i.e. "No Toxicity" while the event $(3, High)$ would give $Y_T = 1$, i.e., "Toxicity." Table 6.1 would be collapsed to a table of the form 6.2, where we have used the mean utilities obtained from the combined pairs

TABLE 6.2: Utilities obtained by dichotomizing Toxicity

Efficacy	No Toxicity	Toxicity
0	37.5	5
1	67.5	10
2	76	13.5
3	87.5	17.5

of columns of Table 6.1. This gives a very different interpretation of the observed clinical outcomes compared to the more refined utilities in Table 6.1, and could lead quite easily to very different conclusions about which dose is "optimal." For example, using the reduced utilities in Table 6.2, $(0, Moderate)$ would be assigned utility 37.5 while $(3, High)$ would be assigned utility 13.5, which says that $(0, Moderate)$ would be considered roughly three times as desirable as $(3, High)$. This disagrees greatly with the original assignment of the same elicited utility 25 to these two events. Taking this simplification a step further by ignoring Efficacy and using a phase I design based on this binary DLT indicator Y_T alone, the eight outcomes in the left two columns of Table 6.1 would be considered equally desirable, despite the fact that their elicited utilities vary from 25 to 100. This illustrates the potential loss of important information when an ordinal variable is dichotomized, or Efficacy is ignored, in the context of a dose-finding trial where both ordinal Efficacy and ordinal Toxicity are observed.

6.2 Subjectivity of Utilities

It may be argued that, because the numerical utilities assigned to the elementary outcomes are subjective, and therefore any statistical inferences based on a given utility must be subjective, such inferences should not be trusted. We disagree strongly with this viewpoint, and believe that the subjectivity of the utilities is a strength of any utility-based comparison, not a weakness. This is because the utilities must be elicited from the physicians planning the trial, and thus their numerical values are based on the physicians' experience treating the disease and observing the good and bad effects of treatment on their patients. As explained earlier, consideration of potential risks and benefits of treatment underlies all clinical decision making. We have found that, invariably, practicing physicians planning a clinical trial are very happy to assign numerical utilities to the clinical outcomes that they have specified, since it gives them the opportunity to explicitly quantify the risk–benefit considerations that underlie their thinking and clinical practice. Moreover, when multiple physicians are involved, a utility reflecting the consensus of the group of physicians is elicited, and we have found that, in practice, obtaining a consensus invariably is quite easy.

Another possible criticism is that it would be better to elicit the numerical utilities from each patient at enrollment. The idea that each patient should be asked to assign their own numerical utilities to the possible outcomes and treated with the resulting optimal regimen may seem ethically appealing. However, it is based on the very unrealistic assumption that each patient fully understands how good or bad each possible outcome that they may experience in the future will be, once their treatment has begun. Most patients about to be treated in a phase I–II clinical trial have not experienced the possible clinical outcomes, and thus they have no experiential basis for assigning numerical utilities. The patients enrolled in most phase I–II trials are about to undergo a treatment regimen that may have severe adverse effects, to treat a disease that is life-threatening. While patients certainly understand the general idea that the potential adverse effects of treatment are a trade-off for its possible beneficial anti-disease effects, they have no experience to guide them in assigning numerical utilities to elementary outcomes. A patient about to undergo anti-disease treatment that may cause severe Toxicities, when shown the possible outcomes and asked to assign utilities, is likely to assign utility 100 to the best possible outcome and utility 0 to all other outcomes. Such emotionally motivated behavior is unrealistically optimistic, since the probability of the best possible outcome may be small for any of the available treatment regimes, and it also ignores a great deal of information. Thus, such a utility would serve the patient poorly if used to choose the patient's treatment. Moreover, this would make it impossible to evaluate the design's operating characteristics. This is because a utility-based design must assume one utility only so, for trial design evaluation by computer simulation, that single utility function must be established as a key part of the design before the trial has accrued any patients. A very important exception is a trial of a second line or later stage of therapy, where the patients to be enrolled previously have experienced some of the clinical outcomes from their front line treatment. In such a setting, patients may have a rational basis for specifying values of $U(y)$. However, this sort of elicitation must be done during the design stage, and not as patients are enrolled, so that the design's utility function may be established and it may be simulated.

Defending the subjectivity of utility-based decision making quickly leads to the simple fact that all statistical methods have highly subjective components, although they often are not recognized as such. For example, any typical two-sample comparative test is based on one or more numerical test cut-offs that are computed by assuming a particular Type I error and a particular power at a particular specified numerical alternative for the parameters. These numerical values actually reflect highly subjective utilities that, typically, are not acknowledged. For example, a two-sample binomial test comparing probabilities π_1 and π_2 may be done with specified Type I error 0.05 and power .80, equivalently Type II error .20, to detect a difference $\delta = |\pi_1 - \pi_2| = .25$. These three numbers reflect the belief that a difference of .25 or larger is meaningful in some sense, and that, given this difference, it is far more important to avoid a Type I error than to avoid a Type II error, since Pr(Type II Error at δ = .25)/ Pr(Type I Error) = .20/.05 = 4. This sort of consideration typically is ignored when specifying Type I and Type II error probabilities for a test of hypotheses. The choice of δ = .25, rather than .20 or .30, also is very subjective. These numerical values often are chosen as a device to obtain a desired sample size. Additionally, for any given data structure, many different test statistics may be used, which also is an inherently subjective choice.

6.3   Utility-Based Sequential Decision Making

6.3.1   Utility Elicitation

In practice, once the trial's entry criteria, treatment regimes, and outcomes all have been established, the utilities may be elicited. For many trials, this may be done by simply explaining what the utilities represent to the Principal Investigator (PI) during the design process, and asking the PI to specify all necessary values of $U(y)$. We have found that, with bivariate outcomes anywhere between 2×2 and 4×4, the process is quite easy and natural. After an initial specification has been written down, comparing outcomes that have the same or similar numerical utilities often motivates the PI to modify the the initial numerical values. In our experience, oncologists quickly understand what the utilities mean, since they reflect actual clinical practice. It is almost as if the oncologists have been waiting for someone to ask them their utilities. After completing this process, and simulating the trial design, it then may be examined by the PI's colleagues in their department. In some cases, the resulting discussion may motivate slight modification of some of the numerical $U(y)$ values, although such modifications typically have little or no effect on the design's OCs.

More formal methods to obtain consensus utilities from the start certainly can be used, and this is especially appropriate for multi-institution studies. The so-called Delphi method (Dalkey and Helmer, 1963; Dalkey, 1969; Brook et al., 1986) begins by performing a series of interrogations, usually by means of a questionnaire, asking the group of individuals whose opinions matter to specify their values of $\{U(y), y \in \mathcal{Y}\}$. After the first stage, each subsequent interrogation is accompanied by the results of the preceding round, including the average utility values and usually presented anonymously. Each individual is given the opportunity to reconsider their utilities on that basis and possibly change their previous values in light of the replies from the other members of the group. This usually is completed with a consensus reached after two or three rounds, and the consensus utility is the group mean. Other formal methods for eliciting and establishing consensus utilities are discussed by Cooke (1991); Swinburn et al. (2010); Hunink et al. (2014). In the context of treating renal cell cancer, Wong et al. (2012) conducted interviews with cancer patients in an attempt to establish patient priorities for assigning weights to prolonged PFS versus the risk of multiple toxicities that may occur with second-line therapy. This last approach may be useful, in general, for settings where the treatment being studied is a second line or later stage of therapy, so the patients have experience with clinical outcomes, including Toxicity, from their front line treatment, and consequently they have a meaningful basis for specifying values of $U(y)$.

A technical complication may arise when eliciting the utilities of joint (Y_E, Y_T) outcomes if one or both outcomes are continuous valued variables. This problem may be solved by partitioning the domain of each continuous variable into intervals and proceeding as if both Y_E and Y_T were discrete. Examples of this approach will be given in trial designs discussed in Chapters 11 and 13.

6.3.2   Computing Mean Utilities

In the Bayesian framework, there are two different but closely related expressions that may be called the "mean utility of a treatment regime ρ." The first is the mean of the numerical utility values over the parametric distribution of $[Y \mid \rho, \theta]$,

$$\overline{U}(\rho, \theta) \;=\; \sum_y U(y)\, \pi(y \mid \rho, \theta). \tag{6.2}$$

The values of this mean utility function are unknown because they depend on the parameter vector θ. One could assume values of the probabilities $\pi(y \mid \rho)$ for all possible outcomes y of Y to examine how the mean utility behaves, but to make adaptive decisions during trial conduct one must use the available data to estimate $\overline{U}(\rho, \theta)$ for each ρ. Given data $\mathcal{D}_n$ at some point in the trial, inference may be done by obtaining a frequentist estimator $\hat{\theta}_n$ and using it to compute the plug-in estimator $\overline{U}(\rho, \hat{\theta}_n)$ for each ρ. Alternatively, one may assume a Bayesian model and compute the posterior mean of $\overline{U}(\rho, \theta)$ for each ρ, which is the approach that will take in all of our applications. The *posterior mean utility of ρ* is

$$\begin{aligned}
u(\rho, \mathcal{D}_n) &= E_\theta\{\overline{U}(\rho, \theta) \mid \mathcal{D}_n\} \\
&= \int_\theta \overline{U}(\rho, \theta)\, p(\theta \mid \mathcal{D}_n)\, d\theta \\
&= \int_\theta \sum_y U(y)\, \pi(y \mid \rho, \theta) p(\theta \mid \mathcal{D}_n)\, d\theta. \tag{6.3}
\end{aligned}$$

Thus, the first mean (6.2) is obtained by averaging over the distribution of $[Y \mid x, \theta]$ to obtain $\overline{U}(\rho, \theta)$, and one then averages this mean utility over the posterior of θ to obtain the posterior mean utility (6.3) of ρ. If Y is continuous, the same computation is carried out with a probability density function, say $f(y \mid \rho, \theta)$ in place of the probabilities $\pi(y \mid \rho, \theta)$ for discrete valued Y, and the sum over y becomes an integral. Given this structure, the *optimal regime given* $\mathcal{D}_n$ at any point in the trial is

$$\rho_n^{opt} = \underset{\rho}{\operatorname{argmax}} \; u(\rho, \mathcal{D}_n).$$

Because $U(y)$ is a patient outcome utility, maximizing $u(\rho, \mathcal{D}_n)$ is very different from the common Bayesian approach of choosing ρ to optimize some posterior function of the Fisher information matrix (cf. Haines et al., 2003; Dragalin and Fedorov, 2006).

An interesting and useful interpretation of $u(\rho, \mathcal{D}_n)$ is obtained by reversing the order of the integral over θ and sum over y in (6.3). Denote the posterior predictive probability

$$\pi(y \mid \rho, \mathcal{D}_n) = \int_\theta \pi(y \mid \rho, \theta) p(\theta \mid \mathcal{D}_n) d\theta$$

for each value y of Y and regime ρ, which is what one would predict the probability of outcome $Y = y$ to be for a future patient treated with ρ, given the current data. This gives

$$
\begin{aligned}
u(\rho, \mathcal{D}_n) &= \int_\theta \sum_y U(y) \, \pi(y \mid \rho, \theta) p(\theta \mid \mathcal{D}_n) d\theta \\
&= \sum_y U(y) \int_\theta \pi(y \mid \rho, \theta) p(\theta \mid \mathcal{D}_n) d\theta \\
&= \sum_y U(y) \, \pi(y \mid \rho, \mathcal{D}_n).
\end{aligned}
\tag{6.4}
$$

Thus, $u(\rho, \mathcal{D}_n)$ may be interpreted as the mean utility of treating a future patient with ρ, obtained by averaging the patient's future clinical outcome Y over its posterior predictive distribution given the current data.

6.3.3 Regime Acceptability Criteria

As with the EffTox design, when doing utility-based decision making in a clinical trial, we do not rely on ρ_n^{opt} alone to choose the regime for each new cohort. That is, motivated by ethical considerations, maximizing the posterior mean of a utility-based objective function, *per se*, is not enough to allow a regimen to be administered to patients. While the optimal regimen under a given utility function is mathematically well-defined, it is only an indirect solution of an optimization in expectation. An important case is that where it has been determined, based on $\mathcal{D}_n$, that no regime is acceptably safe and efficacious, so it is not ethical to treat any patient using any regime, and the trial must be stopped. For example, simply maximizing $u(\rho, \mathcal{D}_n)$ ignores the undesirable but important possibility that all regimes are too toxic. In some applications, the decision-theoretic solution might turn out to have undesirable properties that were not anticipated when specifying the outcomes, model, and numerical utilities. This problem is one reason why many researchers are reluctant to use formal decision-theoretic methods for clinical decision making. Discussions of this issue are given by Spiegelhalter et al. (2004, Chapter 3.14) and Lee et al. (2015, Section 3.3). We thus include additional acceptability criteria that place limits on the probabilities of Efficacy and Toxicity.

For bivariate ordinal outcomes, the following regime acceptability criteria may be used. These generalize the two criteria used by EffTox for binary outcomes. Indexing the outcomes by $y = 1, \cdots, m_k$ for $k = E, T$, denote the marginal probabilities $\pi_k(y|\rho, \theta) = \Pr(Y_k = y \mid \rho, \theta)$, and $\bar{\pi}_k(y|\rho, \theta) = \Pr(Y_k \geq y \mid \rho, \theta)$. To control the risk of Toxicity, one must elicit a level y_T^* of Toxicity considered by the physicians to be suitably high, and an accompanying fixed *upper* limit π_T^* on the probability $\bar{\pi}_T(y^*|\rho, \theta)$ of Toxicity at or above y_T^*. We say that *a regime ρ is unacceptably toxic* if

$$\Pr\{\bar{\pi}_T(y_T^*|\rho, \theta) > \pi_T^* \mid \mathcal{D}_n\} > p_T, \qquad (6.5)$$

where p_T is an upper probability cut-off. Expression (6.5) says it is likely that the probability of Toxicity at level y_T^* or higher is above π_T^*.

Similarly, one may elicit a level y_E^* of Efficacy from the physicians and an accompanying fixed *lower* limit π_E^* on the probability $\bar{\pi}_{E,y^*,\rho}$ of Efficacy at or above y_E^*. We say that *a regime ρ is unacceptably inefficacious* if

$$\Pr\{\bar{\pi}_E(y_E^*|\rho, \theta) < \pi_E^* \mid \mathcal{D}_n\} > p_E, \qquad (6.6)$$

where p_E is an upper probability cut-off similar to p_T. This is essentially a futility rule of the sort used in phase II trials. In the simplest case where Y_E and Y_T are binary, these rules reduce to the criteria used by EffTox.

We will limit regime assignments to *the set of acceptable regimes, $\mathcal{A}_n$,* defined to be all $\rho \in \mathcal{R}$ for which neither (6.5) nor (6.6) is true. In some trials, only the safety rule (6.5) is used. These rules are similar to the dose acceptability criteria used by Thall and Cook (2004), the safety requirements given by Braun et al. (2007), and "escalation with overdose control" proposed by Babb et al. (1998) for phase I trials. Additional data-based rules also may be used to limit the regimes that may be included in $\mathcal{A}_n$, and we will discuss some of these in the illustrations of utility-based designs to follow.

6.3.4   Design Evaluation Criteria

To evaluate how well a design performs in picking a regime to optimize a given utility function, we define the following two summary statistics. In a simulation study, under a scenario defined by the assumed true outcome probabilities $\pi^{true}(y \mid \rho)$ for each ρ, these give the corresponding true mean utility of treating a patient with regime ρ,

$$u^{true}(\rho) = \sum_y U(y)\pi^{true}(y \mid \rho).$$

Given a utility function $U(y)$, in practice it is not intuitively obvious what numerical values of $\{u^{true}(\rho), \rho \in \mathcal{R}\}$ will be obtained under an assumed simulation scenario specified in terms of $\pi^{true}(y \mid \rho)$. This is because the mean utility $u^{true}(\rho)$ reduces a set of many probabilities $\{\pi^{true}(y \mid \rho), y \in \mathcal{Y}\}$ to a single number. However, examining the values of the following two summary statistics for each $\rho \in \mathcal{R}$ on the basis of preliminary computer simulations provides a straightforward way to evaluate design performance, and, if necessary, to adjust design parameters on that basis.

Let $u^{true}(\rho^{select})$ denote the true utility of the final selected regime, and let u_{max} and u_{min} denote the largest and smallest possible true mean utilities among all $\rho \in \mathcal{R}$ under the scenario. A statistic that quantifies how well the method selects a final regime, for benefiting future patients, is

$$R_{select} = 100 \times \frac{u^{true}(\rho^{select}) - u_{min}}{u_{max} - u_{min}}.$$

This is the proportion, rescaled to the domain $[0, 100]$, of the difference between the true mean utilities of the best and worst possible choices that is achieved by ρ^{select}. A similar statistic, that quantifies how well the method assigns doses to the patients enrolled in the trial, is

$$R_{treat} = 100 \times \frac{\frac{1}{N}\sum_{i=1}^{N} u^{true}(\rho_{[i]}) - u_{min}}{u_{max} - u_{min}},$$

where $u^{true}(\rho_{[i]})$ denotes the true mean utility of the regime given to the ith patient, and N is the achieved final sample size. For both statistics, a larger value corresponds to better overall performance. In addition to evaluating R_{select} and R_{treat}, it also is useful to record the numbers of patients treated, and also the distributions of Y_E and Y_T, for each regime.

6.3.5 Utility Sensitivity Analyses

Utilities are subjective, and it may not be obvious how a design will behave for a given $U(y)$. Two useful ways to assess the effect of the utility function on the design are as follows. Two different types of sensitivity analyses may be carried out, one after the trial has been completed and the other before it is begun. The first addresses the concern of subjectivity by anticipating how the trial results may be interpreted by others after its completion. One may conduct the trial using the elicited consensus utility, but analyze the final data using each of the several alternative utilities. These alternative utilities should numerically reflect the viewpoints that, compared to the consensus utility, place greater or less importance on particular outcomes. For each alternative, several numerical values of $U(y)$ should differ substantially from the corresponding values of the consensus utility. For the second sensitivity analysis, one may simulate the trial conducted using each alternative utility in place of the consensus utility. This assesses how acceptable the trial results based on the consensus utility should be for a wide audience who may have differing opinions. These two types of utility sensitivity analysis will be done in the context of the trial design that will be discussed in Chapter 14.

Simulating the design using alternative numerical utilities may provide the physicians with additional insights into how their utilities translate into design performance, which may motivate them to modify their utilities. In the 2×2 case, this may be done easily by changing the values of $U(0,0)$ and $U(1,1)$. For example, an alternative utility that places more value on achieving Efficacy would have a larger value of $U(1,1)$ and a smaller value of $U(0,0)$, while an alternative utility that places more value on avoiding Toxicity would have a smaller value of $U(1,1)$, and a larger value of $U(0,0)$. However, using extreme values that may give pathological trade-offs, as explained above, should not be used. In the example where $U(0,0) = 40$ and $U(1,1) = 70$ an alternative utility favoring $Y_E = 1$ more strongly might have $U(0,0) = 30$ or 25 and $U(1,1) = 75$ or 80. An alternative utility favoring $Y_T = 0$ more strongly might have $U(0,0) = 50$ and $U(1,1) = 60$. For more complex outcomes, such as the 4×4 (Y_E, Y_T) in the trial of RT for brain tumors, this same approach to obtaining alternative utilities to be studied may be applied by adjusting the intermediate values of $U(y_E, y_T)$ in a similar fashion.

6.3.6   More Elaborate Utilities

More complex utilities that account for more than patient outcome may be formulated. As a simple example, suppose that one wishes to incorporate trial cost, with $c_1 =$ the fixed cost of conducting the trial and $c_2 =$ the cost per patient. The utility function could be expanded to

$$U(y, c_1, c_2) = \sum_{i=1}^{N} U(Y_{[i]}) - \lambda(c_1 + c_2\, N),$$

where the parameter λ quantifies the relative value or utility of patient outcome and financial cost of the trial. This formalizes the notion that the attempt to achieve patient benefit has an economic cost. There is an immense literature on utility functions in medical research. For the interested reader, some useful references are Berger (1985); Anand (1995); Sox et al. (1988).

6.4 Optimizing Radiation Dose for Brain Tumors

Our first illustration of utility-based phase I–II design methodology is the design used for the trial of RT for DIPGs, discussed earlier. For $k =$ E,T, let $Y_k = 0, 1, \cdots, m_k$ denote the ordinal outcome levels. For Toxicity, $Y_T = 0$ is the least severe and m_T the most severe level, while $Y_E = 0$ is the worst and m_E the best level of Efficacy. In the RT trial, $m_1 = m_2 = 3$. The RT trial utility, given in Table 6.1, has the required admissibility property that $U(y_E, y_T)$ increases as either toxicity severity level decreases or efficacy increases. It may seem counterintuitive that outcomes with Efficacy score $Y_E = 0$ should be given positive utilities. In general, achieving a lower level of Toxicity must be more desirable for any level of Efficacy. This is especially true in the RT trial, because patient prognosis is very poor and treatment is palliative. Thus, even when $Y_E = 0$, the utility is higher if lower toxicity severity levels are achieved.

We first develop a general model. Index doses by $x = 1, \cdots, J$, and denote the conditional probabilities

$$\lambda_{k,y,x} = \Pr(Y_k \geq y \mid Y_k \geq y - 1, x, \theta_k)$$

and the unconditional probabilities

$$\pi_{k,y,x} = \Pr(Y_k = y \mid x, \theta_k)$$

for $y = 1, \cdots, m_k$ and $k =$ E,T. Given a monotone increasing link function g, the marginal model assumption is

$$g(\lambda_{k,y,x}) = \theta_{k,y,x}, \quad y = 1, ..., m_k, \ k = 1, 2, \tag{6.7}$$

with all $\theta_{k,y,x}$ real-valued. For example, under a logit link

$$\lambda_{k,y,x} = \frac{e^{\theta_{k,y,x}}}{1 + e^{\theta_{k,y,x}}}.$$

Denote $\theta_k = (\theta_{k,1}, \cdots, \theta_{k,m_k})$, and $\theta_{k,y} = (\theta_{k,y,1}, \cdots, \theta_{k,y,J})$. This marginal model is saturated since it has m_k parameters for each x, with $\dim(\theta_k) = Jm_k$, which equals the number of $\pi_{k,y,x}$'s needed to specify the J marginals of Y_k for all x.

Equation (6.7) ensures that the distribution $\{\pi_{k,y,x}, y = 0, 1, \cdots, m_k\}$ is well defined for each k and x. This follows from the fact that, denoting $\bar{\pi}_{k,y,x} = \Pr(Y_k \geq y \mid x, \theta_k)$, the unconditional and conditional probabilities are related by the recursive formula

$$\bar{\pi}_{k,y,x} = \prod_{r=1}^{y} \lambda_{k,r,x} = \prod_{r=1}^{y} g^{-1}(\theta_{k,r,x}), \quad y = 1, \cdots, m_k. \tag{6.8}$$

Consequently, $\bar{\pi}_{k,y,x}$ is decreasing in y for each x, Jm_k-dimensional real-valued θ_k, and monotone link g. The marginal probabilities are

$$\pi_{k,y,x} = (1 - \lambda_{k,y+1,x}) \prod_{r=1}^{y} \lambda_{k,r,x}, \qquad y = 1, \cdots, m_k - 1,$$

$$\pi_{k,m_k,x} = \prod_{r=1}^{m_k} \lambda_{k,r,x}. \tag{6.9}$$

Given the marginals, we obtain a joint distribution of $[Y_1, Y_2 \mid x]$ by using a bivariate Gaussian copula, $C_\rho(v_1, v_2) = \Phi_\rho\{\Phi^{-1}(v_1), \Phi^{-1}(v_2)\}$ for $0 \leq v_1, v_2 \leq 1$, where Φ_ρ is the bivariate standard normal cdf with correlation ρ, and Φ is the univariate standard normal cdf. This gives the joint distribution by the formula

$$\pi(y \mid x, \theta) = \Pr(Y = y \mid x, \theta) = \sum_{a=1}^{2} \sum_{b=1}^{2} (-1)^{a+b} C_\rho(u_{1,a}, u_{2,b})$$

where we denote $u_{k,1} = \Pr(Y_k \leq y_k \mid x, \theta_k)$ and $u_{k,2} = \Pr(Y_k \leq y_k - 1 \mid x, \theta_k)$. The likelihood is the product

$$\mathcal{L}(\mathcal{D}_n \mid \theta) = \prod_{i=1}^{n} \prod_{y_E=0}^{m_E} \prod_{y_T=0}^{m_T} \left\{ \pi(y_E, y_T \mid x_{[i]}, \theta) \right\}^{I(Y_{i,E}=y_E, Y_{i,T}=y_T)}.$$

The full model parameter vector $\theta = (\theta_E, \theta_T, \rho)$ has dimension $p = J(m_E + m_T) + 1$, and characterizes $J(m_E + m_T + m_E m_T)$ bivariate probabilities. This parameterization is feasible for many cases arising in practice. The triples $(J, m_E, m_T) = (3,2,2), (3,3,3), (4,3,2), (4,3,3), (5,2,2), (5,3,2), (5,3,3)$ give corresponding model dimensions $p = 13, 19, 21, 25, 21, 26, 31$. For $m_E = m_T = 1$, which gives the bivariate binary outcome case, $p = 2J + 1$ and $\theta_k = (\theta_{k,1}, \cdots, \theta_{k,J})$, for $k = E, T$. For the RT trial, $\{\pi_k(y \mid x, \theta), y_E, y_T = 0, 1, 2, 3\}$ is determined by 15 probabilities for each x. Since $J = 3$, there are $J(m_E m_T + m_E + m_T) = 45$ bivariate probabilities. For each outcome $k = E, T$ and dose x, the marginals are

$$\pi_{k,0,x} = 1 - \lambda_{k,1,x}$$
$$\pi_{k,1,x} = \lambda_{k,1,x} - \lambda_{k,1,x} \lambda_{k,2,x}$$
$$\pi_{k,2,x} = \lambda_{k,1,x} \lambda_{k,2,x} - \lambda_{k,1,x} \lambda_{k,2,x} \lambda_{k,3,x}$$
$$\pi_{k,3,x} = \lambda_{k,1,x} \lambda_{k,2,x} \lambda_{k,3,x}.$$

We assume a logit link, so $\lambda_{k,y,x} = e^{\theta_{k,y,x}} / (1 + e^{\theta_{k,y,x}})$. For each k and $y = 1, 2, 3$, $\theta_{k,y} = (\mu_{k,y}, \gamma_{k,y,2}, \gamma_{k,y,3})$, so $\dim(\theta_k) = 9$ and $p = \dim(\theta) = 19$.

In general, how $\bar{\pi}_{E,y,x}$ and $\bar{\pi}_{T,y,x}$ vary with x depends on the therapeutic modality and the definitions of Toxicity and Efficacy. In most cases, it is appropriate to assume that $\bar{\pi}_{k,y,x}$ increases in x for one or both outcomes.

However, while this assumption is appropriate for both cytotoxic agents and RT, it may not be realistic for some cytostatic or biologic agents. For the RT trial design, we impose the constraints $\theta_{k,y,1} \leq \theta_{k,y,2} \leq \cdots \leq \theta_{k,y,J}$ to ensure that $\bar{\pi}_{k,y,x}$ increases in x, for each $y = 1, \cdots, m_k$, which follows from the monotonicity of g by equation (6.8). Rather than fitting the model (6.7) with real-valued $\theta_{k,y,x}$'s subject to these constraints, a computationally simpler way to obtain monotonicity of $\bar{\pi}_{k,y,x}$ in x is to re-parameterize the model as

$$\theta_{k,y,x} = \mu_{k,y} + \sum_{z=2}^{x} \gamma_{k,y,z} \qquad \text{for all } x = 2, \cdots, J \qquad (6.10)$$

with real-valued $\mu_{k,y} \equiv \theta_{k,y,1}$ and $\gamma_{k,y,x} \geq 0$ for all k, y, and $x = 2, \cdots, J$. This gives $\theta_{k,y} = (\mu_{k,y}, \gamma_{k,y,2}, \cdots, \gamma_{k,y,J})$, and, collecting terms, $\theta = (\mu, \gamma)$. The parameterization (6.10) borrows strength between doses very strongly because, for any two distinct doses x and z, $\theta_{k,y,x}$ and $\theta_{k,y,z}$ share many parameters.

For the methodology to work, the probability model $\pi(y \mid x, \theta)$ must have sufficient structure to accurately reflect how $u(x, \mathcal{D}_n)$ changes with x. It may seem that a model with the number of parameters in the range 13 to 31 is impractically complex for dose-finding trials with small sample sizes. This is not the case here, essentially because the information in a bivariate ordinal outcome is much greater than that provided by a single ordinal Y or a binary outcome. Because the goal is to find a dose that maximizes the posterior mean utility $u(x, \mathcal{D}_n)$, if the model is tractable then the value of p is irrelevant. For example, in the case $(J, m_1, m_2) = (5,3,3)$ where $p = 31$, the algorithm for computing a prior from elicited values and the MCMC algorithm for computing posteriors both work well, and the design has good performance across a large set of dose-outcome scenarios.

When using a utility $U(Y)$ to quantify the desirability of a bivariate ordinal outcome Y, conventional generalized linear models (GLMs, McCullagh and Nelder, 1972) for the marginals may not be sufficiently refined to distinguish reliably between doses. This is most problematic when a middle dose has the highest utility, which very easily can be the case if both $\bar{\pi}_{E,y,x}$ and $\bar{\pi}_{T,y,x}$ increase with x. The commonly used family of GLMs for ordinal Y_k given by $g(\bar{\pi}_{k,y,x}) = \alpha_{k,y} + \beta_k x$ with $\alpha_{k,y}$ decreasing in y, which is the proportional odds model if g is the logit link, in general are not sufficiently flexible for dose-finding. This is because a single dose effect β_k is assumed for all ordinal levels of Y_k. The more general form $g(\lambda_{k,y,x}) = \alpha_{k,y} + \beta_{k,y} x$, subject to appropriate monotonicity constraints, provides the needed additional flexibility.

An alternative model may be obtained by replacing $\lambda_{k,y,x}$ in (6.7) with the unconditional probability $\bar{\pi}_{k,y,x}$, so that $g(\bar{\pi}_{k,y,x}) = \theta'_{k,y,x}$. However, this requires that $\theta'_{k,y,x}$ and hence $\bar{\pi}_{k,y,x}$ must increase in y for each $k = E, T$ and x. In this case, one must impose two sets of monotonicity constraints, one in dose x and the other in outcome level y, which limits the model's tractability.

For the RT trial, no minimal efficacy requirement was imposed, but the

TABLE 6.3: Elicited prior mean marginal toxicity severity and efficacy score probabilities for the model used in the radiation therapy trial

		Y_1 = Toxicity Severity				Y_2 = Efficacy Score			
x	BED	Low	Moderate	High	Severe	0	1	2	3
1	40.00	0.65	0.20	0.12	0.03	0.20	0.40	0.35	0.05
2	45.76	0.55	0.25	0.15	0.05	0.10	0.30	0.45	0.15
3	53.39	0.40	0.30	0.23	0.07	0.10	0.20	0.50	0.20

dose safety constraint (6.5) was used with the physicians specifying $y^* = 3$ (severe toxicity) with upper limit $\pi_T^* = 0.10$. Thus, using the conservative upper probability cut-off $p_U = 0.80$, a dose x is considered it be *unacceptably toxic* if $\Pr(\pi_{T,3,x} \geq .10 \mid \mathcal{D}_n) > .80$. The set $\mathcal{A}_n$ of acceptable doses based on $\mathcal{D}_n$ is defined as those not unacceptably toxic.

To reduce stickiness in the RT trial, as explained in Section 2.6, we used AR. While AR may be implemented using many different criteria, one ethically attractive approach is to define the AR probabilities in terms of a set of nominally "good" outcomes. In the RT trial, these were defined as $G = \{y : U(y) \geq \underline{U}\}$, where the lower utility limit $\underline{U} = 25$ was elicited from the physicians. Given G, the *probability of a good outcome for a patient treated with dose x* is $\Pr(Y \in G \mid x, \theta)$. Denoting the posterior means $\mu_G(x, \mathcal{D}_n) = \mathrm{E}\{\Pr(Y \in G \mid x, \theta) \mid \mathcal{D}_n\}$, the AR procedure randomizes a patient to dose $x \in \mathcal{A}_n$ with probability

$$r(x, \mathcal{D}_n) = \frac{\mu_G(x, \mathcal{D}_n)}{\sum_{z \in \mathcal{A}_n} \mu_G(z, \mathcal{D}_n)}. \tag{6.11}$$

Thus, the dose-finding method uses both the safety requirement and the good outcome set G to determine the AR probabilities (6.11). This AR method is similar to an "epsilon-decreasing" multi-armed bandit strategy (cf. Auer et al., 2002) that assigns the optimal treatment with probability $1 - \epsilon_n$ and chooses a suboptimal treatment with probability ϵ_n, where ϵ_n decreases with n. or an adaptive "epsilon-greedy" reinforcement learning algorithm.

To establish a prior, $p(\theta \mid \tilde{\theta})$, it was assumed that $\mu_{k,y} \sim \mathrm{N}(\tilde{\mu}_{k,y}, \tilde{\sigma}_{\mu,k,y}^2)$ and $\gamma_{k,y,x} \sim \mathrm{N}_0(\tilde{\gamma}_{k,y,x}, \tilde{\sigma}_{\gamma,k,y,x}^2)$, independently. The numerical values of the hyperparameters were established using the pseudo sampling algorithm, based on the elicited values in Table 6.3. In this application, 1000 pseudo samples were simulated, each of size 300 with 100 patients in each pseudo sample assigned to each dose. For each simulated dataset, a pseudo posterior was computed starting with a pseudo-prior on θ with each $\theta_{k,y,x} \sim N(0, 60^2)$. The means of the 1000 pseudo posterior means were used as the prior means $\tilde{\mu}_{k,y}$ and $\tilde{\gamma}_{k,y,x}$. The standard deviations of the $\theta_{k,y,x}$'s were calibrated using a beta approximation. Setting all $\tilde{\sigma}_{\mu,k,y} = \tilde{\sigma}_{\gamma,k,y,x} = \tilde{\sigma} = 6$ gave ESS values ranging from 0.31 to 0.70, with mean ESS = 0.42.

The trial is conducted with the first cohort of 3 patients treated at $x = 1$

(BED = 40.00), with subsequent cohorts of size 1 and the AR started at the 4th patient. For all subsequent cohorts, once the posterior is updated based on the observed outcomes of previous patients, if $\mathcal{A}_n$ is empty then the trial is stopped and no dose is chosen. Otherwise, patients are randomized among the doses in $\mathcal{A}_n$ using the updated AR probabilities given by (6.11), subject to the usual requirement that no untried dose may be skipped when escalating. In this case, the middle dose $x = 2$ may not be skipped. At the end of the trial, if $\mathcal{A}_n$ is not empty, then x_N^{opt} is selected. A maximum of 30 patients will be treated.

With this design, the trial was simulated under six scenarios, each determined by a set of assumed true probabilities, $\{\pi_{k,y,x}^{true}\}$. In each simulation scenario, the true marginal probabilities $\{\pi_{k,y,x}^{true}\}$ do not depend on the assumed model, although the copula was used to induce association, with correlation parameter $\rho^{true} = 0.10$ used throughout. The true utilities $u^{true}(x)$ are determined by the assumed $\{\pi_{k,y,x}^{true}\}$, ρ^{true}, and the elicited utilities. Scenario 1 is based on the elicited prior means, which give equal utility 64.6 to $x = 1$ and 2 and utility 57.0 to $x = 3$. Scenario 2 has steeply increasing utility, with $x = 3$ best. Scenario 3 has steeply decreasing utility with $x = 1$ best, the middle dose $x = 2$ is best in Scenario 4, and the utility is V-shaped in Scenario 5 with $x = 3$ best. In Scenario 6, no dose is acceptably safe.

The simulation results are summarized in Table 6.4. Additional details of the simulation study design are given in Thall and Nguyen (2012). In each of Scenarios 1–5, the selection probabilities follow the utilities quite closely. The algorithm's selection reliability is quite striking in Scenario 5, which has a V-shaped utility with the middle dose $x = 2$ least desirable. In all scenarios, the sample size distribution is biased toward lower doses, reflecting the initial cohort of 3 patients at $x = 1$, the do-not-skip rule, and the fact that the prior was biased toward the lower doses, which favors AR to these doses early in the trial. In Scenario 6, where no dose is acceptably safe and the true severe toxicity probabilities are 0.25, 0.28, 0.30 at the three doses, compared to the specified upper limit .10 in the safety rule, the method correctly stops early and chooses no dose 91% of the time, on average treating 14.6 patients. Modifying Scenario 6 so that the true severe toxicity probabilities at the three doses are the slightly higher values .30, .35, .40, the stopping probability becomes 98% and the mean sample size drops to 11.6 patients.

It is useful to illustrate how the utility function $U(y)$ maps the assumed outcome probabilities into a single number. This is done in Figure 6.2 for three of the simulation scenarios. The figure also includes the selection percentages and percent of patients treated for each dose. This figure gives a graphical representation of the mapping $(\pi_E^{true}(d), \pi_T^{true}(d)) \to u^{true}(d)$. It also shows that the design does a good job of selecting the doses with the highest utilities, and that the patient subsample size distribution also follows this pattern. When interpreting Table 6.4 and Figure 6.2, it should be kept in mind that these simulation results are based on a maximum sample size of only $N = 30$.

To assess the effect of AR on the method's performance, we simulated an

TABLE 6.4: Simulation results for the RT trial. Under each scenario, each tabled dose selection % and sample size is the mean from 5000 simulated trials. "None" means that no dose was selected

Dose	$u^{true}(x)$	% Sel	# Pats	$u^{true}(x)$	% Sel	# Pats
		Scenario 1			Scenario 2	
$x = 1$	64.6	50	15.7	51.1	13	11.3
$x = 2$	64.6	32	8.5	58.6	22	8.8
$x = 3$	57.0	17	5.6	63.7	61	9.5
None		1			4	
		Scenario 3			Scenario 4	
$x = 1$	65.2	63	17.2	61.7	31	13.5
$x = 2$	60.8	20	7.2	66.2	51	10.4
$x = 3$	54.6	14	5.0	53.1	15	5.7
None		4			3	
		Scenario 5			Scenario 6	
$x = 1$	60.7	35	14.7	37.6	6	10.3
$x = 2$	54.3	9	6.6	37.6	2	2.9
$x = 3$	65.7	54	8.4	33.4	1	1.4
None		3			91	

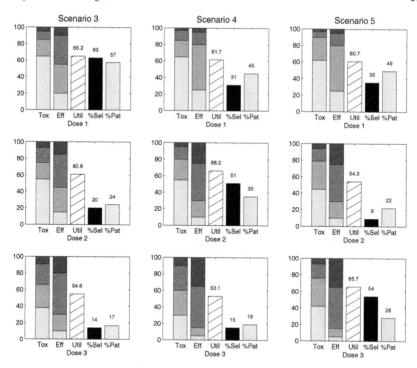

FIGURE 6.2: Outcome probabilities, utilities, and operating characteristics under scenarios 3, 4, and 5 of the radiation therapy trial simulation.

alternative version of the design that did not use AR. The results are given in Table 6.5. Scenario 6 is not included since, in this case where all doses are too toxic, the design stops early with high probability regardless of whether AR is used. Table 6.5 shows that, across all five scenarios, the design with AR has R_{select} values between 72 and 89. In sharp contrast, when AR is not used, the R_{select} values vary much more widely, from 12 to 100. In particular, R_{select} drops from 79 to 12 in Scenario 2 and from 76 to 54 in Scenario 5 when AR is not used. Similar drops are seen for R_{treat}. It thus appears that AR acts as an insurance policy against scenarios where the method gets stuck at a suboptimal dose. This insurance policy comes with a price, however. For example, in Scenarios 1 and 3 the design without AR has higher R_{select} and R_{select} values, essentially because it gets lucky.

Our motivating application is somewhat atypical in that most phase I–II trials have more than 3 dose levels. To more fully illustrate the methodology, we also include a simulation study with $J = 5$ doses. The model, which now has $p = 31$ parameters, and the design used for this simulation are very similar to those of the RT trial, but we assume the larger maximum sample size 40. For choosing maximum sample size in practice, one should keep in mind that a phase I–II trial replaces the conventional approach of first conducting a

TABLE 6.5: Simulations to assess the effect of using adaptive randomization (AR). The numbers in parentheses after R_{select} are the percentages of the trial being stopped with no dose selected

Scenario	AR		No AR	
	R_{select}	R_{treat}	R_{select}	R_{treat}
1	81 (1)	77	100 (2)	100
2	79 (1)	42	12 (5)	10
3	76 (4)	65	99 (5)	99
4	72 (1)	62	68 (2)	67
5	76 (1)	50	54 (3)	53

phase I trial based on Toxicity only, and then a phase II based on Efficacy only. Thus, maximum $N = 40$ is reasonable for a phase I–II trial, and larger values often are much more desirable in terms of design reliability. Figure 6.3 illustrates how the values of R_{select} could be increased if larger N could be used in the RT trial. Maximum sample sizes of 120 to 240 often are not feasible or are considered unrealistic in dose-finding trials, especially for rare diseases. However, Figure 6.3 shows that the reliability of the design increases dramatically as N increases from 30 to 240. It thus appears that, if optimizing the dose of an experimental treatment matters, then phase I–II trials with several hundred patients should be considered, if this is feasible.

All numerical values in the prior and model corresponding to the new doses $x' \in \{1, 2, 3, 4, 5\}$ were obtained by the matching values for $x' = 1, 3, 5$ to the original doses $x = 1, 2, 3$, respectively, and interpolating to obtain dose values for $x' = 2$ and $x' = 4$. The simulation is summarized in Table 6.6, which shows that the qualitative behavior of the design for $J = 5$ dose levels is very similar to what was seen for $J = 3$.

A final question pertains to model complexity. According to the principle of *Occam's Razor*, if the design would work as well assuming a simpler, more conventional model with fewer parameters, then our assumed model is not needed. To address this issue, we simulated the trial assuming a bivariate model with PO marginals defined by $\text{logit}(\bar{\pi}_{k,y,x}) = \alpha_{k,y} + \beta_k x$ with $\alpha_{k,1} > \alpha_{k,2} > \alpha_{k,3}$ so $\theta = (\alpha_{1,1}, \alpha_{1,2}, \alpha_{1,3}, \alpha_{2,1}, \alpha_{2,2}, \alpha_{2,3}, \beta_1, \beta_2, \rho)$ and $p = 9$. The prior for this model was obtained similarly to that of the 31-parameter model, using the pseudo sampling method. The results are summarized in Table 6.7, which shows that the simpler 9-parameter model gives a design with greatly inferior performance in Scenarios 1 and 4, superior performance in Scenarios 2 and 5, and the comparative results are mixed in Scenario 3. This illustrates the point that, in the present setting, no model is uniformly best. Using the 31-parameter model gives R_{select} values in range $[64, 87]$, whereas the PO model has much wider corresponding range $[32, 92]$. Thus, the saturated model performs much more consistently across a diverse set of scenarios, with far better worst-case results than the simpler PO model.

TABLE 6.6: Simulation results for the 5-dose elaboration of the radiation therapy trial

Dose	$u^{true}(x)$	% Sel	# Pats	$u^{true}(x)$	% Sel	# Pats
		Scenario 1			*Scenario 2*	
$x = 1$	64.6	44	15.4	51.1	10	12.0
$x = 2$	64.6	21	8.8	54.9	10	7.8
$x = 3$	64.6	16	6.7	58.6	15	7.3
$x = 4$	60.8	10	5.1	61.2	24	6.8
$x = 5$	57.0	7	3.9	63.7	39	5.8
None		1			2	
		Scenario 3			*Scenario 4*	
$x = 1$	65.2	58	16.9	61.7	27	13.9
$x = 2$	63.0	18	8.5	64.0	22	8.9
$x = 3$	60.8	10	6.1	66.2	30	7.7
$x = 4$	57.7	7	4.5	59.8	15	5.4
$x = 5$	54.6	5	3.4	53.1	6	3.8
None		3			1	
		Scenario 5			*Scenario 6*	
$x = 1$	60.7	36	15.3	37.6	4	10.5
$x = 2$	57.5	11	7.8	37.7	1	3.2
$x = 3$	54.3	5	5.7	37.6	1	1.6
$x = 4$	60.0	13	5.8	35.5	0	0.8
$x = 5$	65.7	34	5.2	33.4	0	0.4
None		1			94	

TABLE 6.7: Comparison of performance under the simplified 9-parameter bivariate proportional odds model ($p=9$) versus the model with saturated marginals ($p=31$) in the 5-dose trial. The numbers in parentheses after R_{select} are the percentages of the trial being stopped with no dose selected

Scenario	Prop. odds marginals		Saturated marginals	
	R_{select}	R_{treat}	R_{select}	R_{treat}
1	55 (3)	79	87 (1)	84
2	92 (8)	55	71 (2)	45
3	67 (8)	82	82 (3)	72
4	32 (9)	47	74 (1)	68
5	84 (4)	66	64 (1)	47

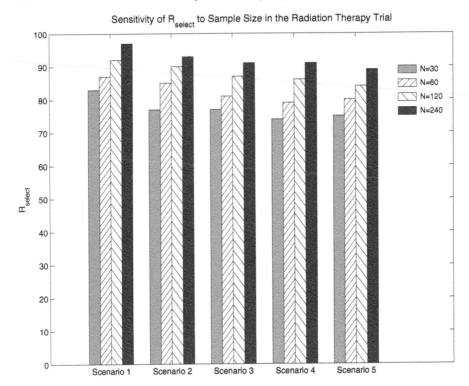

FIGURE 6.3: Sensitivity of R_{select} to N in the radiation therapy trial design.

A computer program named "UAROET" for implementing this utility-based dose-finding method for bivariate ordinal (Y_E, Y_T) is available at https://biostatistics.mdanderson.org/SoftwareDownload/.

7

Personalized Dose Finding

CONTENTS

7.1   The EffTox Design with Covariates 129
7.2   Biomarker-Based Dose Finding 137

7.1   The EffTox Design with Covariates

A useful extension of the EffTox design accounts for the effects of patient baseline covariates, $Z = (Z_1, \cdots, Z_q)$, as well as dose, x, on the probabilities of Toxicity and Efficacy. This methodology is given by Thall et al. (2008). The marginal probabilities of the two outcomes now are written as $\pi_E(x, Z, \theta_E)$ and $\pi_T(x, Z, \theta_T)$ to account for their dependence on both x and Z. For example, accounting for Z addresses the well-known problem that a patient's risk of Toxicity from a cytotoxic agent increases with age, number of prior therapies, and worse performance status. More generally, in addition to these common prognostic variables, Z may include biomarkers, provided that all elements of Z may be measured quickly enough so that Z may be included in the adaptive decision rules for each patient. Using each patient's Z to help choose x is called "personalized" dose-finding. If Z includes a biomarker, it may be called "precision medicine." Such methods have been discussed extensively in phase I designs (Babb and Rogatko, 2001; Ratain et al., 1996; Wijesinha and Piantadosi, 1995; O'Quigley et al., 1999). Phase I designs for finding optimal doses within ordinal prognostic subgroups have been proposed by O'Quigley and Paoletti (2003); Yuan and Chappell (2004); Ivanova and Wang (2003). The use of modern models and methods aside, it should be kept in mind that physicians have been practicing individualized medicine for thousands of years.

For individualized dose-finding in phase I–II, after identifying each new patient's Z, the general objective is to choose x to obtain a desirably large value of $\pi_E(x, Z, \theta_E)$ while also controlling $\pi_T(x, Z, \theta_T)$ for that patient. The extended EffTox method that accounts for each patient's Z, which we call EffToxCovs, focuses on the probability pair, $\pi(x, Z, \theta) = (\pi_E(x, Z, \theta_E), \pi_T(x, Z, \theta_T))$, which will be denoted by π for brevity when no meaning is lost. A major point of departure from EffTox is that EffToxCovs requires an informative prior on covariate effect parameters, obtained from a preliminary fit of historical data. The model is generalized to account for effects of both Z and historical treatments, as well as the dose x of the agent being studied in the planned trial, on (Y_E, Y_T). EffToxCovs generalizes the model and decision rules of EffTox to incorporate Z into its dose acceptability criteria and adaptive dose assignment rules. One also must account for possible interactions between Z and x in their joint effect on π_E and π_T. Simulations show that, if interactive effects between Z and x exist but they are not included in the model, then the methodology can have poor properties. This is a general way of saying that, for example, the model and method must account for the possibility that a given dose x is more likely to result in Toxicity in patients who are older or who have poor performance status. It also accounts for the possibility that a given dose x may be more likely to result in Efficacy in patients who are positive for a particular biomarker.

For standardized doses $x_1 < x_2 < \cdots < x_J$, the data from the first n patients in the trial now takes the form $\mathcal{D}_n = \{(Y_i, Z_i, x_{[i]}), i = 1, \cdots, n\}$. Denote the data from n_H historical patients by $\mathcal{H} = \{(Y_i, Z_i, \rho_{[i]}), i = 1, \cdots, n_H\}$, where $\{\rho_1, \cdots, \rho_m\}$ are historical treatments in $\mathcal{H}$ and $\rho_{[i]}$ denotes the ith historical patient's treatment. Denote either a dose in the trial or a historical treatment by unsubscripted ρ. The joint outcome probabilities of a patient with covariates Z treated with ρ is denoted $\pi_{a,b}(\rho, Z, \theta) = \Pr(Y_E = a, Y_T = b \mid \rho, Z, \theta)$, for $a, b \in \{0, 1\}$.

As done with EffTox, the modeling strategy is to first specify the marginals in terms of $\eta_E = g(\pi_E)$ and $\eta_T = g(\pi_T)$ for link function g, and use a copula to obtain a joint distribution. Tractable models may be obtained using the FGM copula, as in Chapter 4, or the Gaussian copula, given by

$$C_\psi(u, v) = \Phi_\psi(\Phi^{-1}(u), \Phi^{-1}(v)), \qquad 0 \le u, v \le 1, \qquad (7.1)$$

where Φ_ψ denotes the bivariate standard normal cdf with correlation ψ and unsubscripted Φ denotes the univariate standard normal cdf. For bivariate binary outcomes,

$$\pi_{0,0} = \Phi_\psi(\Phi^{-1}(1 - \pi_E), \Phi^{-1}(1 - \pi_T)), \qquad (7.2)$$

and this determines the remaining $\pi_{a,b}$'s as $\pi_{1,0} = 1 - \pi_E - \pi_{0,0}$, $\pi_{0,1} = 1 - \pi_T - \pi_{0,0}$, and $\pi_{1,1} = \pi_E + \pi_T + \pi_{0,0} - 1$. Under the probit link $\pi_k = \Phi(\eta_k)$, the model 7.2 takes the simpler form $\pi_{0,0} = \Phi_\psi(-\eta_E, -\eta_T)$.

Given the assumed copula and link function, the model is determined by specific parametric forms for the linear terms $\eta_E(\tau, Z, \theta)$ and $\eta_T(\tau, Z, \theta)$. These must provide a basis for using historical data to estimate covariate effects while also accounting for joint effects of x and Z on π_E and π_T in the trial. A general model that accommodates this is defined as follows. Let $I_\rho(\rho')$

denote the indicator that $\rho = \rho'$. For $k = E, T$, the general form is

$$\eta_k(\rho, Z, \theta) = \beta_k Z + \left\{ \sum_{j=1}^{m} (\mu_{k,j} + \xi_{k,j} Z) \right\}^{I_\rho(\rho_j)} \left\{ f_k(x, \alpha_k) + \gamma_k Z \right\}^{I_\rho(x)},$$

(7.3)

denoting the linear combinations

$$\beta_k Z = \sum_{r=1}^{q} \beta_{k,r} Z_r \quad \text{and} \quad \gamma_k Z = \sum_{r=1}^{q} \gamma_{k,r} Z_r.$$

The main dose effects are characterized by the functions $f_E(x, \alpha_E)$ and $f_T(x, \alpha_T)$, historical treatment main effects are $\mu_k = (\mu_{k,1}, \cdots, \mu_{k,m})$, covariate main effects are $\beta_k = (\beta_{k,1}, \cdots, \beta_{k,q})$, interactions between Z and historical treatment ρ_j are $\xi_{k,j} = (\xi_{k,j,1}, \cdots, \xi_{k,j,q})$, and dose-covariate interactions are $\gamma_k = (\gamma_{k,1}, \cdots, \gamma_{k,q})$. For each $k = E, T$, for the historical data the general expression (7.3) takes the form

$$\eta_k(\rho_j, Z, \theta) = \mu_{k,j} + \beta_k Z + \xi_{k,j} Z,$$

(7.4)

for $j = 1, \cdots, m$ and for data obtained during the trial (7.3) is

$$\eta_k(x, Z, \theta) = f_k(x, \alpha_k) + \beta_k Z + x \gamma_k Z.$$

(7.5)

This model, and the methodology described below, rely on the key assumption that, given the functional form of the linear terms, the covariate main effects $\beta = (\beta_E, \beta_T)$ in the trial are the same as their historical effects. This formalizes the idea that the covariates Z are prognostic, that is, that they are known to be associated with the observed Y for any treatment.

Denoting $\alpha = (\alpha_E, \alpha_T)$, $\mu = (\mu_E, \mu_T)$, $\gamma = (\gamma_E, \gamma_T)$ and $\xi = (\xi_{E,1}, \xi_{T,1}, \cdots, \xi_{E,k}, \xi_{T,k})$, the vector of all model parameters is $\theta = (\mu, \beta, \xi, \psi, \alpha, \gamma)$. To establish a prior on θ, the first step is to fit the model to $\mathcal{H}$ to obtain the posterior $p(\mu, \beta, \xi, \psi \mid \mathcal{H})$. For the purpose of dose-finding, historical treatment main effects μ and covariate interactions ξ are nuisance parameters, but the informative marginal posterior

$$p(\beta, \psi \mid \mathcal{H}) = \int p(\mu, \beta, \xi, \psi \mid \mathcal{H}) d\mu d\xi$$

plays a key role in the method, since it is used as the prior on (β, ψ) at the start of the trial. In contrast, since α and γ account for experimental agent effects, their priors must be non-informative. Prior means are established by setting $E(\gamma) = \mathbf{0}$, and obtaining $E(\alpha)$ by eliciting means of $\pi_E(x_j, Z^*, \theta)$ and $\pi_T(x_j, Z^*, \theta)$ at selected values x_j and Z^*, and solving for $E(\alpha)$. If the number of elicited means is larger than $\dim(\alpha)$, then pseudo sampling or least squares may be used to solve for $E(\alpha)$. Prior variances may be obtained by assuming that all entries of α have variance $\tilde{\sigma}_\alpha^2$, and all entries of γ have variance $\tilde{\sigma}_\gamma^2$, and calibrating these to control the ESS of the priors $p\{\pi_k(x_j, Z^*, \theta)\}$ for all combinations of $k = E, T$, x_j, and Z^*. As before, this may be done by matching the first two moments of each prior distribution with a beta, and using ESS to calibrate $\tilde{\sigma}_\alpha^2$ and $\tilde{\sigma}_\gamma^2$.

At any interim point in the trial when a patient's dose must be chosen, the likelihood for the current trial data is the product

$$\mathcal{L}(\mathcal{D}_n \mid \theta) = \prod_{i=1}^{n} \prod_{a=0}^{1} \prod_{b=0}^{1} \{\pi_{a,b}(x_{[i]}, Z_i, \theta)\}^{1\{Y_i=(a,b)\}}.$$

Adaptive decisions during the trial are based on the posteriors

$$p(\alpha, \gamma, \beta, \psi \mid \mathcal{H} \cup \mathcal{D}_n) \propto \mathcal{L}(\mathcal{D}_n \mid \theta) \, p(\alpha, \gamma) \, p(\beta, \psi \mid \mathcal{H}) \qquad (7.6)$$

To account for both x and Z, the EffTox dose acceptability criteria are generalized to so that the upper limit on π_T and the lower limit on π_E vary as functions of Z. This is done using the following construction. To begin, first specify a representative set of covariate vectors, $\{Z^{(1)}, \cdots, Z^{(K)}\}$ that, together, vary widely over the domain of Z. For each $Z^{(j)}$, elicit the smallest probability of Efficacy, $\underline{\pi}_E^{(j)}$, and the largest probability of Toxicity, $\overline{\pi}_T^{(j)}$, that the physician will allow for a patient with covariates $Z^{(j)}$. These $2K$ elicited limits are used to construct functions of Z that provide a lower bound on $\pi_E(x, Z)$ and an upper bound on $\pi_T(x, Z)$ for a patient with covariates Z. While a general requirement is $K > q$, one must keep K small enough so that the elicitation process is practical. Denote $\zeta_k(Z) = \mathrm{E}(\beta_k Z \mid \mathcal{H})$, the posterior mean effect of Z in the real-valued domain of the linear term η_k, given the historical data. To construct a bounding function for $\pi_E(x, Z, \theta)$, treat the K pairs $(\zeta_E(Z^{(1)}), \underline{\pi}_E^{(1)}), \ldots, (\zeta_E(Z^{(K)}), \underline{\pi}_E^{(K)})$ like a regression dataset, and fit a curve to these points using least squares (LS) with $\zeta_E(Z^{(j)})$ the predictor and $\underline{\pi}_E^{(j)}$ the outcome variable. Any simple monotone function may be used, provided that $0 \le \hat{\underline{\pi}}_E(\zeta_E) \le 1$ on the domain of ζ_E values considered. In practice, a linear function $\underline{\pi}_E(\zeta_E) = a + b\zeta_E$ or quadratic $a + b\zeta_E + c\zeta_E^2$ works quite well. The *Efficacy lower bounding function* is

$$\underline{\pi}_E(Z) = \hat{\underline{\pi}}_E(\zeta_E(Z)).$$

For example, if the fitted LS curve is $\hat{\underline{\pi}}_E(\zeta_E) = \hat{a} + \hat{b}\zeta_E + \hat{c}\zeta_E^2$ then the estimated Efficacy lower bound at Z is $\underline{\pi}_E(Z) = \hat{a} + \hat{b}\zeta_E(Z) + \hat{c}\{\zeta_E(Z)\}^2$. The Toxicity bounding function is constructed similarly, by fitting a curve to the K pairs $\{\zeta_T(Z^{(1)}), \overline{\pi}_T^{(1)}\}, \ldots, \{\zeta_T(Z^{(K)}), \overline{\pi}_T^{(K)}\}$, obtaining a LS estimate $\hat{\overline{\pi}}_T(\zeta_T)$, and defining the *Toxicity upper bounding function*

$$\overline{\pi}_T(Z) = \hat{\overline{\pi}}_T(\zeta_T(Z)).$$

When constructing these functions, it is useful to plot the scattergram of $(\zeta_E^{(1)}, \underline{\pi}_E^{(1)}), \cdots, (\zeta_E^{(K)}, \underline{\pi}_E^{(K)})$ with a smooth line for its fitted function $\hat{\underline{\pi}}_E(\zeta_E)$, and likewise plot $(\zeta_T^{(1)}, \bar{\pi}_T^{(1)}), \cdots, (\zeta_T^{(K)}, \bar{\pi}_T^{(K)})$ with a line for $\hat{\bar{\pi}}_T(\zeta_T)$. Since the goal is to obtain bounds on $\pi_E(x, Z, \theta)$ and $\pi_T(x, Z, \theta)$ as Z is varied that fulfill the physician's requirements, these plots provide a visual guide to allow the physician to adjust any $\underline{\pi}_E^{(j)}$ or $\bar{\pi}_T^{(j)}$ values, if desired. Figure 7.1 gives the fitted bounds for the illustrative PR104 trial, to be described below. In the figure, the elicited values for $K = 4$ representative $Z^{(j)}$ values are plotted. The estimated values of $\underline{\pi}_E(Z)$ and $\bar{\pi}_T(Z)$ for a poor and good prognosis patient are identified by a triangle and square, respectively, in the two plots.

The bounding functions yield the following dose acceptability criteria. Given current trial data $\mathcal{D}_n$ and fixed probability cut-offs p_T and p_E, *the set $\mathcal{A}_n(Z)$ of acceptable doses for a patient with covariates Z is all doses such that*

$$\Pr\{\pi_E(x, Z, \theta) > \underline{\pi}_E(Z) \mid \mathcal{D}_n \cup \mathcal{H}\} > p_E \tag{7.7}$$

and

$$\Pr\{\pi_T(x, Z, \theta) < \bar{\pi}_T(Z) \mid \mathcal{D}_n \cup \mathcal{H}\} > p_T . \tag{7.8}$$

For a patient with covariates Z, (7.7) says that x is likely to be efficacious. and (7.8) says that x is likely to have acceptable Toxicity. If $\mathcal{A}_n(Z)$ is empty, then no dose is acceptable for that patient. If $\mathcal{A}_n(Z)$ consists of a single dose, then that dose is given by default. If $\mathcal{A}_n(Z)$ contains more than one dose, then a patient-specific criterion for choosing a dose from $\mathcal{A}_n(Z)$ is needed.

An Efficacy–Toxicity trade-off contour $\mathcal{C}$ is constructed exactly as done for EffTox, using a desirability function such as $\phi(\pi) = 1 - \|\pi - (1, 0)\|_r$. For a patient with covariates Z, the desirabilities of the J doses are computed using $\mu_{k,x_j,n}(Z) = E(\pi_k(x_j, Z, \theta) \mid \mathcal{H} \cup \mathcal{D}_n)$. The desirability of giving dose x_j to a patient with covariates Z is $\phi(\mu_{E,x_j,n}(Z), \mu_{T,x_j,n}(Z))$, for $j = 1, \cdots, J$. A patient with covariates Z is treated with the dose in $\mathcal{A}_n(Z)$ that maximizes this desirability function.

The steps for constructing a design are as follows:

Step 1. Analyze the historical data to compute the marginal posterior $p(\beta, \psi \mid \mathcal{H})$, and use this as an informative prior on (β, ψ).

Step 2. Elicit means of $\pi_E(x_j, Z^*, \theta)$ and $\pi_T(x_j, Z^*, \theta)$ at selected x_j's and Z^*, and solve for $E(\alpha)$ by LS or pseudo sampling. Set $E(\gamma) = \mathbf{0}$. Solve for prior variances using ESS and beta moment matching so that $p(\alpha, \gamma)$ is non-informative.

Step 3. Determine the doses to be studied, maximum trial sample size, N, and the set $\{Z^{(1)}, \cdots, Z^{(K)}\}$, of representative covariate vectors. Use these to compute the dose acceptability criteria (7.7) and (7.8).

Step 4. Establish the trade-off contour $\mathcal{C}$ and desirability function $\phi(\pi)$

Step 5. Simulate the trial and adjust any parameters as necessary to obtain a design with good OCs.

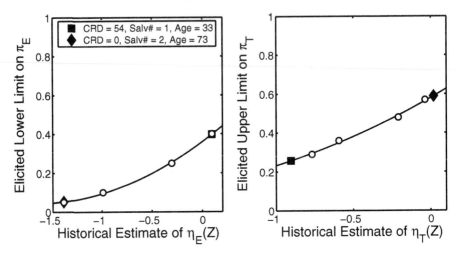

FIGURE 7.1: Covariate-dependent dose acceptability bounds.

The steps for trial conduct are as follows:

Step 1. During the trial, when a new patient with covariates Z is enrolled, compute $\mathcal{A}_n(Z)$ based on the current posterior.

1.1. If $\mathcal{A}_n(Z)$ is empty, do not treat the patient on protocol.

1.2. If $\mathcal{A}_n(Z)$ contains at least one dose, treat the patient using the dose x in $\mathcal{A}_n(Z)$ that maximizes $\phi(\mu_{E,x,n}(Z), \mu_{T,x,n}(Z))$.

Step 2. If $\mathcal{A}_n(Z^{(j)})$ is empty for all $j = 1, \cdots, K$, that is, no doses are acceptable for any of the representative covariate vectors, stop the trial and declare the new agent unacceptable for any patient at any dose.

If the trial is not stopped early, use the final data $\mathcal{D}_N$ and final acceptability and desirability criteria based on $p(\theta \mid \mathcal{H} \cup \mathcal{D}_N)$ to select Z-specific doses for future patients.

In practice, if no dose is acceptable for a patient with covariates Z then the patient must either be given a different treatment off protocol or may have such poor prognosis that no treatment can be given. This formalizes decisions that often are made subjectively by physicians. A major departure from conventional designs is that different patients may have different optimal doses at the same point in the trial, as a consequence of covariate-specific dose-finding. Another key point is that, because, the acceptability criteria (7.7) and (7.8) depend on Z, x, and $\mathcal{D}_n$, whether a patient with a particular Z has any acceptable dose, or what the optimal dose is, may change with $\mathcal{D}_n$ over the course of the trial. Thus, a given x_j that was unacceptable for a patient with given Z at some point in the trial may later become acceptable, or conversely.

The methodology was applied to design a trial of the hypoxia-activated prodrug PR104 in patients with refractory or relapsed AML or ALL (Konopleva et al., 2015) The trial was designed to study the four doses 1.1, 1.5, 1.2, 3.0 grams/m^2 using the EffToxCovs method. Efficacy was defined as CR or CRp (CR without the requirement of platelet recovery) by day 42, and Toxicity was defined as regimen-related death or any grade 3 or 4 non-hematologic Toxicity within 42 days for the start of therapy. Preliminary analysis of historical data on 274 patients who satisfied the trials entry criteria included consideration of multiple models and different covariate combinations. Goodness-of-fit analyses, including computation of the Bayes Information Criterion (BIC, Schwarz, 1978) for each model, led to use of a Gaussian copula with probit link, and three covariates. Denoting the patient's first CR duration prior to enrollment in the trial by CRD and number of prior salvage therapies by SALV, the covariates in the model were the binary indicator [CRD≥52] of the favorable history that the patient's first CR duration was at least 52 weeks, the binary indicator [SALV=2] of the unfavorable history the patient had 2 (versus 1) previous salvage therapies, and Age. The covariate vector was $Z = (Z_1, Z_2, Z_3)$ = ([CRD≥52], [SALV=2], (Age-56)/100), and the linear terms were

$$\eta_E(Z, \beta_E) = \beta_{E,0} + \beta_{E,1}[CRD \geq 52] + \beta_{T,2}[SALV = 2]$$

and

$$\eta_T(Z, \beta_T) = \beta_{T,0} + \beta_{T,1}[CRD \geq 52] + \beta_{T,2}(Age - 56)/100$$

Table 7.1 summarizes posterior values of $[\pi_E(Z, \beta_E) \mid \mathcal{H}]$ and $[\pi_T(Z, \beta_T) \mid \mathcal{H}]$ for selected covariate vectors, and also gives covariate-specific acceptability limits. Figure 7.2 plots the corresponding posteriors $p(\pi_E(Z, \beta_E) \mid \mathcal{H})$ and $p(\pi_T(Z, \beta_E) \mid \mathcal{H})$. The figure illustrates that $\pi_E(Z, \beta_E)$ increased with [$CRD \geq 52$] and decreased with [SALV=2], while $\pi_T(Z, \beta_T)$ decreased with [$CRD \geq 52$] and increased with Age.

The trial was designed to have a maximum of 36 patients, trade-off contour based on the three probability pairs $(\pi_E, \pi_T) = (.50, .28), (.25, 0), (1, .55)$, and dose acceptability probability cut-offs $p_E = p_T = .90$. It is easily seen that the resulting trade-off contour was too shallow, and could have been fixed easily by changing (1, .55) to (1, .75). A hypothetical trial outcome is summarized in Table 7.3.

The trial played out very differently from the hypothetical example. As noted in Konopleva et al. (2015), the EffToxCovs design was used only for the first 17 patients enrolled in the trial. As shown by Table 7.3, after 17 patients

TABLE 7.1: Posterior values from the model fit to historical data on 274 patients, and acceptability bounds

CRD$\geq$52	SALV	Age	Mean (sd) of $\pi_E(Z, \beta_E)$	$\underline{\pi}_E(Z)$
No	1	–	0.16(0.03)	0.10
No	2	–	0.09(0.04)	0.05
Yes	1	–	0.54(0.07)	0.40
Yes	2	–	0.39(0.12)	0.25

CRD$\geq$52	SALV	Age	Mean (sd) of $\pi_T(Z, \beta_T)$	$\overline{\pi}_T(Z)$
No	–	48	0.42(0.03)	0.48
No	–	67	0.49(0.04)	0.57
Yes	–	48	0.23(0.03)	0.29
Yes	–	67	0.28(0.04)	0.36

TABLE 7.2: Hypothetical final recommended covariate-specific doses for the PR104 Trial

Age	CRD < 52 Weeks SALV=2	SALV=1	CRD $\geq$ 52 Weeks SALV=2	SALV=1
18 - 33	1.6	2.2	3.0	3.0
34 - 42	1.6	2.2	2.2	3.0
43 - 58	1.6	2.2	2.2	2.2
59 - 66	1.1	1.6	1.6	2.2
> 66	None	1.1	1.6	1.6

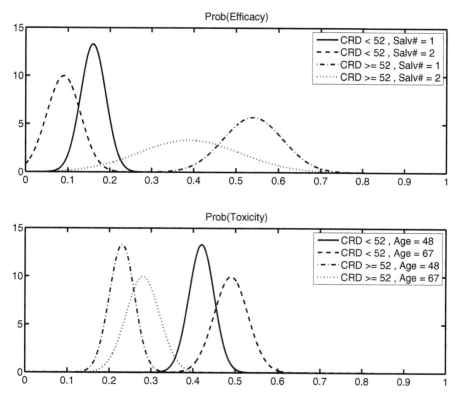

FIGURE 7.2: Posteriors of π_E and π_T for different values of first CR duration, number of previous salvage therapies, and age, based on historical data from 274 patients.

had been treated at doses in the set $\{1.1, 1.6, 1.2, 3.0\}$ mg/m^2 and evaluated, none had experienced the Efficacy event [CR or CRp], 2 had experienced Toxicity, and the design did not consider any of the four doses 1.2, 1.6, 2.2, or 3.0 acceptable for any patient. This was due to the fact that even the highest dose was inefficacious for any Z. The fact that the trade-off contour was not sufficiently steep did not play a role in this decision, since the dose unacceptability was based on the investigator's elicited covariate-specific dose acceptability bounds. Subsequently, the EffToxCovs design was abandoned, the trial protocol was amended per IRB approval to also include the higher dose 4.0 mg/m^2, and an additional 33 patients were treated at dose either 3.0 or 4.0. Among a total of 41 patients treated at these two doses, 6 (14.6%) achieved CR or CRp (Konopleva et al., 2015, Table 4). Assuming the very simple model that ignores Z, as was done for most of the trial, and assuming the simple uninformative prior $\pi = \Pr(\text{CR or CRp at dose 3.0 or 4.0}) \sim$ beta(.50, .50), the posterior of π has mean .16 and 95% credible interval 0.06 – 0.28, with $\Pr(\pi > .20 \mid 6/41) = .20$.

TABLE 7.3: Interim decisions made by the design in the PR104 trial

After n=8, all (No Eff, No Tox)

CRD≥52	SALV=2	Age	Dose/Decision
No	No	< 82	3.0
No	No	≥ 82	2.2
No	Yes	< 42	3.0
No	Yes	≥ 42	2.2
Yes	No	All	3.0
Yes	Yes	All	3.0

After n=17, 15 (No Eff, No Tox) + 2 (No Eff, Tox)

CRD≥52	SALV=2	Age	Dose/Decision
No	No	All	None
No	Yes	All	None
Yes	No	All	None
Yes	Yes	All	None

7.2 Biomarker-Based Dose Finding

The EffToxCovs design is useful for trials with binary Toxicity and Efficacy and a small number of well-established patient baseline prognostic covariates. If one wishes to account for biomarkers that may affect the dose-response relationships, including dose-biomarker interactions, the resulting covariate vector may easily become too large for use by the EffToxCovs design. Additionally, unlike established prognostic covariates like age or number of previous therapies, it usually is not known whether a given biomarker is related to clinical outcomes, since typically there are no historical data to estimate biomarker effects on Y_E and Y_T for establishing a prior. A third problem is that biomarkers may be highly correlated, which produces collinearity in any dose-response regression model. In such settings, the EffToxCovs design becomes impractical due to the curse of dimensionality (Bellman, 1957), especially given the small to moderate sample sizes typical of early-phase trials.

To account for patient heterogeneity introduced by biomarkers in phase I–II settings, so that one may choose biomarker-specific doses, we first describe a motivating example. This is a phase I–II trial to find the optimal doses of a novel molecularly targeted agent in patients with locally advanced or metastatic solid tumors. Each patient's tumor may harbor molecular alterations in any of five genes, denoted by the acronyms *NTRK1*, *NTRK2*, *NTRK3*, *ROS1*, and *ALK*. The types of possible molecular alterations include gene rearrangements, single-nucleotide polymorphisms, insertions, deletions, splice variants, and gene amplifications. Molecular alterations in these target genes have been detected in various cancers, including non-small cell lung cancer, colorectal cancer, thyroid cancer, pancreatic cancer, and neuroblastoma. These alterations are expected to be predictive markers that may influence the treatment effect of the agent. In the study, the status of each target gene is coded as positive (the alteration is present) or negative (no alteration), and is evaluated for each patient using next-generation sequencing. Patients receive the treatment agent orally, once daily in the morning for 28 consecutive days in repeated 4-week cycles. Adverse events are graded according to the NCI Common Terminology Criteria for Adverse Events Version 4.03, and coded as a three-level ordinal variable: grade 1 or 2, grade 3, or grade ≥ 4 hematologic, non-hematologic, or gastrointestinal toxicities. Efficacy is evaluated using the Response Evaluation Criteria In Solid Tumors (RECIST), and coded as a three-level ordinal variable: progressive disease (PD), stable disease (SD), or partial or complete remission (PR/CR). Five daily doses are evaluated, 100, 300, 500, 700, and 900 mg/m^2/day. The primary objective is to find an optimal dose that is safe and efficacious for each patient according to the patient's specific pattern of molecular alterations of the five genes. For this trial, the straightforward approach that directly includes gene alterations and their interactions with the dose as covariates in the EffToxCovs model would result in 11 covariates, consisting of the dose, 5 gene alteration indicators, and 5 dose-gene alteration interactions.

The following Bayesian phase I–II personalized dose-finding method accommodates settings of the sort described in the above illustration. For brevity, we will use "biomarkers" and "covariates," interchangeably. To deal with the curse of dimensionality and potential high correlations among biomarkers, the design employs the canonical partial least squares (CPLS) method to extract a small number of components from the covariate matrix consisting of dose, biomarker profile, and dose by biomarker interactions. These CPLS components capture most of the covariate information that is predictive of response (Garthwaite, 1994) and will be used to model relationships between dose/biomarker and Toxicity/Efficacy outcomes.

Partial least squares (PLS) is a dimension-reduction technique for modeling the relationship between one or more response variables and a vector of covariates in regression (Stone and Brooks, 1990; Frank and Friedman, 1993; Garthwaite, 1994). PLS can be applied for univariate regression with one response variable or multivariate regression with a vector of responses. The basic idea is to construct a small number of PLS components, each a linear combination of the covariates, to capture most of the information contained in the covariate vector for predicting the responses. The PLS components are used in place of the original high-dimensional covariate vector in the regression model. Unlike principal component analysis, which determines principal components as linear combinations of the covariates without using the response variables, PLS determines components using both the responses and covariates. Therefore, PLS is more relevant for regression and provides better prediction. PLS was originally developed for continuous responses (Garth-waite, 1994). To handle categorical responses, Indahl et al. (2009) proposed the CPLS method, which integrates the PLS methodology with canonical cor-relation analysis. These authors showed that CPLS extracts more information from the first few components than the ordinary PLS approach that applies multivariate PLS with dummy coded responses indicating group membership. Since CPLS models are parsimonious with fewer components, this approach is particularly attractive for early-phase clinical trials with small sample sizes.

First suppose that there is one response variable, with $s \geq 2$ categories, and there are p biomarkers. Below, we will provide the necessary elaboration to accommodate the two ordinal categorical variables Y_E and Y_T in the mo-tivating example given above. For sample size n, let Z be the $n \times p$ covariate matrix with each covariate centered at its mean, Y the $n \times 1$ categorical re-sponse vector, and A_Y the $n \times s$ group membership indicator matrix for Y, with $A_Y[i, j] = 1$ if $Y_i = j$, and 0 otherwise. The CPLS algorithm is a se-quential procedure that iteratively computes components of Z, each a linear combination of the original covariates, in such a way that the first compo-nent contains the most information for predicting Y, the second component contains less information than the first, and so on.

To begin, CPLS first transforms the Z matrix to $R = ZQ$, where $Q = Z'A_Y$. A CPLS component for predicting A_Y is found by maximizing the canonical correlation between R and A_Y. Specifically, the CPLS method finds s-dimensional vectors a and b to maximize the correlation between Ra and A_Yb, given by

$$\text{cor}(Ra, A_Yb) = \frac{a'R'A_Yb}{\sqrt{a'R'Ra}\sqrt{b'A_Y'A_Yb}}. \tag{7.9}$$

This optimization problem is the canonical correlation analysis with respect to R and A_Y, so in this sense CPLS combines PLS and canonical correlation analysis. Maximizing the objective function (7.9) is equivalent to maximizing

$$f(r, t) = r'(R'R)^{-\frac{1}{2}}R'A_Y(A_Y'A_Y)^{-\frac{1}{2}}t$$

over unit vectors r and t (Indahl et al., 2009). The solutions r and t are the dominant left and right singular vectors, with unit length, correspond-ing to the largest singular value in the singular value decomposition of the matrix $(R'R)^{-\frac{1}{2}}R'A_Y(A_Y'A_Y)^{-\frac{1}{2}}$. The values of a and b that maximize the objective function (7.9) are given by $a = (R'R)^{-\frac{1}{2}}r$ and $b = (A_Y'A_Y)^{-\frac{1}{2}}t$, and the resulting CPLS component is $c_1 = Zw$, a linear combination of the original covariates, where $w = Qa/\|Qa\|$ is a vector of the weights. This is the first CPLS component. Subsequent CPLS components are extracted similarly, in sequence, by replacing Z and A_Y with their deflated matrices. For example, the second CPLS component c_2 is obtained by maximizing the objective function (7.9) with Z and A_Y replaced by their deflated matrices $\tilde{Z} = Z - (c_1'c_1)^{-1}c_1c_1'Z$ and $\tilde{A}_Y = A_Y - (c_1'c_1)^{-1}c_1c_1'A_Y$. The deflation ensures that subsequent components contain information that is not explained by ear-lier components. The CPLS components can be extracted using the NIPALS algorithm (Burnham et al., 1996), or the SIMPLS algorithm (de Jong, 1993). When the response variable Y has only two categories, the CPLS reduces to traditional PLS.

Consider a phase I–II clinical trial with standardized doses $x_1 < \cdots < x_J$ of a molecularly targeted agent, as follows. Denote the levels of ordinal Y_E and Y_T by $y_k = 1, 2, \cdots, m_k$ for $k = E, T$, indexed in order of increasing severity of Toxicity, and increasingly desirable levels of Efficacy. In many trials, ordinal variables provide a more refined evaluation of clinical outcomes, and reflect the actual way that Toxicity and Efficacy are measured. In particular, 3-level or 4-level ordinal scales often contain much more information than the dichotomized Toxicity and Efficacy outcomes for decision making (Yuan et al., 2007; Houede et al., 2010; Lee et al., 2016; Thall et al., 2016). To see why using binary Toxicity and Efficacy may be inadequate, consider a binary Efficacy outcome defined as CR/PR, so that PD/SD is a nonresponse. While this dichotomization may be sensible for many conventional cytotoxic agents that work by shrinking the tumor, many targeted agents are cytostatic, with the aim to stabilize the tumor rather than shrinking it. For these agents, SD often is regarded as a favorable outcome, although not as desirable as CR/PR, and certainly more favorable than PD.

The CPLS algorithm is applied to construct a personalized dose-finding method as follows. Let n denote the number of patients enrolled in the trial at an interim decision time, $Z = (Z_1, \cdots, Z_p)'$ a vector of binary biomarkers. Define the $n \times (2p+1)$ covariate matrix $V = (x, Z_1, \cdots, Z_p, xZ_1, \cdots, xZ_p)$, where $xZ_1, \cdots, xZ_p$ are dose-biomarker interactions. In the motivating trial, there are 5 genes so $p = 5$ and V is $n \times 11$. With small phase I–II sample sizes, directly regressing (Y_T, Y_E) on V suffers from the curse of dimensionality and also potential collinearity, which may result in highly unstable estimates. To address these issues, we first apply CPLS to reduce the dimension of V, and then regress (Y_T, Y_E) on the reduced covariate matrix. Specifically, we extract the first q_E CPLS components $W_E(x, Z) = (W_{E,1}(x, Z), \cdots, W_{E,q_E}(x, Z))$ for predicting Y_E, and the first q_T CPLS components $W_T(x, Z) = (W_{T,1}(x, Z), \cdots, W_{T,q_T}(x, Z))$ from V for predicting Y_T, where in general $q_E, q_T < 2p + 1$. In a cancer classification experiment using PLS with gene expression profiles, Nguyen and Rocke (2002) showed that 3 to 5 PLS components often are adequate, even in applications starting with thousands of genes. To accommodate the small sample sizes of early-phase trials, we recommend $2 \leq q_E, q_T \leq 4$. Each CPLS component is a linear combination of biomarkers Z, dose x, and their interactions. Since biomarkers that are predictive of Y_T may differ from those that are predictive of Y_E, the CPLS components should be extracted separately for the two marginals. The jth component of $W_T(x, Z)$ thus is not necessarily the same as that of $W_E(x, Z)$. For notational brevity, we suppress the arguments x and Z in $W_T(x, Z)$ and $W_E(x, Z)$ when it does not cause confusion.

A computationally convenient approach to modeling the relationship between W_k and ordinal Y_k is to use latent variables. Let $Y_{T,i}^*$ and $Y_{E,i}^*$ be two latent normal variables for patient i treated at dose $x_{[i]}$, following the linear models

$$Y^*_{T,i}|W_{T,i},\beta_T,\zeta_i,\tau^2_{T,i} \sim N(\zeta_i + W_{T,i}\beta_T, \tau^2_{T,i})$$
$$Y^*_{E,i}|W_{E,i},\beta_E,\zeta_i,\tau^2_{E,i} \sim N(\zeta_i + W_{E,i}\beta_E, \tau^2_{E,i}),$$

where β_T and β_E are vectors of regression coefficients, and $\zeta_i \overset{iid}{\sim} N(0,\sigma^2)$ are patient-specific random effects that account for correlation between $Y^*_{T,i}$ and $Y^*_{E,i}$ and between-patient variability. Integrating out ζ_i, the above model implies that $Y^*_{T,i}$ and $Y^*_{E,i}$ follow a bivariate normal distribution

$$Y^*_{T,i}, Y^*_{E,i}|W_{T,i}, W_{E,i}, \theta_i, \sim N_2 \left(\begin{pmatrix} W_{T,i}\beta_T \\ W_{E,i}\beta_E \end{pmatrix}, \begin{pmatrix} \tau^2_{T,i}+\sigma^2 & \sigma^2 \\ \sigma^2 & \tau^2_{E,i}+\sigma^2 \end{pmatrix} \right),$$

where $\theta_i = (\beta_T, \beta_E, \tau^2_{T,i}, \tau^2_{E,i}, \sigma^2)$. Thus, the random patient effects inflate the variances and induce correlation between the latent variables. The observed Toxicity and Efficacy outcomes $Y_{T,i}$ and $Y_{E,i}$ for the ith patient are expressed in terms of $Y^*_{T,i}$ and $Y^*_{E,i}$ by the equations

$$Y_{T,i} = l \quad \text{if} \quad \gamma_{T,l-1} < Y^*_{T,i} \le \gamma_{T,l}$$
$$Y_{E,i} = r \quad \text{if} \quad \gamma_{E,r-1} < Y^*_{E,i} \le \gamma_{E,r}$$

where $l = 1, \cdots, m_T$, $r = 1, \cdots, m_E$, $-\infty \equiv \gamma_{T,0} < \gamma_{T,1} < \cdots < \gamma_{T,m_T} \equiv \infty$ and $-\infty \equiv \gamma_{E,0} < \gamma_{E,1} < \cdots < \gamma_{E,m_E} \equiv \infty$ are unknown cut-offs. Thus, ζ_i induces association between the observable $Y_{E,i}$ and $Y_{T,i}$.

This model for $(Y_{E,i}, Y_{T,i})$ is not identifiable because, using $Y_{T,i}$ as an example, the scale parameter $\tau_{T,i}$ of the latent variable $Y^*_{T,i}$ is fully confounded with β_T and the cut-offs $\gamma_{T,l}$. This follows from the fact that the same likelihood is obtained if β_T, $\tau_{T,i}$ and $\gamma_{T,l}$ are multiplied by a constant. The same problem arises with $Y_{E,i}$. To identify the model for Toxicity, we fix the scale of the latent variable $Y^*_{T,i}$ by setting $\tau^2_{T,i} = 1$ (Albert and Chib, 1993), which gives the familiar cumulative probit model,

$$\Phi^{-1}[\Pr(Y_{T,i} \le l|W_{T,i},\beta_T,\zeta_i,\gamma_{T,l})] = \gamma_{T,l} - \zeta_i - W_{T,i}\beta_T \qquad (7.10)$$

for $l = 1, \cdots, m_T - 1$. Although one may simply assume the above model for Y_T, taking the latent variable approach greatly simplifies the posterior sampling using the Gibbs sampler (Albert and Chib, 1993).

It may appear that one may take the same approach for Efficacy by defining a cumulative probit model for Y_E and setting $\tau^2_{E,i} = 1$. However, the cumulative probit model (7.10) implies a stochastic ordering of the effects of the covariates on the outcome. That is, $\Pr(Y_{T,i} \le l|W_T(x,Z))$ is either increasing or decreasing in x. While such a monotonicity assumption typically is reasonable for Toxicity, it is problematic for Efficacy because effects of molecularly targeted agents on Y_E may be non-monotonic. To accommodate this, we set $\tau_{E,i} = \exp(\tau x_{[i]})$, resulting in the following generalized cumulative probit model (McCullagh, 1980; Agresti, 2002),

$$\Phi^{-1}[\Pr(Y_{E,i} \le r | W_{E,i}, \beta_E, \zeta_i, \gamma_{E,r})] = \frac{\gamma_{E,r} - \zeta_i - W_{E,i}\beta_E}{\exp(\tau x_{[i]})}, \quad r = 1, \cdots, m_E - 1.$$

The dispersion parameter τ causes the variance to change with x, and thus the model does not impose the stochastic ordering of the dose effect on Efficacy (Agresti, 2002). When $\tau = 0$, the model reduces to the standard cumulative probit model.

With this formulation, the likelihood for patient i is

$$\Pr(Y_{T,i} = y_{T,i}, Y_{E,i} = y_{E,i})$$

$$= \Pr\left(\gamma_{T,y_{T,i}-1} < Y_{T,i}^* \le \gamma_{T,y_{T,i}}, \gamma_{E,y_{E,i}-1} < Y_{E,i}^* \le \gamma_{E,y_{E,i}}\right)$$

$$= \int_{\gamma_{T,y_{T,i}-1}}^{\gamma_{T,y_{T,i}}} \int_{\gamma_{E,y_{E,i}-1}}^{\gamma_{E,y_{E,i}}} \phi_2(y_{T,i}^*, y_{E,i}^* | \boldsymbol{\mu}_Y, \boldsymbol{\Sigma}_Y) dy_{T,i}^* dy_{E,i}^*$$

where $\phi_2(\cdot | \boldsymbol{\mu}, \boldsymbol{\Sigma})$ denotes the density of a bivariate normal distribution with mean vector $\boldsymbol{\mu}$ and covariance matrix $\boldsymbol{\Sigma}$. Here,

$$\boldsymbol{\mu}_Y = \left(\begin{array}{c} W_{T,i}\beta_T \\ W_{E,i}\beta_E \end{array} \right) \text{ and } \boldsymbol{\Sigma}_Y = \left(\begin{array}{cc} 1 + \sigma^2 & \sigma^2 \\ \sigma^2 & \exp(\tau x_{[i]}) + \sigma^2 \end{array} \right).$$

The model parameter vector is $\theta = (\gamma_{T,1}, \cdots, \gamma_{T,m_T}, \beta_T, \gamma_{E,1}, \cdots, \gamma_{E,m_E}, \beta_E, \tau, \sigma^2)$, and the data from n patients takes the form $\mathcal{D}_n = \{(Y_{T,i}, Y_{E,i}, x_{[i]}, W_i), i = 1, \cdots, n\}$.

Under the probit model, a change of 2.5 on the probit scale moves a probability of Y_T or Y_E located in one category from 0.10 to 0.89. It is very unlikely that the effect of a covariate or biomarker will be this large. To avoid such unduly large effects, we scale each covariate in W_T and W_E to have mean 0 and standard deviation 0.5, and then assign the independent normal prior distribution $N(0, 1.25^2)$ to each element of β_T and β_E. This implies that a change in a covariate from one standard deviation below the mean to one standard deviation above the mean will result in a change likely to be within the range of $(0, 2.5)$, i.e., a change of 2 standard deviations for the prior on the probit scale. For the intercepts $\gamma_{T,l}$ and $\gamma_{E,r}$, the same normal priors can be used with the constraints that $\gamma_{T,1} < \cdots < \gamma_{T,m_T}$ and $\gamma_{E,1} < \cdots < \gamma_{E,m_E}$. The priors for σ^2 and τ are chosen to be $InvGamma(a,b)$ and $Uniform(-c,c)$ distributions, respectively. The hyper-parameters are set to be $a = 0.1$ and $b = 0.1$ so that a priori the probability that the correlation between Toxicity and Efficacy is between 0.045 and 1 is 99%, and $c = 4$ to make the prior distribution of τ weakly informative.

Dose acceptability criteria are defined as follows. Denote $\pi_T(3) \equiv \Pr(Y_T = 3 | x, Z)$, $\pi_E(3) \equiv \Pr(Y_E = 3 | x, Z)$, and $\pi_E(2,3) \equiv \Pr(Y_E = 2 \text{ or } 3 | x, Z)$.

Given data $\mathcal{D}_n$, for a patient with biomarker vector Z, a dose x has *acceptable Toxicity* if

$$\Pr\big(\pi_T(3) \geq \bar{\pi}_T | W(x, Z), \mathcal{D}_n\big) \leq p_T, \tag{7.11}$$

and *acceptable Efficacy* if

$$\Pr\big(\pi_E(3) \leq \underline{\pi}_{E,3} | W(x, Z), \mathcal{D}_n\big) \leq p_{E,3} \tag{7.12}$$

or

$$\Pr\big(\pi_E(2, 3) \leq \underline{\pi}_{E,2} | W(x, Z), \mathcal{D}_n\big) \leq p_{E,2}, \tag{7.13}$$

where $\bar{\pi}_T$, $\underline{\pi}_{E,3}$ and $\underline{\pi}_{E,2}$ are upper and lower bounds on the probabilities of Toxicity and Efficacy elicited from physicians, and $p_{E,3}$, and $p_{E,2}$ and p_T are probability cut-offs. The definition of acceptable Efficacy (7.12) and (7.13) accounts for the practical consideration that, for a molecularly targeted agent, a dose is considered promising if it can achieve a minimal rate of CR/PR or a minimal rate of SD or better.

The desirability of each outcome (y_E, y_T) is quantified using the utility function given in Table 7.4.

TABLE 7.4: Utilities for the solid tumor trial of the cytostatic agent

	$y_E=1$	$y_E=2$	$y_E=3$
$y_T=1$	10	50	100
$y_T=2$	5	20	60
$y_T=3$	0	10	20

For a patient with biomarker profile Z, if θ were known the optimal personalized dose would be the acceptable dose maximizing the mean utility

$$\bar{U}(x, Z, \theta) = \sum_{y_T=1}^{3} \sum_{y_E=1}^{3} u(y_T, y_E) \Pr(y_T, y_E | x, Z, \theta).$$

Proceeding as in Chapter 6, the *optimal personalized dose for a patient with biomarkers Z* is defined as the acceptable dose maximizing the posterior mean utility

$$u(x, Z, \mathcal{D}_n) = E\{\bar{U}(x, Z, \theta) \mid \mathcal{D}_n\}.$$

The trial is conducted using the following two-stage algorithm. In stage I, dose escalation is done for N_1 patients based only on Y_T, without using either Y_E or Z, with Toxicity dichotomized as dose-limiting Toxicity (DLT) or not. The two objectives are to evaluate the safety of the doses while also collecting preliminary (Y_E, Y_T, Z) data to facilitate model fitting in stage II. A wide variety of phase I methods may be used. The Bayesian optimal interval (BOIN) design (Liu and Yuan, 2015) is an attractive choice because the dose escalation and de-escalation rules can be prespecified, and its performance is substantially superior to that of the 3+3 algorithm.

Personalized dose finding is done in stage II with a maximum sample size of N_2 patients. As with EffToxCovs, in stage II patients must be treated in cohorts of size 1 since their selected dose depends on Z. The dose assigned to the nth patient with biomarker profile Z_n is determined as follows.

1. Given data $\mathcal{D}_{n-1}$, extract the CPLS components, fit the model, and determine the acceptable dose set $\mathcal{A}(Z_n)$.

2. If $\mathcal{A}(Z_n)$ is empty, no dose is acceptable for that patient, and the patient is treated off protocol.

3. If $\mathcal{A}(Z_n)$ is not empty, use AR to choose a dose in $\mathcal{A}(Z_n)$, randomizing the patient to dose $x_j \in \mathcal{A}(Z_n)$ with probability w_n proportional to its posterior expected utility,

$$w_n = \frac{u(x_j, Z_n, \mathcal{D}_{n-1})}{\sum_{x_{j'} \in \mathcal{A}(Z_n)} u(x_{j'}, Z_n, \mathcal{D}_{n-1})}.$$

4. Regardless of Z_n, do not skip an untried dose when escalating.

5. Repeat steps 1-4 until the maximum sample size of N_2 is reached.

The design may be modified by pre-specifying a number of patients treated off protocol that motivates termination of the trial and with the conclusion that no dose is acceptable for any Z.

The following simulation study gives the operating characteristics of the design. The 5 doses are $(x_1, \cdots, x_5) = (0.1, 0.3, 0.5, 0.7, 0.9)$, with 5 binary biomarkers. A high correlation of 0.9 between Z_1 and Z_2 is assumed, with Z_3, Z_4, and Z_5 independent of each other and of Z_1 and Z_2. The assumed probabilities of being positive for the 5 biomarkers were 0.50, 0.55, 0.50, 0.70, and 0.30. The Toxicity upper bound was $\bar{\pi}_T = 0.3$, and the Efficacy lower bounds were $\pi_{E,2} = 0.4$ and $\pi_{E,3} = 0.25$. The maximum sample size was 60, with stage I sample size $N_1 = 21$ and stage II sample size $N_2 = 39$. The Bayesian optimal interval design was used to conduct the stage I dose escalation with a cohort size of 3. In stage II, two CPLS components were extracted to fit the regression models for Toxicity and Efficacy.

Two scenarios are presented, chosen to differ in their main effects of the 5 biomarkers and their interactions with the dose. As shown by Figure 7.3, in Scenario 1, biomarkers 1 and 5 have main effects on Toxicity and biomarkers 1, 2, 4, and 5 interact with the dose to affect Toxicity. Biomarkers 1 and 3 have main effects on Efficacy, and biomarkers 1 and 4 interact with the dose to affect Efficacy. In Scenario 2, the interaction between biomarker 5 and the dose is the main contributor to Toxicity, and four biomarkers and four interactions affect the Efficacy probability. Because the Efficacy and Toxicity probabilities depend on the biomarkers, the shape of the dose-utility relationship varies with Z. There were $2^5 = 32$ possible biomarker patterns. Figure 7.4 shows the shapes of the dose-utility curves for 6 selected biomarker patterns under the 2 scenarios.

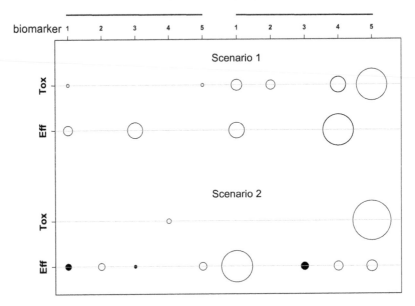

FIGURE 7.3: Main effects and dose-biomarker interactions on Toxicity probabilities for the two scenarios. The radius of a circle is proportional to the absolute value of the coefficient. Empty and black circles represent positive and negative coefficients, respectively.

The biomarker-based personalized dose finding (PDF) design is compared to a modified version of the EffToxCovs design that includes dose, biomarkers, and dose-biomarker interactions in the regression model. In the original EffToxCovs design, Toxicity and Efficacy are treated as binary variables and logistic regression is used for the marginals. To make the comparison meaningful, the same latent-variable models, utility, and a dose-finding algorithm were used in the two designs to ensure that they have the same target doses. Since it is not feasible to include all five biomarkers and their interactions with the dose, a total of 11 covariates, in the model, the modified EffToxCovs design included the dose, two randomly selected biomarkers, Z_1 and Z_3, and their interactions with dose in the model.

Reporting the simulation results is not straightforward for personalized dose finding because, under each scenario, there are 32 different biomarker patterns, and each pattern is associated with a set of dose-Toxicity and dose-Efficacy curves and optimal doses. Table 7.5 reports the selection percentage for each dose, given two representative biomarker patterns, in each scenario. Under each representative biomarker pattern, the first three rows show the true marginal probabilities of $Y_T = 3$ and $Y_E = 2$ or 3, which determine the acceptability of the dose. The fourth row shows the true utility of each dose,

TABLE 7.5: Selection percentage for each dose and the percentage of correct selection for two representative biomarker patterns under the personalized dose-finding (PDF) design and modified EffToxCovs design. The numbers in boldface are target doses

		Dose level					Percentage of
		1	2	3	4	5	correct selection
				Scenario 1			
				$Z = (+ + + + +)$			
$P(Y_T = 3)$		**0.100**	**0.229**	0.419	0.631	0.809	
$P(Y_E = 2)$		**0.197**	**0.117**	0.052	0.017	0.004	
$P(Y_E = 3)$		**0.773**	**0.875**	0.946	0.982	0.996	
True utility		**54.39**	**49.50**	42.49	34.48	27.57	
Sel %	PDF	**0.720**	**0.139**	0.069	0.031	0.037	0.859
	EffToxCovs	**0.524**	**0.144**	0.124	0.076	0.132	0.668
				$Z = (- - - - +)$			
$P(Y_T = 3)$		**0.051**	0.071	0.096	0.126	0.164	
$P(Y_E = 2)$		**0.407**	0.393	0.331	0.236	0.142	
$P(Y_E = 3)$		**0.183**	0.099	0.043	0.015	0.004	
True utility		**25.75**	18.72	13.20	9.38	6.93	
Sel %	PDF	**0.923**	0.000	0.001	0.001	0.062	0.923
	EffToxCovs	**0.572**	0.008	0.008	0.013	0.399	0.572
				Scenario 2			
				$Z = (+ + + + -)$			
$P(Y_T = 3)$		0.027	0.031	0.035	**0.040**	**0.045**	
$P(Y_E = 2)$		0.416	0.507	0.391	**0.187**	**0.056**	
$P(Y_E = 3)$		0.148	0.296	0.554	**0.803**	**0.943**	
True utility		27.31	40.12	55.81	68.18	**74.18**	
Sel %	PDF	0.001	0.003	0.009	**0.107**	**0.880**	0.987
	EffToxCovs	0.000	0.002	0.012	**0.122**	**0.864**	0.986
				$Z = (+ + - + +)$			
$P(Y_T = 3)$		0.040	**0.091**	**0.177**	**0.300**	0.458	
$P(Y_E = 2)$		0.444	**0.295**	**0.078**	**0.009**	0.000	
$P(Y_E = 3)$		0.350	**0.672**	**0.920**	**0.991**	1.000	
True utility		40.89	**53.29**	**57.07**	**51.68**	43.60	
Sel %	PDF	0.025	**0.100**	**0.378**	**0.308**	0.189	0.786
	EffToxCovs	0.001	**0.000**	**0.037**	**0.184**	0.778	0.221

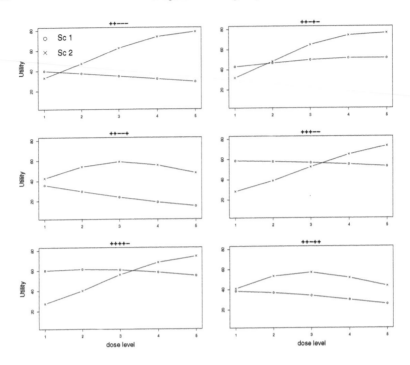

FIGURE 7.4: Utility of the five doses for 6 biomarker patterns under the two scenarios. Each graph shows the utility for one biomarker pattern. The symbols consisting of "+" and "−" above each graph indicate the status for the 5 biomarkers.

which determines the target doses. Here, the target doses are defined as the doses for which the utility values are at least 90% of that of the optimal dose.

The PDF design outperformed the modified EffToxCovs design. In Scenario 1, for both representative biomarker patterns, the utility decreases with dose. The target doses are dose levels 1 and 2 for the first pattern, and dose level 1 for the second pattern. The target dose selection percentages were 20% and 35% higher under the PDF design than under the modified EffToxCovs design for the two patterns. In Scenario 2, for biomarker pattern $(+ + - + +)$, the PDF design yielded a 56% higher percentage of target dose selection than the EffToxCovs design. Across all 32 possible biomarker patterns, the average percentages of correct selection of the target doses were 0.697 and 0.775 in Scenarios 1 and 2, respectively, for the PDF design, while those for the EffToxCovs design were 0.589 and 0.637.

8

Combination Trials

CONTENTS

8.1   Bivariate Binary Outcomes 150
8.2   Bivariate Ordinal Outcomes 159
    8.2.1   Generalized Continuation Ratio Model 159
    8.2.2   Generalized Aranda–Ordaz Link Model 160
    8.2.3   An mTOR Inhibitor Chemo Combination Trial 166
    8.2.4   Parametric Dose Standardization 168
    8.2.5   mTOR Inhibitor Trial Design 173
    8.2.6   Alternative Models 177

Treating patients with a combination of two agents is quite common in cancer therapy. Advantages of giving combinations include the potential to induce a synergistic treatment effect, target different drug susceptibilities of cancer cells, or achieve a higher overall dose intensity with non-overlapping toxicities. Trial designs for drug-combination studies involve several distinct features that are beyond the scope of methods for single-agent studies. In single-agent trials, it often is assumed that $\pi_T(d)$ and $\pi_E(d)$ increase with dose d, resulting in a simple ordering of each probability. Under this assumption, one can escalate to higher, more toxic doses or de-escalate to lower, safer doses in the one-dimensional dose domain. In contrast, when a trial involves two agents, the probabilities of π_E and π_T for drug combinations are not fully ordered in the two-dimensional dose pair space. For example, let $(d_{1,j}, d_{2,l})$ denote the combination of drug A at dose level j and drug B at dose level l. When no meaning is lost, we will use the notation $(j, l) = (d_{1,j}, d_{2,l})$. While the combination $(2, 3)$ is more toxic than $(2, 2)$, there is no obvious ordering of either $\pi_T(d)$ or $\pi_E(d)$ between $d = (2, 3)$ and $d = (3, 2)$.

An important feature of drug-combination trials is the outcome-probability-equivalent contour in the two-dimensional dose-Toxicity and dose-Efficacy spaces. Thinking of the dose pairs $(d_{1,j}, d_{2,l})$ as varying smoothly over a rectangular set, the probabilities $\pi_k(d_{1,j}, d_{2,l})$ may be represented by a surface over the rectangle for each $k = E, T$. For each outcome $k = E, T$, the set $\{(d_{1,j}, d_{2,l}) : \pi_k(d_{1,j}, d_{2,l}) = p\}$ is that outcome's *probability contour* of dose pairs with common outcome k and probability p. Because dose pairs on the same Toxicity contour may have different Efficacy probabilities, they may have different desirabilities. Therefore, phase I–II combination trials are much more complicated and more difficult than phase I trials that only account for Toxicity as a function of $(d_{1,j}, d_{2,l})$.

In what follows, we describe several phase I–II designs that adopt different modeling and decision making strategies. The first design, described in Section 8.1, models (Y_E, Y_T) as binary outcomes and aims to find the most efficacious drug combination that satisfies a safety requirement. The second set of designs, described in Section 8.2, model (Y_E, Y_T) as ordinal outcomes, with the goal to find the dose combination having highest posterior mean utility.

8.1   Bivariate Binary Outcomes

Consider a trial to study J doses $d_{1,1} < \cdots < d_{1,J}$ of agent A, and L doses $d_{2,1} < \cdots < d_{2,L}$ of agent B, with bivariate binary (Y_T, Y_E). Denote $\pi_k(d_{1,j}, d_{2,l}) = \Pr(Y_k = 1 \mid d_{1,j}, d_{2,l})$, $k = E, T$, the joint Toxicity and Efficacy probabilities of drug combination $(d_{1,j}, d_{2,l})$. The objective of the trial is to find the optimal dose pair that has the highest $\pi_E(d_{1,j}, d_{2,l})$ with the $\pi_T(d_{1,j}, d_{2,l})$ below a prespecified upper limit $\bar{\pi}_T$.

In most combination trials, before the two drugs are combined a requirement is that each drug should have been investigated when administered alone. Given the relatively large dose-pair space and the limited sample size in drug-combination trials, it is useful to utilize prior information from previous single-agent trials for dose finding. Let $x_{1,j}$ be the estimated Toxicity probability of $d_{1,j}$ when agent A is administered alone, and $x_{2,l}$ the estimated Toxicity probability of $d_{2,l}$ when agent B is administered alone. Typically, the maximum dose for each drug in the combination trial is either the individual MTD determined in the single-agent trial or a dose below the MTD. Therefore, prior values of $x_{1,j}$ and $x_{2,l}$ have the MTDs as respective upper bounds $x_{1,J}$ and $x_{2,L}$. Probabilities $x_{1,j}$ and $x_{2,l}$ can be viewed as standardized or "effective" doses of $d_{1,j}$ and $d_{2,l}$.

The joint Toxicity probability at the dose combination $(d_{1,j}, d_{2,l})$ can be modelled using the copula-type regression model (Yin and Yuan, 2009a)

$$\pi_T(d_{1,j}, d_{2,l}) = 1 - \{(1 - x_{1,j}^\alpha)^{-\gamma} + (1 - x_{2,l}^\beta)^{-\gamma} - 1\}^{-1/\gamma}, \qquad (8.1)$$

where $\alpha, \beta, \gamma > 0$ are unknown model parameters. This model satisfies natural constraints for drug-combination trials. For example, if the Toxicity probabilities of both drugs are zero at $d_{1,j}$ and $d_{2,l}$ then the joint Toxicity probability $\pi_T(d_{1,j}, d_{2,l}) = 0$. If the Toxicity probability of either drug A at $d_{1,j}$ or drug B at $d_{2,l}$ is one, then $\pi_T(d_{1,j}, d_{2,l}) = 1$. Another attractive feature of model (8.1) is that if only one drug is tested, it reduces to the model typically used with the CRM.

Suppose that, at an interim decision time, among n_{jl} patients treated at the dose pair $(d_{1,j}, d_{2,l})$, m_{jl} have experienced DLT. The likelihood given the observed data $\mathcal{D} = \{(m_{jl}, n_{jl}); j = 1, \cdots, J, l = 1, \cdots, L\}$ is

$$\mathcal{L}(\alpha, \beta, \gamma | \mathcal{D}) \propto \prod_{j=1}^{J} \prod_{l=1}^{L} \pi_T(d_{1,j}, d_{2,l})^{m_{jl}} (1 - \pi_T(d_{1,j}, d_{2,l}))^{n_{jl} - m_{jl}}.$$

The trial design has two stages, with stage I carried out as follows. Let c_d and c_e be fixed probability cut-offs.

1. The first cohort of patients is treated at the lowest dose pair $(1, 1)$.

2. During the trial, at the current dose pair (j, l):

    (i) If $\Pr(\pi_T(d_{1,j}, d_{2,l}) < \bar{\pi}_T | \mathcal{D}) > c_e$, the dose pair for treating the next cohort of patients is chosen from an adjacent dose combination $\{(j+1, l), (j+1, l-1), (j-1, l+1), \text{ or } (j, l+1)\}$, having Toxicity probability higher than the current dose pair and closest to $\bar{\pi}_T$. If the current dose combination is (J, L), the dose pair stays at the same levels.

    (ii) If $\Pr(\pi_T(d_{1,j}, d_{2,l}) < \bar{\pi}_T | \mathcal{D}) < c_d$, the dose pair for treating the next cohort of patients is chosen from an adjacent dose combination chosen from $\{(j-1, l), (j-1, l+1), (j+1, l-1), (j, l-1)\}$, having Toxicity probability lower than the current pair and closest to $\bar{\pi}_T$. If the current dose combination is $(1, 1)$, the trial is terminated.

    (iii) Otherwise, the next cohort is treated at the current dose combination.

3. Repeat step 2 until the stage I maximum sample size, N_1, is reached.

At the end of stage I, the admissible dose set $\mathcal{A}$ is defined as the dose combinations satisfying $\Pr(\pi_T(d_{1,j}, d_{2,l}) < \bar{\pi}_T | \mathcal{D}) > p_T$, where p_T is a fixed probability cut-off. As usual, the cut-offs c_e, c_d and p_T should be calibrated through simulation to obtain desirable operating characteristics. Although the main purpose of stage I is to identify a set of admissible doses satisfying the safety requirements, Efficacy data also are collected for the N_1 patients.

Stage II is conducted to find the optimal dose combination in $\mathcal{A}$ based on both Efficacy and Toxicity. AR is used in stage II to avoid getting stuck at a suboptimal dose pair. If $\mathcal{A}$ contains S admissible dose pairs, denote their Efficacy probabilities by $(\pi_{E,1}, \cdots, \pi_{E,S})$. Assume that, among n_s patients treated in treatment arm (or dose pair) s, o_s subjects have experienced Efficacy. We assume the following Bayesian hierarchical model for Efficacy to borrow information across multiple treatment arms or doses:

$$\begin{aligned}
o_s | \pi_{E,s} &\sim Binom(n_s, \pi_{E,s}) & (8.2) \\
\pi_{E,s} &\sim Beta(\zeta, \xi) \\
\zeta &\sim Ga(0.01, 0.01) \\
\xi &\sim Ga(0.01, 0.01)
\end{aligned}$$

where $Binom(n, p)$ denotes a binomial distribution, and $Beta(\zeta, \xi)$ denotes a beta distribution with shape parameter ζ and scale parameter ξ. The posterior full conditional distribution of p_s is $Beta(\zeta + o_s, \xi + n_s - o_s)$, but the posteriors of ζ and ξ do not have closed forms.

A common practice is to make the AR probability proportional to the estimated response rate of each arm/dose, for example, using the posterior means of $\pi_{E,s}$ for $s = 1, \cdots, S$. However, such an AR scheme does not account for the variability of the estimated response rates. For example, the estimated response rates of arms 1 and 2, say $\hat{\pi}_{E,1} = 0.5$ and $\hat{\pi}_{E,2} = 0.6$, should not play a dominant role in patient assignment, because more data are needed to confirm that arm 2 is truly superior to arm 1. Thus, in addition to point estimates of the $\pi_{E,s}$'s, their variance estimates also are critical when determining AR probabilities.

To address this issue, Huang et al. (2007) used one study treatment arm as the reference, say the first treatment arm, and randomized patients based on $R_s = \Pr(\pi_{E,s} > \pi_{E,1} | \mathcal{D})$ for $s > 1$ while setting $R_1 = 0.5$. For convenience, we refer to this method as fixed-reference adaptive randomization (FRAR), since each arm is compared with the same fixed reference to determine AR probabilities. Unfortunately, FRAR cannot fully resolve the problem described above. For example, in a three-arm trial if $\pi_{E,1}$ is low but $\pi_{E,2}$ and $\pi_{E,3}$ are high, say $\pi_{E,1} = 0.1$, $\pi_{E,2} = 0.4$ and $\pi_{E,3} = 0.6$, FRAR may have difficulty distinguishing arm 2 and arm 3, because both R_2 and R_3 would be very close to 1. Even with a sufficient amount of data to support the finding that arm 3 is the best treatment, the probabilities of assigning a patient to arms 2 or 3 still are close. This reveals one limitation of FRAR that is due to the use of a fixed reference. The reference (arm 1) is adequate to distinguish arm 1 from arms 2 and 3, but it may not be helpful to compare arms 2 and 3. In addition, because $R_1 = 0.5$, no matter how inefficacious arm 1 is, it has an assignment probability of at least 1/5, if we use $R_1/(R_1 + R_2 + R_3)$ as the randomization probability to arm 1. Even worse, in the case of a two-arm trial with $\pi_{E,1} = 0.1$, and $\pi_{E,2} = 0.6$, arm 1 has a lower bound of the assignment probability 1/3, which is true even if $\pi_{E,1} = 0$ and $\pi_{E,2} = 1$. This illustrates another limitation of FRAR that is due to the use of one arm as the reference for comparison. Moreover, the performance of FRAR depends on the chosen reference, with different reference arms leading to different randomization probabilities.

The following Bayesian moving-reference adaptive randomization (MRAR) method addresses these issues. MRAR accounts for both the magnitude and uncertainty of the estimates of the $\pi_{E,s}$'s. Unlike FRAR, the reference in MRAR is adaptive and varies according to the set of treatment arms under consideration. One important feature of MRAR is that the set of treatments in comparison is continuously reduced, because once an arm has been assigned a randomization probability, it will be removed from the comparison set. Assigning AR probabilities to treatment arms on a one-by-one basis provides a reliable basis for distinguishing between different treatments. Based on the posterior samples of the $\pi_{E,s}$, we diagram the Bayesian MRAR in Figure 8.1 and describe it as follows.

1. Let $\bar{\mathcal{S}}$ and $\mathcal{S}$ denote the sets of indices of the treatment arms that have and have not been assigned randomization probabilities, respectively. Start with $\bar{\mathcal{S}} = \{\cdot\}$ an empty set, and $\mathcal{S} = \{1, 2, \cdots, S\}$.

2. Compute the mean response rate for the arms belonging to the set $\mathcal{S}$, $\bar{\pi}_E = \sum_{s \in \mathcal{S}} \pi_{E,s}/|\mathcal{S}|$, and use $\bar{\pi}_E$ as the reference to determine $R_s = \Pr(\pi_{E,s} > \bar{\pi}_E | \mathcal{D})$, for $s \in \mathcal{S}$. Identify the arm s^* with smallest R_s, i.e., $R_{s^*} = \min_{s \in \mathcal{S}} R_s$.

3. Assign arm s^* randomization probability ω_{s^*},

$$\omega_{s^*} = \frac{R_{s^*}}{\sum_{s \in \mathcal{S}} R_s} \left(1 - \sum_{s' \in \bar{\mathcal{S}}} \omega_{s'} \right),$$

and update $\mathcal{S}$ and $\bar{\mathcal{S}}$ by moving arm s^* from $\mathcal{S}$ into $\bar{\mathcal{S}}$. Note that ω_{s^*} is the fraction of the remaining probability $1 - \sum_{s' \in \bar{\mathcal{S}}} \omega_{s'}$ because the assignment probability $\sum_{s' \in \bar{\mathcal{S}}} \omega_{s'}$ has already been "spent" in the previous steps.

4. Repeat steps 2 and 3, and keep spending the rest of the randomization probability until all of the arms are assigned randomization probabilities, $(\omega_1, \cdots, \omega_S)$, and then randomize the next cohort of patients to the sth arm with probability ω_s.

The proposed MRAR scheme has a desirable limiting property as given below.

Theorem 8.1.1 *In a randomized trial with L treatments, asymptotically, MRAR assigns patients to the most efficacious arm with a limiting probability of 1.*

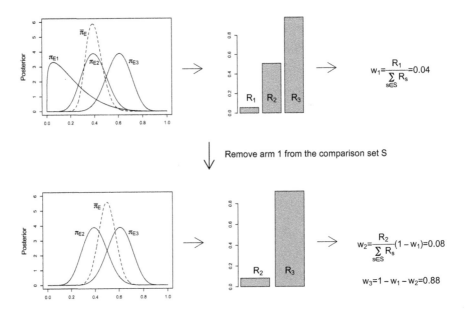

FIGURE 8.1: Diagram of moving-reference adaptive randomization for a three-arm trial. The top panels, from left to right, show that posterior distributions of $\pi_{E,1}, \pi_{E,2}, \pi_{E,3}$ and $\bar{\pi}_E$ first are computed; then $R_s = \Pr(\pi_{E,s} > \bar{\pi}_E | \mathcal{D})$ is calculated for $s = 1, 2, 3$. The arm with the smallest value of R_s (i.e., arm 1) is assigned randomization probability w_1. After spending w_1, arm 1 is removed from the comparison set and the remaining randomization probability is distributed to the remaining arms (i.e, arms 2 and 3) in a similar manner, as demonstrated in the bottom panels.

After stage I is completed and the admissible dose set $\mathcal{A}$ is identified, stage II is conducted, using the following dose finding algorithm. Let π_E be the fixed lower Efficacy bound on $\pi_{E,s}$, and p_E the fixed probability cutoff.

1. Randomize each new cohort of patients to the S dose pairs in $\mathcal{A}$ using MRAR.

2. At any point of the trial, given observed data $\mathcal{D}$, if

$$\Pr(\pi_{T,s} < \bar{\pi}_T | \mathcal{D}) < p_T \quad \text{(overly toxic)},$$

or

$$\Pr(\pi_{E,s} > \underline{\pi}_E | \mathcal{D}) < p_E \quad \text{(inefficacious)},$$

dose s will be closed and not eligible for treating patients, for $s = 1, \cdots, S$. Because data accumulate along the trial, a dose closed at a certain time point may be reopened subsequently if the updated data indicate that the dose is safe and not inefficacious.

3. Once the maximum stage II sample size, N_2, is reached, the dose combination with highest posterior mean of Efficacy is selected as the optimal one.

In the design, response is assumed to be observable quickly so that each incoming patient can be randomized immediately based on the Efficacy outcomes of previously treated patients. This assumption can be partially relaxed by using a group sequential AR approach, if response is delayed. Group sequential AR updates the AR probabilities after each groups' outcomes become available, rather than after each individual outcome (Jennison and Turnbull, 1999). Therefore, within groups, patients can be enrolled continuously, but between groups, one still must suspend accrual and wait for enrolled patients' data to mature before enrolling the next new group of patients. A more systematic, and more preferable approach to handling delayed Efficacy outcomes that does not require suspending patient accrual is provided in Chapter 5.

The above phase I–II design is suitable for trials with a small number of dose combinations, because all dose combinations satisfying the safety threshold would be taken to phase II. If a trial starts with a large number of dose combinations, many more doses could go to phase II, possibly some with Toxicity much lower than the upper bound. From a practical point of view, one could tighten the admissibility criteria by choosing only those satisfying the condition

$$\Pr\{\pi_T(d_{1,j}, d_{2,l}) \in (\bar{\pi}_T - \delta, \bar{\pi}_T) | \mathcal{D}\} > p_T,$$

where δ is a prespecified margin. That is, one moves combinations to stage II that have Toxicity close to and lower than the upper limit $\bar{\pi}_T$.

As an illustrative application, consider a cancer clinical trial at M. D. Anderson Cancer Center for patients diagnosed with malignant melanoma. The experimental agents to be combined were decitabine, a DNA methyltransferase inhibitor that has shown clinical activity in patients with leukemia or myelodysplastic syndrome, and a derivative of recombinant interferon which has been used to treat cancer patients with advanced solid tumors. The primary objective was to find the most effective, safe dose pairs of the two drugs when used in combination. The trial examined three doses of decitabine (drug A) and two doses of the derivative of recombinant interferon (drug B). Toxicity was defined as any grade 3 or 4 non-hematologic Toxicity, grade 4 thrombocytopenia, or grade 4 neutropenia lasting more than 2 weeks or associated with infection. Efficacy was defined as partial or complete response. The Toxicity upper limit was $\bar{\pi}_T = 0.33$, and the Efficacy lower limit was $\underline{\pi}_E = 0.2$. The maximum sample size was 80, with $N_1 = 20$ for stage I, and $N_2 = 60$ for stage II. In the copula-type Toxicity model, the prior Toxicity probabilities of drug 1 were $x_1 = (0.05, 0.1, 0.2)$, and those of drug 2 were $x_2 = (0.1, 0.2)$. We elicited prior distributions $Ga(0.5, 0.5)$ for α and β, and $Ga(0.1, 0.1)$ for γ.

In this trial, it took up to 2 weeks to assess both Y_E and Y_T, and the accrual rate was 2 patients per month. Thus, no accrual suspension was needed to wait for patients' responses in order to assign doses to new patients, and the AR was feasible. It took approximately 10 months to conduct the stage I portion and 30 months to complete the stage II portion of the trial. We used $c_e = 0.8$ and $c_d = 0.45$ to direct dose escalation and de-escalation, and $p_T = 0.45$ and $p_E = 0.1$ to define the admissible doses. The decisions on dose assignment and AR were made after observing the outcomes of every individual patient.

Operating characteristics of the design are given in Table 8.1. In each

TABLE 8.1: Selection probability and number of patients treated at each dose combination, with the target dose combinations in boldface

	Drug A						Simulation results					
Drug	True Pr(Toxicity)			True Pr(Efficacy)			Selection			Number of		
B	1	2	3	1	2	3	percentage			patients		
						Scenario 1						
2	0.1	0.15	0.45	0.2	0.4	0.6	1.0	25.2	18.3	8.8	17.0	15.3
1	0.05	0.15	**0.2**	0.1	0.3	**0.5**	0.0	10.7	**42.8**	8.5	11.3	**18.0**
						Scenario 2						
2	0.1	**0.2**	0.5	0.2	**0.4**	0.55	4.0	**44.5**	2.8	11.3	**21.2**	8.1
1	0.05	0.15	0.4	0.1	0.3	0.5	0.3	24.0	19.2	9.7	15.8	11.4
						Scenario 3						
2	0.1	0.15	**0.2**	0.2	0.3	**0.5**	1.7	7.0	**67.1**	8.3	10.9	**31.3**
1	0.05	0.1	0.15	0.1	0.2	0.4	0.0	1.9	19.8	8.2	7.9	11.9
						Scenario 4						
2	0.1	0.4	0.6	0.3	0.5	0.6	16.3	25.4	0.2	16.1	15.1	3.7
1	0.05	**0.2**	0.5	0.2	**0.4**	0.55	3.9	**46.2**	3.1	14.2	**22.3**	5.7

scenario, the target dose-combination is defined as that maximizing Efficacy

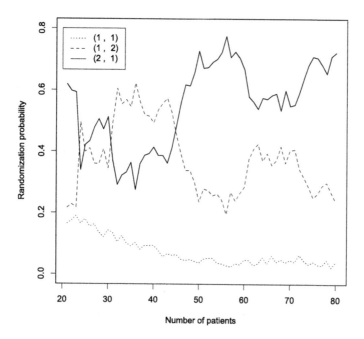

FIGURE 8.2: Adaptive randomization probabilities for the three admissible dose combinations in the melanoma clinical trial.

in $\mathcal{A}$. We present the selection percentages and the numbers of patients treated at each dose combination. Scenarios 1–4 represent common cases in which both $\pi_E(d)$ and $\pi_T(d)$ increase with d, with target doses located differently in the two-dimensional space. The target dose pair is $(3, 1)$ in Scenario 1, and $(2, 2)$ in Scenario 2, which not only had the highest selection probability, but also was the arm to which most of the patients were randomized. In Scenario 3, the target dose is the combination of the highest doses of drug A and drug B, for which the selection probability was close to 70%, and more than 30 patients were treated at the most efficacious dose. In Scenario 4, the design had a high selection probability of selecting the target dose pair.

To illustrate the performance of stage I of the design, Table 8.2 displays the selection percentages for the admissible set, and the average number of admissible doses, $\bar{S}$, at the end of stage I. In most of the cases, the selection percentages of the admissible doses were higher than 90%, and the average number of admissible doses was close to the true value. For example, in Scenario 1, the true number of admissible doses is 5, and the design, on average, selected 5.4 admissible doses for further study in phase II.

TABLE 8.2: Selection percentage of each dose combination to the admissible set and the average size of the admissible set (i.e., $\bar{S}$) in Stage I. The true admissible doses are given in the box

% of admissible		$\bar{S}$	% of admissible		$\bar{S}$
Scenario 1			Scenario 2		
97.8 95.2	67.9	5.4	97.9 92.2	38.2	4.9
98.1 98.0	91.9		98.8 98.2	72.6	
Scenario 3			Scenario 4		
99.6 99.0 91.8		5.9	93.3	75.9 14.6	4.2
99.7 99.7 98.3			96.5 94.9	52.1	

The trial played out as follows. After 20 patients had been treated in stage I, three dose combinations $(1, 1)$, $(2, 1)$ and $(1, 2)$ were identified as admissible and carried forward to stage II for further evaluation of Efficacy. During Stage II, the MRAR procedure was used to allocate the remaining 60 patients to the three dose combinations. Figure 8.2 displays the adaptively changing randomization probabilities for the three treatment arms as the trial proceeded. In particular, the randomization probability of $(2, 1)$ first decreased, and then increased. That of $(1, 2)$ first increased and then decreased, and that of $(1, 1)$ kept decreasing as the trial progressed. At the end of the trial, the dose combination $(2, 1)$ was selected as most desirable, with the highest estimated Efficacy rate of 0.36.

The problem of optimizing the doses of a two-agent combination based on bivariate binary (Y_E, Y_T) outcomes also has been addressed by Wages and Conaway (2014). They take a different approach based on partial orderings of the two-dimensional dose domain.

8.2   Bivariate Ordinal Outcomes

For two ordinal outcomes, let $Y_T = \{0, 1, \cdots, L_T\}$ be indices of the Toxicity outcomes, corresponding to increasing levels of severity, and let $Y_E = \{0, 1, \cdots, L_E\}$ be the Efficacy outcome indices corresponding to increasing desirability. The first two-agent combination dose-finding design for bivariate ordinal outcomes that we will discuss accounts for the possibility that Y_E may not be evaluated. This is done by defining $\epsilon = I(Y_E$ is evaluated), with $\zeta = \Pr(\epsilon = 1)$. For example, in some trials severe Toxicity may preclude evaluation of Y_E. Thus, the outcome pair $Y = (Y_E, Y_T)$ is observed if $\epsilon = 1$, but only Y_T is observed if $\epsilon = 0$. For dose pair $d = (d_{1.j}, d_{2,l})$, denote the joint pdf by $\pi(y \mid d, \theta) = \Pr(Y = y \mid \epsilon = 1, d, \theta)$, and denote the marginal of Y_k by $\pi_k(y_k, d, \theta) = \Pr(Y_k = y_k \mid d, \theta)$. Assuming that ϵ does not affect the marginal distribution of Toxicity, $\pi_T(y_T, d, \theta) = \Pr(Y_T = y_T \mid \epsilon, d, \theta)$. Denoting $\delta(y) = I(Y = y)$ if $\epsilon = 1$ and $\delta_T(y_T) = I(Y_T = y_T)$, the likelihood is

$$\mathcal{L}(Y, Z \mid d, \theta) = \left[\zeta \prod_y \{\pi(y \mid d, \theta)\}^{\delta(y)} \right]^\epsilon \left[(1-\zeta) \prod_{y_T} \{\pi_T(y_T, d, \theta)\}^{\delta_T(y_T)} \right]^{1-\epsilon}.$$

$$(8.3)$$

8.2.1   Generalized Continuation Ratio Model

We define a generalized continuation ratio (GCR) model in terms of the conditional probabilities

$$\gamma_k(y, d, \theta_k) = \Pr(Y_k \geq y \mid Y_k \geq y - 1, d, \theta_k). \qquad (8.4)$$

The marginal probabilities are denoted by

$$\pi_k(y, d, \theta_k) = \Pr(Y_k = y \mid d, \theta_k)$$

and

$$\pi_k^+(y, d, \theta_k) = \Pr(Y_k \geq y \mid d, \theta_k).$$

For a given link function g and linear term $\eta(y, d, \theta_k)$, a GCR model may be obtained by first defining

$$\gamma_k(y, d, \theta_k) = g^{-1}\{\eta(y, d), \theta_k\}.$$

The marginal probabilities then take the forms

$$\pi_k(0, d, \theta_k) = 1 - \gamma_k(1, d, \theta_k)$$

$$\pi_k(y, d, \theta_k) = \{1 - \gamma_k(y+1, d, \theta_k)\} \prod_{r=1}^{y} \gamma_k(r, , \theta_k), \qquad y = 1, \cdots, L_k,$$

$$\pi_k^+(y, d, \theta_k) = \prod_{r=1}^{y} \gamma_k(r, d, \theta_k), \quad y = 1, \cdots, L_k.$$

Since

$$P(Y_k \geq y \mid Y_k \geq y - 1, d, \theta_k) = 1 - \frac{P(Y_k = y - 1 \mid d, \theta_k)}{P(Y_k \geq y - 1 \mid d, \theta_k)},$$

the GCR model may be specified equivalently by the equations

$$\frac{\Pr(Y_k = y \mid d, \theta_k)}{\Pr(Y_k \geq y \mid d, \theta_k)} = 1 - \gamma_k(y+1, d, \theta_k), \qquad y = 0, \cdots, L_k - 1.$$

This model generalizes the continuation ratio (CR) model (Fienberg, 1980, Cox, 1988).

8.2.2 Generalized Aranda–Ordaz Link Model

The parametric link function given by Aranda–Ordaz (AO) (1981) defines a probability p in terms of a real-valued linear term η and parameter $\phi > 0$ by the equation

$$p = 1 - (1 + \phi e^\eta)^{-1/\lambda}. \tag{8.5}$$

The AO link gives a very flexible model for p as a function of η, with $\lambda = 1$ corresponding to the logit link and the complementary log-log link obtained as a limiting case, since $\lim_{\lambda \to 0} p(\eta(d, \alpha), \lambda) = 1 - \exp\{-e^{\eta(d,\alpha)}\}$. In the AO model with linear term formulated in terms of log dose, $\eta(d, \alpha) = \alpha_0 + \alpha_1 \log(d)$, if $d = 0$, then $p = 0$, which says that the outcome is impossible if no treatment is given. If, instead, $\eta(d, \alpha) = \alpha_0 + \alpha_1 d$, then $d = 0$ implies that

$$p\{\eta(0, \alpha), \lambda\} = 1 - (1 + \lambda e^{\alpha_0})^{-1/\lambda}.$$

For example, if p is the probability of Toxicity, then this says that even with no treatment there is a non-zero baseline Toxicity probability, possibly due to other agents given at fixed doses in combination with the agent whose dose d is varied.

A generalization of the AO link function to account for the joint effects of the two doses $d = (d_1, d_2)$ on each entry of Y, with each marginal distribution modeled as a function of d, is given in Houede et al. (2010). This generalized AO model accounts for effects of the two-agent dose pair $d = (d_1, d_2)$ by including two linear terms, $\eta_a = \eta_a(d_a, \alpha_a)$ for agents $a = 1, 2$. The generalized AO (GAO) model probability function is

$$\xi\{\eta_1, \eta_2, \lambda, \gamma\} = 1 - \{1 + \lambda(e^{\eta_1} + e^{\eta_2} + \gamma e^{\eta_1 + \eta_2})\}^{-1/\lambda}. \quad (8.6)$$

In this extended model, γ parameterizes interaction between the two agents. Values of $\gamma > 0$ ensure that p is a probability, and $0 > \gamma > -(e^{-\eta_1} + e^{-\eta_2})$ for all α allows a negative interaction.

Marginals for Y_E and Y_T are determined by first defining agent-specific linear terms and then incorporating them into a GAO model for $\gamma_k(y_k) = \Pr(Y_k \geq y_k \mid Y_k \geq y_k - 1)$. We assume that, for each outcome $k = E, T$, agent $a = 1, 2$ at dose d_a, and outcome $y = 1, ..., L_k$, the linear terms of the marginal distribution of Y_k are

$$\eta_k^{(a)}(y_k, d_a, \alpha_k^{(a)}) = \alpha_{k,y_k,0}^{(a)} + \alpha_{k,y_k,1}^{(a)} d_a. \quad (8.7)$$

Thus, $\alpha_{k,y_k,0}^{(1)}$, $\alpha_{k,y_k,0}^{(2)}$ are intercepts and $\alpha_{k,y_k,1}^{(1)}$, $\alpha_{k,y_k,1}^{(2)}$ are dose effects (slopes). To stabilize variances, each d_j is centered at the mean of its possible values. Denoting $\alpha_k^{(a)} = (\alpha_{k,1,0}^{(a)}, \alpha_{k,1,1}^{(a)}, \alpha_{k,2,0}^{(a)}, \alpha_{k,2,1}^{(a)})$, the marginal of Y_k is parameterized by the 10-dimensional vector $\theta_k = (\alpha_k^{(1)}, \alpha_k^{(2)}, \lambda_k, \gamma_k)$. The linear terms are incorporated into the marginals by assuming that, for each $y = 1, ..., L_k$,

$$\begin{aligned}
\gamma_k(y_k, d, \theta_k) &= \Pr(Y_k \geq y_k \mid Y_k \geq y_k - 1, d, \theta_k) \\
&= \xi\{\eta_k^{(1)}(y_k, d_1, \alpha_k^{(1)}), \eta_k^{(2)}(y_k, d_2, \alpha_k^{(2)}), \lambda_k, \gamma_k\},
\end{aligned}$$

which we denote for brevity by $\xi_k(y_k, d, \theta_k)$. The marginal probabilities take the form

$$\pi_k(y_k, d, \theta_k) = \{1 - \xi_k(y_k + 1, d, \theta_k)\} \prod_{r=1}^{y_k} \xi_k(r, d, \theta_k), \quad (8.8)$$

for all $y_k \geq 1$, with $\pi_k(0, d, \theta_k) = 1 - \xi_k(1, d, \theta_k)$. We will refer to this as the GCR-GAO model.

A joint distribution for Y is obtained using a Gaussian copula. Let Φ_r denote the cdf of a bivariate standard normal distribution with correlation R_{select}, and let Φ denote the univariate standard normal cdf. A Gaussian copula (Nelsen, 2006) is defined by

$$C_r(u, v) = \Phi_r\{\Phi^{-1}(u), \Phi^{-1}(v)\} \qquad \text{for} \quad 0 \leq u, v \leq 1. \quad (8.9)$$

In the three-level ordinal outcome setting of the application we will consider below, this copula structure is applied by noting first that the cdf of an ordinal outcome with support $\mathcal{Y}_k = \{0, 1, 2\}$ is

$$F_k(y_k \mid d, \theta_k) = \begin{cases} 0 & \text{if } y_k < 0 \\ 1 - \pi_k(1, d, \theta_k) - \pi_k(2, d, \theta_k) & \text{if } 0 \leq y_k < 1 \\ 1 - \pi_k(2, d, \theta_k) & \text{if } 1 \leq y < 2 \\ 1 & \text{if } y_k \geq 2. \end{cases}$$

This is computed by using the fact that $\pi_k(1, d, \theta_k) + \pi_k(2, d, \theta_k) = \xi_k(1, d, \theta_k)$ and $\pi_k(2, d, \theta_k) = \xi_k(1, d, \theta_k)\xi_k(2, d, \theta_k)$. The joint pdf of Y is then

$$\pi(y \mid d, \theta) \;=\; \sum_{a=1}^{2}\sum_{b=1}^{2}(-1)^{a+b}C_\rho(u_a, v_b) \tag{8.10}$$

where $u_1 = F_1(y_1 \mid d, \theta)$, $v_1 = F_2(y_2 \mid d, \theta)$, $u_2 = F_1(y_1 - 1 \mid d, \theta)$, and $v_2 = F_2(y_2 - 1 \mid d, \theta)$ with u_2, v_2 the left-hand limits of F_k at y_k. The model parameter vector is $\theta = (\theta_1, \theta_2, l)$, and $\dim(\theta) = 21$. Suppressing the arguments (d, θ), expanding this expression gives

$$\begin{aligned}
\pi(y) \;=\;& \Phi_\rho\{\Phi^{-1} \circ F_1(y_1), \; \Phi^{-1} \circ F_2(y_2)\} \\
&- \Phi_\rho\{\Phi^{-1} \circ F_1(y_1 - 1), \; \Phi^{-1} \circ F_2(y_2)\} \\
&- \Phi_\rho\{\Phi^{-1} \circ F_1(y_1), \; \Phi^{-1} \circ F_2(y_2 - 1)\} \\
&+ \Phi_\rho\{\Phi^{-1} \circ F_1(y_1 - 1), \; \Phi^{-1} \circ F_2(y_2 - 1)\}.
\end{aligned}$$

Bivariate probabilities for which one or both of the y_k's equal 0 are slightly simpler since $F_k(-1) = 0$, $\Phi^{-1}(0) = -\infty$ and $\Phi_\rho(x, y) = 0$ if either of its arguments is $-\infty$. Simulations, below, will show that this model works well for 3×3 outcomes. For four or more levels of either Efficacy or Toxicity, however, a more parsimonious modeling scheme is needed. Such a model will be discussed in Section 8.2.2.

For the motivating solid tumor trial, both outcomes are three-level ordinal variables, with $Y_T = 0$ if Toxicity does not occur, 1 if mild or moderate Toxicity occurs, and 2 if severe Toxicity occurs. For Efficacy, $Y_E = 0$ if progressive disease occurs, 1 if the patient has stable disease, and 2 if partial or complete response is achieved. The standardized dose values are $\{-1.5, -0.5, 0.5, 1.5\}$ for d_1 and $\{-1.0, 0, 1.0\}$ for d_2. In the three-level outcome case, the marginal probabilities are

$$\pi_k(1, d, \theta_k) = \xi_k(1, d, \theta_k) \{1 - \xi_k(2, d, \theta_k)\}$$

and

$$\pi_k(2, d, \theta_k) = \xi_k(1, d, \theta_k) \, \xi_k(2, d, \theta_k).$$

Prior means of $\pi_k(1, d, \theta)$ and $\pi_k(2, d, \theta)$ were elicited for each k and dose pair d, given in Table 8.3.

An extension of the least squares method of Thall and Cook (2004) was applied to solve for prior means of the 20 model parameters (θ_1, θ_2). Prior variances were calibrated to obtain a suitably non-informative prior in terms of ESS of the prior of each $\pi_k(y, d, \theta_k)$. This was done by matching means and variances beta priors and solving for the approximate ESS values, as described in Chapter 3. We assumed that the $\alpha_{k,y,r}^{(a)}$'s and γ_k's were normally distributed, that each λ_k was log normal, and that $\rho \sim Unif[-1, +1]$. Setting $\mathrm{var}(\alpha_{k,y,r}^{(a)}) = 100$ and $\mathrm{var}\{\log(\lambda_k)\} = \mathrm{var}(\gamma_k) = 2.25$ gave priors for all $\pi_{k,y}(d, \theta)$'s with

TABLE 8.3: Elicited prior means $\mu_{T,1}(d)^{(e)}, \mu_{T,2}(d)^{(e)}$ of $\pi_k(1, d)$, $\pi_k(2, d)$ for each dose pair $d = (d_1, d_2)$ and outcome $k = E, T$

		d_1			
		1	2	3	4
$d_2 = 1$	T	.70, .02	.70, .03	.70, .04	.70, .06
	E	.45, .25	.45, .25	.50, .27	.55, .30
$d_2 = 2$	T	.80, .04	.80, .05	.80, .06	.80, .08
	E	.50, .33	.50, .33	.55, .35	.60, .38
$d_2 = 3$	T	.85, .10	.85, .11	.85, .12	.82, .15
	E	.50, .33	.50, .33	.55, .35	.60, .38

$0.81 \leq$ ESS ≤ 2.86 with overall mean $\overline{ESS} = 1.45$. Utilities of the elementary outcomes, given in Table 8.4, were elicited using the Delphi method.

As usual, safety rules are included to protect patient safety. The first rule constrains escalation so that untried levels of each agent may not be skipped. In the two-dimensional dose setting, this works as follows. If (d_1, d_2) is the current dose pair, then escalation is allowed to untried pairs $(d_1 + 1, d_2)$, $(d_1, d_2 + 1)$, or $(d_1 + 1, d_2 + 1)$, if these are in the matrix of dose pairs being studied. For example, after the current cohort is treated at $(2,2)$, allowable higher dose pairs for the next cohort are $(3,2)$, $(2,3)$ and $(3,3)$ but not $(4,2)$ or $(4,3)$. There is no constraint on de-escalation. The second safety rule is defined by a stopping rule. Let $\bar{\pi}_{T,2}$ be a fixed upper limit on the probability of the most severe level of Toxicity, $Y_T = 2$. For fixed upper probability cut-off $p_{T,U}$, the trial will be stopped early if

$$\min_d \Pr\{\pi_{T,2}(d, \theta) > \bar{\pi}_{T,2} \mid \mathcal{D}_n\} > p_{T,U}. \tag{8.11}$$

This rule says that the trial will be stopped if, given the current data, there is a high posterior probability for all dose pairs that the most severe level of Toxicity exceeds the pre-specified limit $\bar{\pi}_{1,2}$. In the solid tumor trial, the starting dose pair was $(2,2)$, with each cohort's dose pair chosen to maximize $u(d|data_n)$ subject to the safety rule with $\bar{\pi}_{1,2} = .33$ and $p_{T,U} = .80$.

MCMC with Gibbs sampling (Robert and Cassella, 1999) was used to compute all posterior quantities. The integral $\int \pi(y \mid d, \theta)d\theta$ was computed by generating a series $\theta^{(1)}, \cdots, \theta^{(N)}$ distributed proportionally to the posterior integrand, using the two-level algorithm described in the Appendix of Braun et al. (2007). MCMC convergence was determined by a ratio $< 3\%$ of the Monte Carlo standard error (MCSE) to the standard deviation of the utilities of the four corner dose pairs. For each $\theta^{(i)}$, all linear terms $\eta_{k,y}^{(a)}(\theta^{(i)})$ associated with each agent first were computed. For each outcome $k = 1, 2$ and level $y = 1, 2$, $xi(\eta_{k,y}^{(1)}, \eta_{k,y}^{(2)}, \lambda_k, \gamma_k)$ was evaluated at $\theta^{(i)}$, to obtain $\pi_{k,1}(d, \theta_k^{(i)})$ and

TABLE 8.4: Elicited consensus utilities for outcomes in the solid tumor trial

	$Y_E = 0$ Progressive Disease	$Y_E = 1$ Stable Disease	$Y_E = 2$ Tumor Response
$Y_T = 0$	25	76	100
$Y_T = 1$	10	60	82
$Y_T = 2$	2	40	52

$\pi_{k,2}(d, \theta_k^{(i)})$. The Gaussian copula values were then computed to obtain the joint probabilities $\pi(y \mid d, \theta^{(i)})$ and averaged over the $\theta^{(i)}$'s to obtain the posterior means.

For the simulation study of the design, a maximum sample size of $N = 48$ was chosen based on preliminary simulations examining the design's sensitivity to values of N in the range 36 to 60. Each simulation scenario was determined by true probability values $\{\pi_k^{true}(1,d), \pi_k^{true}(2,d)\}$ for $k = E, T$ and each $d = (d_1, d_2)$, not derived from the assumed model, and true correlation ρ^{true}. Scenario 1 corresponds to the prior. In Scenario 2, the intermediate dose pairs $d = (1,2), (2,2), (3,2)$ have the highest utilities, with $d = (2,2)$ optimal. Scenario 3 has lower Toxicity and higher interactions between the agents compared to Scenario 1. Scenario 4 has the same toxicities as Scenario 1, but antagonistic effects on $\pi_{2,y}^{true}$ between the agents. In Scenario 5 no dose pair is safe, with $.60 \leq \pi_{1,2}^{true}(d) \leq .75$ for all d.

The simulations for Scenarios 1–4 are summarized in Table 8.5. The method performs well in all scenarios, with dose pair selection probabilities following the true utilities and d pairs with $u^{true}(d)$ close to the maximum likely to be chosen. In Scenario 2, the two-dimensional utility surface as a function of $d = (d_1, d_2)$ has a hill shape with largest $u^{true}(d)$ in the middle of the dose domain at $d = (1,2), (2,2)$, and $(3,2)$. The method correctly selects one of these pairs with high probability, and the best pair $(2,2)$ with highest probability. In Scenario 4, the method is very likely to correctly select a high utility dose pair with $d_1 = 1$, in the left column. In Scenario 5, where all pairs were excessively toxic, the method correctly stops the trial early and chooses no dose pair 85% of the time. Additional simulations, given in Houede et al. (2011), showed that R_{select} is insensitive to cohorts size using $c = 1$ versus $c = 3$, and that R_{select} increases with N in all scenarios

As always, prior calibration is critically important. For this design, if a naive, putatively "noninformative" prior is used with all means 0 and prior standard deviations $\sigma(\alpha) = \sigma\{\log(\lambda)\} = \sigma(\gamma) = 1000$, the R_{select} statistic drops substantially, from .81 to .51 under Scenario 1, .85 to .74 under Scenario 2, and .78 to .74 under Scenario 3, but increases from .78 to .89 under Scenario 4. These results show the importance of carefully calibrating the

TABLE 8.5: Simulation results for the GCR-GAO model based design

Scenario	d_2		1	2	3	4	R_{select}
					d_1		
1	3	u^{true}	57.3	56.9	60.4	64.2	0.71
		% Sel	1	2	6	14	
	2	u^{true}	60.5	60.1	63.6	67.4	
		% Sel	4	4	14	29	
	1	u^{true}	54.6	54.2	57.8	61.7	
		% Sel	1	0	2	22	
2	3	u^{true}	47.2	46.2	44.2	42.2	0.81
		% Sel	2	1	2	1	
	2	u^{true}	54.6	65.8	61.8	43.4	
		% Sel	8	44	34	1	
	1	u^{true}	44.6	44.9	45.1	39.1	
		% Sel	3	0	2	1	
3	3	u^{true}	48.6	53.1	59.6	64.9	0.85
		% Sel	1	2	9	23	
	2	u^{true}	43.9	50.8	55.2	63.5	
		% Sel	0	1	4	35	
	1	u^{true}	41.4	48.9	53.4	58.8	
		% Sel	0	0	1	25	
4	3	u^{true}	61.2	51.0	38.0	26.0	0.78
		% Sel	12	2	1	1	
	2	u^{true}	65.4	53.6	45.3	37.3	
		% Sel	19	2	4	4	
	1	u^{true}	73.9	61.9	55.2	44.9	
		% Sel	44	0	1	9	

prior variances, rather than simply choosing large values that appear to be "non-informative."

The method is sensitive to be starting dose pair, (1,1), (2,2), (1,2), or (2,1) under some scenarios, but insensitive to the starting pair under Scenarios 3 and 5. For example, under Scenario 2 starting at (1,1) gives R_{select} = .66 versus R_{select} = .81 when starting at (2,2). For the antagonistic dose effect Scenario 4, starting at (1,1) gives R_{select} = .94 versus R_{select} = .78 when starting at (2,2). So there seems to be a trade-off with regard to choice of starting dose pair.

A computer program named "U2OET" for implementing this methodology is available from the website https://biostatistics.mdanderson.org/SoftwareDownload/.

8.2.3   An mTOR Inhibitor Chemo Combination Trial

The following model and design were motivated by a phase I–II trial of a three agent combination for treating advanced solid tumors with mTOR abnormalities. The investigative treatment was a molecule (M) designed to inhibit the protein kinase complexes mTORC1 and mTORC2, directly targeting the cancer cells by interfering with cell proliferation and survival, among other cancer properties. The molecule was designed to have antiangiogenic properties that deprive the tumor of its blood vessels. The other two treatment components were the common chemotherapeutic agents carboplatin and paclitaxel. Paclitaxel, given weekly, is a known angiogenesis inhibitor, and the property of antiangiogenesis shared by M and weekly paclitaxel motivated this combination regimen. All three drugs also directly target cancer cells through additional, complementary mechanisms. Carboplatin was given at a fixed dose computed based on the patient's age, weight, and kidney function. The doses of the two agents that were varied in the trial thus were d_M = 4, 5, or 6 mg of M given orally each day, and d_P = 40, 60, or 80 mg/m^2 of paclitaxel given IV twice weekly, for a total of nine dose pairs $d = (d_M, d_P)$ to be studied.

Toxicity was defined as an ordinal variable, Y_T, with four possible levels {Mild, Moderate, High, Severe}, represented by the indices 0, 1, 2, 3. Table 8.6 shows that Y_T was defined in terms of the severity grades of many qualitatively different toxicities, with the level of Y_T determined by the highest level of any individual Toxicity experienced by the patient. This sort of detailed structure very often is the case in cancer trials. The process of the oncologist reducing this to a single ordinal categorical Y_T is a non-trivial step in the process.

A possible alternative approach to defining a Toxicity outcome variable in such settings, given by Bekele and Thall (2004), is to ask the physician to assign a numerical severity score to each level of each type of Toxicity. The sum of the scores of all Toxicity types is called the patient's "total Toxicity burden" (TTB). This was used by Bekele and Thall to design a phase I trial with dose-finding based on TTB, using a CRM-like criterion to choose successive doses. The results of this trial were reported by Tseng et al. (2015). A possible

TABLE 8.6: Definition of overall Toxicity levels by individual toxicities. Y_T is scored using the maximum of the individual Toxicity grades

	Overall Toxicity Severity Level (Y_T)			
	Mild	*Moderate*	*High*	*Severe*
Fatigue	Grade 1	Grade 2	Grade 3	Grade 4
Nausea	Grade 1	Grade 2	Grade 3	–
Neuropathy	–	Grade 1	Grade 2	Grade ≥ 3
Hyperglycemia	Grade 2	Grade 3	Grade 4	–
Rash	Grade 1	Grade 2	Grade 3	Grade 4
Diarrhea	Grade 1	Grade 2	Grade 3	Grade 4
Stomatitis	Grade 1	Grade 2	Grade 3	Grade 4
Pneumonitis	Grade 1	Grade 2	Grade 3	Grade 4
Febrile neutropenia	–	–	Grade 3	Grade 4
Other Non-hematologic	Grade 1	Grade 2	Grade 3	Grade 4
Hyperlipidemia	Grade 1	Grade 2	Grade 3	Grade 4
Anemia	Grade 3	Grade 4	–	–
Thrombocytopenia	Grade 2	Grade 3	–	–
Neutropenia	Grade 3	Grade 4	–	–
AST/ALT	Grade 2	Grade 3	Grade 4	–
Blindness	–	–	–	Grade 4
Myocardioal Infarction	–	–	–	Grade 4
Stroke	–	–	–	Grade 4
Regimen-Related Death	–	–	–	Grade 5

extension of this approach that might accommodate a phase I–II setting would be to establish the TTB as described above, and then define Y_T to be an ordinal variable in terms of intervals of TTB values. Given TTB cut-points $0 < t_1 < t_2 < \cdots < t_L$, one could define $Y_T = 0$ for $0 \leq TTB < t_1$, $Y_T = 1$ for $t_1 \leq TTB < t_2$, and so on. Given ordinal Y_E, one then could apply the phase I–II methodology defined here using the pair (Y_E, Y_T).

For the mTOR inhibitor trial, Efficacy was defined as the ordinal variable, Y_E, with possible levels {PD, SD1, SD2, PR/CR}, where PD = [progressive disease] = [> 20% increase in tumor size], SD1 = [stable disease level 1] = [0 to 20% increase in tumor size], SD2 = [stable disease level 2] = [0 to 30% reduction in tumor size], and PR/CR = [partial or complete response] = [> 30% reduction in tumor size]. These are indexed similarly by $Y_E = 0, 1, 2, 3$. Both Y_E and Y_T were scored within 42 days from the start of treatment. The trial had a maximum of 60 patients, treated in 20 cohorts of size 3, starting at $d = (4, 60)$.

Medically and biologically, this trial was very similar to the trial motivating the phase I–II design of Riviere, Yuan, Dubois, and Zohar (2015), since both trials addressed the problem of finding an optimal dose pair of a targeted agent combined with chemotherapy. Two key differences are that Riviere et al. addressed settings where Toxicity is a binary variable and Efficacy is a time-to-event variable and, assuming a proportional hazards model, the dose-Efficacy curve may increase initially but then reach a plateau. This problem will be discussed in Chapter 9.

Defining Efficacy and Toxicity as ordinal variables with three or more levels is more informative than collapsing categories and defining two binary indicators, such as $Y_E = I(\text{SD2 or PR/CR})$ and $Y_T = I(\text{High or Severe/Very Severe Toxicity})$. However, formulating a probability model and adaptive decision rules that take advantage of a 4×4 bivariate ordinal categorical outcome effectively to choose d in a sequentially adaptive phase I–II trial is very challenging. Even if the completed trial's 60 patients were distributed evenly among the 16 possible $y = (y_E, y_T)$ pairs, there would be only about four patients per outcome. Moreover, because the elementary outcomes are not equally likely for any d, and the dose pairs are assigned sequentially and adaptively, the final distribution of 60 patients among the 144 possible (d, y) combinations will be very unbalanced. Consequently, a dose-outcome model $\pi(y \mid d, \theta)$ must be sufficiently flexible to reflect a wide range of possible functional forms, since it must borrow strength across the many possible (d, y) values. Since there are $(16\text{-}1) \times 9 = 135$ probabilities $\pi(y \mid d, \theta)$, as we have done previously we take the practical approach of modeling the marginals of $[Y_E | d]$ and $[Y_T | d]$ and using a bivariate FGM copula to induce association between Y_E and Y_T. Still, each marginal model must account for four outcome level main effects, two dose effects on each outcome level, and possibly complex dose–dose interactions.

8.2.4   Parametric Dose Standardization

In utility-based phase I–II dose selection, a key issue is modeling the effects of intermediate doses on both π_E and π_T. First consider a single agent phase I–II trial. Given lowest dose d_1 and highest dose d_M, with mean dose $\bar{d}$, it may seem that one may use standardized dose $x = d - \bar{d}$ or $d/\bar{d}$ and reasonably flexible parametric models for $\pi_E(x, \theta)$ and $\pi_T(x, \theta)$ to reflect actual dose-outcome effects. However, for each outcome $k = E$ or T, the actual value of $\pi_k(d_j, \theta)$ may be, approximately, close to $\pi_k(d_1, \theta)$, midway between $\pi_k(d_1, \theta)$ and $\pi_k(d_M, \theta)$, or close to $\pi_k(d_M, \theta)$. A problem arises from the fact that the shapes of the two dose-probability curves $\pi_E(d, \theta)$ and $\pi_T(d, \theta)$ may be very different. Thus, for a given intermediate d_j between d_1 and d_M, its desirabilities in terms of Efficacy and Toxicity may be very different. For example, d_j may have desirably low $\pi_T(d_j, \theta)$ close to $\pi_T(d_1, \theta)$, and low, intermediate, or high $\pi_E(d_j, \theta)$. Since any combination of marginal probabilities is possible, and moreover $\pi_T(d_j, \theta)$ and $\pi_E(d_j, \theta)$ are combined in a highly nonlinear fashion to compute the posterior mean utility $u(d_j, \mathcal{D}_n)$ for making decisions, using a single standardized dose for both outcomes may be inadequate. A difficult and important case is one where an intermediate d_j has $\pi_T(d_j, \theta)$ relatively close to $\pi_T(d_1, \theta)$ and $\pi_E(d_j, \theta)$ relatively close to $\pi_M(d_M, \theta)$, so that d_j is optimal for any reasonable utility function. In this case, if the model does not accurately reflect both $\pi_T(d, \theta)$ and $\pi_E(d, \theta)$ as functions of d, then the utility-based method may not select d_j with sufficiently high probability.

Next, consider a phase I–II combination trial. For each of the two agents, $a = 1, 2$, denote the vector of doses by $d_a = (d_{a,1}, \cdots, d_{a,M_a})$ with mean $\bar{d}_a = (d_{a,1} + \cdots + d_{a,M_a})/M_a$. If one standardizes each dose as $x_{a,j} = d_{a,j} - \bar{d}_a$ or $d_{a,j}/\bar{d}_a$, this will suffer from the same limitations described above in characterizing each individual agent's effect. With two agents given together, the additional problem arises of characterizing the joint effects of the two doses $(d_{1,j}, d_{2,l})$ on both Y_E and Y_T. Conventionally, this is done by adding multiplicative "dose–dose interaction" terms of the general form $\beta_{k,12} x_{a,j} x_{a,l}$ to the linear components of the models for π_E and π_T. Unfortunately, in many settings, the particular functional form

$$\eta_k(d_{1,j}, d_{2,l}, \beta_k) = \beta_{k,0} + \beta_{k,1} x_{1,j} + \beta_{k,2} x_{2,l} + \beta_{k,12} x_{a,j} x_{a,l}$$

for the linear terms may not accurately characterize the actual joint effect of the two doses on each outcome. While the goal is optimal dose pair selection, rather than model fitting *per se*, to achieve this goal reliably a more flexible model may be needed.

This problem motivates the use of two parametrically standardized versions of each dose, one version with parameters corresponding to Efficacy and the other with parameters corresponding to Toxicity. In the phase I–II two-agent combination model presented here, outcome-specific parameters are defined for standardizing each of the two doses. An intermediate dose pair for the two agents is any pair $d = (d_{1,j}, d_{2,l})$ that is not located at one of the four corners of the rectangular dose pair domain, i.e., $1 < j < M_1$ and $1 < l < M_2$. Consequently, the problems described above for a single dose are more complex in that they now are elaborated in terms of the two probability surfaces $\pi_E(d_{1,j}, d_{2,l})$ and $\pi_T(d_{1,j}, d_{2,l})$. Finally, since we will address the case of ordinal-valued Y_E and Y_T, the above probabilities of binary outcomes must be elaborated to accommodate the levels of each outcome.

For two agents and ordinal valued Y_E and Y_T, parametrically standardized doses are defined as follows. For each outcome $k = E, T$ and agent a, the *parametrically standardized dose* is given by the formula

$$d^\lambda_{k,a,j} = \frac{d_{a,1}}{\bar{d}_a} + \left(\frac{d_{a,j} - d_{a,1}}{d_{a,M_a} - d_{a,1}} \right)^{\lambda_{k,a}} \left(\frac{d_{a,M_a} - d_{a,1}}{\bar{d}_a} \right),$$

where all entries of the dose standardization parameter vector $\lambda = (\lambda_{E,1}, \lambda_{E,2}, \lambda_{T,1}, \lambda_{T,2})$ are positive-valued. This gives four parametrically standardized versions of each dose, one for each (agent, outcome) combination, mapping $d_{1,j}$ for agent 1 to $(d^\lambda_{E,1,j}, d^\lambda_{T,1,j})$, $j = 1, \cdots, M_1$ and $d_{2,l}$ for agent 2 to $(d^\lambda_{E,2,l}, d^\lambda_{T,2,l})$, $l = 1, \cdots, M_2$. This formula is a two-agent elaboration of that used by Thall et al. (2013) in the model for a design to optimize dose and schedule of one agent, discussed below in Chapter 11. For each agent a, the lowest and highest standardized doses are $d_{k,a,1}^{\lambda} = d_{a,1}/\bar{d}_a$ and $d_{k,a,M_a}^{\lambda} = d_{a,M_a}/\bar{d}_a$, so the parametrically standardized doses at the lower and upper limits of the dose domain are usual standardized doses, and do not depend on λ or k. These anchor the intermediate doses, $1 < j < M_a$, where the standardization involves λ and k, with $d_{k,a,j}^{\lambda}$ a parametric, outcome-specific modification of the commonly used form $d_{a,j}/\bar{d}_a$, that corresponds to $\lambda_{k,a} \equiv 1$. The motivation for using $d_{k,a,j}^{\lambda}$ rather than $d_{a,j}/\bar{d}_a$ is that exponentiating $(d_{a,j}-d_{a,1})/(d_{a,M_a}-d_{a,1})$ by the model parameter $\lambda_{k,a}$ shifts the intermediate dose $d_{a,j}$ either up toward d_{a,M_a} or down toward $d_{a,1}$. This more accurately represents the actual effect of $d_{a,j}$ on Y_k relative to $d_{a,1}$ and d_{a,M_a}. Since λ is updated along with the other model parameters in the posterior, this provides a data-driven refinement of dose effects on the outcomes that is not obtained using the usual standardized values $d_{a,j}/\bar{d}_a$. We will use the acronym PDS to represent parametric dose standardization.

Each intermediate standardized dose $d_{k,a,j}^{\lambda}$ varies between $d_{a,1}/\bar{d}_a$ and $d_{a,M_a}/\bar{d}_a$, and 1 may be considered the middle numerical value around which the doses vary. A final mapping of each $d_{k,a,j}^{\lambda}$ to either $x_{k,a,j}^{\lambda} = \log(d_{k,a,j}^{\lambda})$ or $x_{k,a,j}^{\lambda} = d_{k,a,j}^{\lambda} - 1$ thus has the same effect as centering covariates at their means in a usual regression model to reduce colinearity. Similarly, to improve numerical stability we define $x_{k,a,j}^{\lambda}$, so that it varies around 0 rather than 1. For $x_{k,a,j}^{\lambda} = \log(d_{k,a,j}^{\lambda})$, this implies that

$$e^{\eta_k(y, x_k^{\lambda}, \theta_k)} = e^{\alpha_{k,y}} (d_{k,1,j}^{\lambda})^{\beta_{k,y,1}} (d_{k,2,j}^{\lambda})^{\beta_{k,y,2}},$$

with $\gamma_k(y, x_k^{\lambda}, \theta_k) = 1/2$ obtained if $\eta_k(y, x_k^{\lambda}, \theta_k) = 0$. In this case,

$$e^{\alpha_{k,y}} (d_{k,1,j}^{\lambda})^{\beta_{k,y,1}} (d_{k,2,j}^{\lambda})^{\beta_{k,y,2}} = 1,$$

and if $d_{k,1,j}^{\lambda} = d_{k,2,j}^{\lambda} = 1$ then $\alpha_{k,y} = 0$. Thus, numerical stability is greatest in this dose pair neighborhood, equivalently for $x_{k,1,j}^{\lambda} = x_{k,2,j}^{\lambda} = 0$ and $\gamma_k(y, x_k^{\lambda}, \theta_k) = 1/2$.

Thall et al. (2016) give a different type of generalized CR model for dose-finding with two agents and bivariate ordinal outcomes. For each marginal, the two-agent linear dose-outcome term is additive in the parametrically standardized doses,

$$\eta_k(y_k, x_k^{\lambda}, \theta_k) = \alpha_{k,y_k} + \beta_{k,y,1}\, x_{k,1,j}^{\lambda} + \beta_{k,y_k,2}\, x_{k,2,l}^{\lambda}$$

for $y_k = 1, \cdots, L_k$, with $\eta_k(0, x_k^{\lambda}, \theta_k) = +\infty$. A generalized CR model is completed by defining the conditional probabilities

$$\gamma_k(y_k, d, \theta_k) = g^{-1}\{\eta_k(y_k, x_k^{\lambda}, \theta_k)\}$$

for link function g and $y_k = 1, \cdots, L_k$, with $\eta_k(L_k+1, x_k^{\lambda}, \theta_k) = -\infty$ to ensure that $\gamma_k(L_k + 1, x_k^\lambda, \theta_k) = 0$. We require $\beta_{k,y_k,1}, \beta_{k,y_k,2} > 0$ for each $y_k \geq 1$ to ensure that the conditional probability $\gamma_k(y_k, x_k^\lambda, \theta_k)$ increases in each dose. Writing $\lambda_k = \{\lambda_{k,1}, \lambda_{k,2}\}$, $\alpha_k = \{\alpha_{k,y_k}, y_k = 1, \cdots, L_k, a = 1, 2\}$ and $\beta_k = \{\beta_{k,y_k,a}, y_k = 1, \cdots, L_k, a = 1, 2\}$, each marginal parameter vector is $\theta_k = (\alpha_k, \beta_k, \lambda_k)$.

Denote the marginal probabilities

$$\pi_k(y_k, x_k^\lambda, \theta_k) = \Pr(Y_k = y_k \mid x_k^\lambda, \theta_k)$$

and

$$\pi_k^+(y_k, x_k^\lambda, \theta_k) = \Pr(Y_k \geq y_k \mid x_k^\lambda, \theta_k).$$

Under this generalized CR model, these probabilities take the forms

$$\pi_k(0, x_k^\lambda, \theta_k) = 1 - \gamma_k(1, x_k^\lambda, \theta_k)$$

$$\pi_k(y_k, x_k^\lambda, \theta_k) = \{1 - \gamma_k(y_k + 1, x_k^\lambda, \theta_k)\} \prod_{r=1}^{y_k} \gamma_k(r, x_k^\lambda, \theta_k), \quad y_k = 1, \cdots, L_k,$$

$$\pi_k^+(y_k, x_k^\lambda, \theta_k) = \prod_{r=1}^{y_k} \gamma_k(r, x_k^\lambda, \theta_k), \quad y_k = 1, \cdots, L_k.$$

Figure 8.3 illustrates possible shapes of the probability surface $\gamma_E(1, d, \theta_E)$ $= \Pr(Y_E \geq 1 | \theta_E, d)$ as a function of the pair $d = $ (Dose of Targeted Agent, Dose of Paclitaxel), for each of four different numerical dose standardization parameter pairs $(\lambda_{E,1}, \lambda_{E,2})$. The surface in the upper left for $\lambda_{E,1} = \lambda_{E,2} = 1$ corresponds to the additive model with linear term

$$\eta_E(1, (d_{1,j}, d_{2,l}), \theta_k) = \alpha_{E,1} + \beta_{E,1,1}\frac{d_{1,j}}{\bar{d}_1} + \beta_{E,1,2}\frac{d_{2,l}}{\bar{d}_2},$$

as a basis for visual comparison. Other probability surfaces as functions of d may be drawn similarly, such as $\gamma_E(y, d, \theta_E)$, $\gamma_T(y, d, \theta_T)$, $\pi_E(y, d, \theta_E)$, or $\pi_T(y, d, \theta_T)$, for $y = 1, 2$, or 3. Figure 8.3 shows that PDS gives a very flexible model for the probabilities that are the basis for the dose-finding design.

To obtain a bivariate distribution for $Y = (Y_E, Y_T)$, the marginals are combined assuming a FGM copula. The joint pmf

$$\pi_{E,T}(y_E, y_T \mid d, \theta) =_{def} \Pr(Y_E = y_E, Y_T = y_T \mid d, \theta)$$

of Y is obtained in terms of the marginal cdfs

$$F_k(y_k \mid d, \theta_k) = \Pr(Y_k \leq y_k \mid d, \theta_k) = 1 - \pi_k^+(y_k + 1, x_k^\lambda),$$

for $y_k = 0, \cdots, L_k - 1$ and $k = E, T$, using the same formulae as in Section 8.2.1, but assuming a FGM copula

$$C_\rho(u, v) = uv\{1 + \rho(1 - u)(1 - v)\}, \quad 0 \leq u, v \leq 1,$$

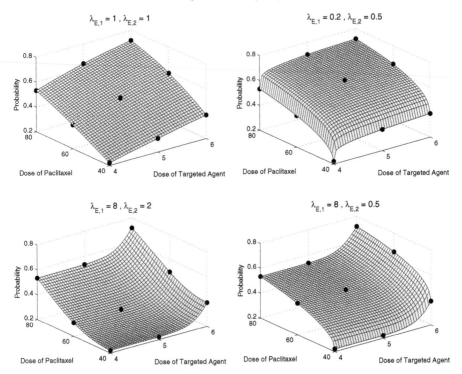

FIGURE 8.3: Illustration of $\gamma(1, \theta_E, d)$ as a function of dose pair and four different values of the dose standardization parameters $(\lambda_{E,1}, \lambda_{E,2})$.

for $-1 \le \rho \le +1$. Collecting terms, for $k = E, T$, $y = 1, 2, 3$, and $a = 1, 2$, the model parameters are $\lambda = \{\lambda_{k,a}\}$ for PDS, the intercepts $\alpha = \{\alpha_{k,y}\}$, the dose effects $\beta = \{\beta_{k,y,a}\}$, and the copula's association parameter ρ. Thus $\theta = (\lambda, \alpha, \beta, \phi, \rho)$.

To enhance robustness, Thall et al. (2016) assume an AO link function for each marginal,

$$\gamma_k(y_k, x_k^\lambda, \theta_k) = 1 - \left[1 + \phi_k\, e^{\eta_k(y_k, x_k^\lambda, \theta_k)}\right]^{-1/\phi_k},$$

which adds the two link parameters $\phi = (\phi_E, \phi_T)$ to θ. The combined acronym GCR-PDS-AO will be used to refer to this model, in order to keep track of the marginal probability model, form of the linear terms, and link function.

Normal priors were assumed for all real-valued parameters $\{\alpha_{k,y_k}\}$ and $\{\beta_{k,12}\}$. The positive-valued dose main effect coefficients $\{\beta_{k,y_k,a}\}$ were assumed to follow normal priors truncated below at 0, with copula parameter $\rho \sim U[-1, +1]$. Each $\lambda_{k,a}$ and the AO link parameters ϕ_k were assumed to be lognormal. Prior means were estimated from the elicited probabilities using the pseudo sampling method, with prior variances calibrated to give $\overline{ESS} = .09$.

TABLE 8.7: Elicited elementary outcome utilities

Toxicity	Disease Status			
	PD	SD1	SD2	CR/PR
Mild	25	55	80	100
Moderate	20	35	70	90
High	10	25	50	70
Severe	0	10	25	40

8.2.5 mTOR Inhibitor Trial Design

The trial's decision criteria were based on the elicited outcome utilities given in Table 8.7. For acceptability criteria, recalling that the Toxicity level indexes are $y_T = 0, 1, 2, 3$ for mild, moderate, high, severe, $\pi_T^+(2 \mid d, \theta)$ is the probability of high or severe Toxicity with d. A dose pair d was *unacceptably toxic* if

$$\Pr\{\pi_T^+(2 \mid d, \theta) > .45 \mid \mathcal{D}_n\} > .90. \tag{8.12}$$

That is, d was considered unsafe if, based on the current data, it was likely that d had a probability of high or severe Toxicity above .45. For the Efficacy rule, similarly indexing the outcomes {PD, SD1, SD2, PR/CR} by $y_E = 0, 1, 2, 3$, $\pi_E^+(2 \mid d, \theta)$ is the probability of SD2 or better with dose pair d. A dose pair d was considered *unacceptably inefficacious* if

$$\Pr\{\pi_E^+(2 \mid d, \theta) < .40 \mid \mathcal{D}_n\} > .90. \tag{8.13}$$

That is, d was considered inefficacious if, given the current data, it was likely that achieving SD2 or better had probability below .40. The set $\mathcal{A}_n$ of acceptable doses was defined as those satisfying neither 8.12 nor 8.13.

To address the problem of stickiness, the following variant of AR was used. Recall the general form for AR probabilities for dose pair d is based on the posterior mean utilities of all acceptable dose pairs $\mathcal{A}_n$,

$$r_n(d) = \frac{u(d \mid data_n)}{\sum_{d' \in \mathcal{A}_n} u(d' \mid \mathcal{D}_n)}.$$

For the two-agent mTOR inhibitor trial, a refinement of this AR criterion was used that only includes the two empirically best acceptable dose pairs. Let d_n^{second} denotes the dose pair having second largest posterior mean utility among acceptable d. The next cohort of patients is treated with dose pair d_n^{opt} with probability

$$r_n = \frac{u(d_n^{opt} \mid data_n)}{u(d_n^{opt} \mid data_n) + u(d_n^{second} \mid data_n)},$$

and treated with dose pair d_n^{second} with probability $1 - r_n$. This particular AR probability was chosen after studying the design's behavior with similar AR probabilities that included the three best, four best, or all acceptable doses in $\mathcal{A}_n$.

The rules for trial conduct were follows, with $N = 60$, and cohort size 3.

1. Treat the first cohort at $d = (d_M, d_P) = (4, 60)$.

2. For each cohort after the first, compute the posterior decision criteria based on $\mathcal{D}_n$.

3. If no d is acceptable, stop the trial and do not select any d.

4. If one d is acceptable, treat the next cohort at that d.

5. If two or more d's are acceptable and the number of patients treated at d_n^{opt} minus the largest number of patients treated at any other acceptable dose is

    (a) ≥ 3, apply AR to choose between d_n^{opt} and d_n^{second}.
    (b) < 3, treat the next cohort at d_n^{opt}.

The cut-off 3 used in 5a and 5b was chosen, based on preliminary simulations, to allow the method to be greedy until enough information had been obtained at the current d^{opt} to make the posterior AR criterion sufficiently reliable.

The design was simulated under 12 scenarios, each specified in terms of fixed true marginal Efficacy and Toxicity outcome probabilities not based on the design's model, with association induced by assuming a Gaussian copula with true association parameter 0.10. A detailed account of the scenarios is given by Thall et al. (2016). For each case studied, the trial was replicated 3000 times, and all posterior quantities were computed using MCMC with Gibbs sampling. Operating characteristics of the design are given for five selected scenarios in Table 8.8. The results show that, in terms of true utilities and selection percentages of the nine dose pairs, the design does a reliable job of selecting acceptable dose pairs having true mean utility at or near the maximum, while also reliably avoiding unacceptable dose pairs.

A natural question is how the design's performance compares to what would be obtained if a model with conventional multiplicative dose–dose interactions in the linear terms were assumed, instead of using additive parametrically standardized doses. This more conventional model formulation is obtained by setting all $\lambda_{k,a} = 1$ and including a multiplicative dose interaction term in the linear component. In this case, the usual standardized doses $x_{a,j} = \log(d_{a,j}/\bar{d}_a)$ are used, and linear components given by the conventional multiplicative dose–dose interaction form 8.2.4.

Table 8.9 summarizes comparisons of the design's performance conducted using these two alternative models, across all 12 scenarios. In the five scenarios $\{2, 4, 5, 6, 8\}$ where d^{opt} is a middle dose pair, not located at one of the four corners of the 3×3 matrix of d pairs, the model with parametrically standardized doses gives R_{select} values that are 9 to 12 larger than the corresponding values given by the conventional model. In the four scenarios $\{1, 3, 7, 9\}$ where d^{opt} is located at one of the four corners of the matrix of d

TABLE 8.8: Operating characteristics of the mTOR inhibitor trial design under the GCR-PDS-AO model. The true utility and (selection %, number of patients treated) are given for each dose pair (d_M, d_P) in each scenario.

Scenario		$d_P=40$	$d_P=60$	$d_P=80$
1	$d_M=4$	56.0	51.8	48.3
		(32, 9.4)	(25, 14.8)	(9 , 8.4)
	$d_M=5$	51.8	47.2	44.7
		(15, 7.4)	(7 , 6.8)	(2 , 3.2)
	$d_M=6$	48.3	44.7	39.4
		(8 , 6.0)	(2 , 2.6)	(0 , 0.9)
2	$d_M=4$	43.2	44.4	37.9
		(8, 3.5)	(17, 12.2)	(3 , 5.3)
	$d_M=5$	49.7	46.8	38.9
		(28, 8.7)	(24 , 10.5)	(2 , 5.2)
	$d_M=6$	45.5	39.7	33.6
		(10 , 6.7)	(5 , 5.6)	(0 , 1.7)
3	$d_M=4$	38.8	37.9	34.5
		(1, 1.0)	(2, 7.9)	(1 , 3.2)
	$d_M=5$	46.7	45.3	40.8
		(16, 6.5)	(19 , 9.0)	(6 , 7.2)
	$d_M=6$	49.7	47.2	42.7
		(25 , 8.7)	(22 , 9.8)	(5 , 5.9)
5	$d_M=4$	30.4	44.4	44.2
		(1, 1.5)	(16, 12.1)	(12 , 7.4)
	$d_M=5$	44.4	51.3	43.0
		(9, 4.7)	(36 , 12.2)	(7 , 7.6)
	$d_M=6$	44.2	43.0	39.1
		(8 , 4.6)	(7 , 6.9)	(1 , 2.6)
8	$d_M=4$	33.8	45.4	48.2
		(1, 0.8)	(9, 10.0)	(15 , 7.6)
	$d_M=5$	37.2	48,9	53.2
		(2, 2.6)	(21 , 9.7)	(33 , 12.6)
	$d_M=6$	41.3	45.9	45.6
		(3 , 2.5)	(9 , 6.2)	(6 , 7.9)

† The highest utility is given in a box.
‡ Utilities of unacceptable d have a gray background.

TABLE 8.9: Comparative summary statistics for alternative dose-outcome models

		Parametrically Standardized Doses			Multiplicative Dose-Dose Interactions		
Scenario	d^{opt}	R_{select}	R_{treat}	% None	R_{select}	R_{treat}	% None
1	(4,40)	76	65	2	83	69	1
2	(5,40)	77	63	2	67	60	3
3	(6,40)	77	62	3	80	62	4
4	(4,60)	80	69	2	69	65	2
5	(5,60)	77	69	1	65	63	1
6	(6,60)	78	67	7	69	64	6
7	(4,80)	78	70	2	84	73	2
8	(5,80)	78	70	1	68	68	1
9	(6,80)	78	67	2	87	68	2
10[†]	Three	89	85	0	92	86	0
11[‡]	None	–	79	95	–	80	91
12[‡]	None	–	67	96	–	68	94

[†] Acceptable $d = (6, 40), (5, 60), (4, 80)$ all have maximum $u^{true} = 51.4$.
[‡] Scenarios 11 and 12 have no acceptable d.

pairs, the conventional model gives R_{select} values that are larger by 3 to 9. The R_{treat} values also follow this pattern, but with much smaller differences. Scenario 10 corresponds to the prior, and has three acceptable dose pairs all having the same maximum true utility. With either model, the design reliably stops the trial early if no d pairs are acceptable, in Scenarios 11 and 12. It thus appears that using parametrically standardized doses additively may be regarded as insurance against a very large loss in R_{select} for the harder cases where d^{opt} is a middle dose pair, with the price being a smaller loss in R_{select} for the easier cases where d^{opt} is located at a corner of the dose pair domain.

A study of the design's sensitivity to maximum sample size N in the range 30 to 300 showed that the design's OCs improve greatly as N increases. For example, in Scenario 1, for $N = 30, 60, 300$, the corresponding R_{select} values are 67, 76, 95 and the corresponding R_{treat} values are 61, 76, 78. The same pattern is seen for all other scenarios with acceptable dose pairs. Figure 8.4 illustrates the combination trial design's R_{select} value sensitivity to maximum sample size N in the range 60 to 240. Like the similar study in the single dose trial of RT for brain tumors discussed in Chapter 7, the design's reliability increases dramatically with N.

These numerical values suggest that, in cases where an optimal acceptable dose pair exists, R_{select} may converge to 100 for sufficiently large N. In the two Scenarios 11 and 12 with no acceptable d, the simulated probability that no pair is selected is 1 for $N \geq 120$. These results provide an empirical validation

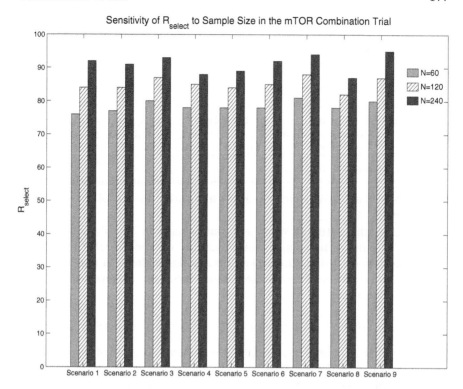

FIGURE 8.4: Sensitivity of R_{select} to N in the mTOR combination trial design.

of the method's consistency, in terms of both optimal dose pair selection and stopping the trial early for futility or safety in cases where this should be done. These numerical results also show that the $N = 60$ cannot reliably achieve R_{select} values of 80 or larger across the scenarios studied, at least in this particular setting, and that $N = 90$ is needed to achieve $R_{select} \geq 80$, with N roughly 200 to 240 if $R_{select} \geq 90$ is desired. More generally, if optimizing the dose pair matters, these results imply that much larger phase I-II combination trials, with $N > 200$, are needed. For phase I-II trials in oncology as they currently are conducted, sample sizes this large seldom are considered feasible. These results suggest that larger sample sizes are worthwhile in such phase I-II studies, especially since d^{opt} may be used as the basis for a subsequent large-scale phase III trial of the two-agent combination.

8.2.6 Alternative Models

Because the generalized CR model links the conditional probability $\gamma_k(y, x_k^\lambda, \theta_k)$ to the linear term $\eta_k(y, x_k^\lambda, \theta_k)$, it has the computational advantage that no order constraints need to be imposed on the intercept parameters

$\alpha_{k,1}, \cdots, \alpha_{k,L_k}$. An alternative model may be defined by

$$\pi_k^+(y, x_k^\lambda, \theta_k) = 1 - \left[1 + \phi_k\, e^{\eta_k(y, x_k^\lambda, \theta_k)}\right]^{-1/\phi_k},$$

which generalizes the proportional odds (PO) model (McCullagh, 1980) by replacing the logit link with the AO link. Aside from the link, because the PO model links the unconditional probability $\pi_k^+(y, x_k^\lambda, \theta_k)$ to the linear term, it requires the order constraints $\alpha_{k,1} > \cdots > \alpha_{k,L_k}$ in order for the probabilities to be well defined. For dose-finding, the need to impose these constraints on each parameter vector $\alpha_k = (\alpha_{k,1}, \cdots, \alpha_{k,L_k})$, $k = E, T$ makes MCMC computations to obtain posteriors much more difficult, especially for small amounts of data. This is an important motivation for use of the generalized CR model.

Several other alternative model formulations can be obtained by changing one or more of its components. A natural question is whether adding a multiplicative dose–dose interaction term to the model with parametric dose standardization would improve the design's behavior. This model would have linear components

$$\eta_k(y, x_k^\lambda, \theta_k) \;=\; \alpha_{k,y} + \beta_{k,y,1}\, x_{k,1,j}^\lambda + \beta_{k,y,2}\, x_{k,2,l}^\lambda + \beta_{k,12} x_{k,1,j}^\lambda x_{k,2,l}^\lambda,$$

and a total of 27 parameters. It may be considered a hybrid of the two models considered previously. Simulations show that, compared to the original model without the interaction term $\beta_{k,12} x_{k,1,j}^\lambda x_{k,2,l}^\lambda$, the hybrid model has R_{select} values 1 to 3 smaller in eight scenarios, 1 to 3 larger in two scenarios, and slightly larger incorrect early stopping probabilities. Thus, on average, this hybrid model produces a design with slightly worse performance.

9

Optimizing Molecularly Targeted Agents

CONTENTS

9.1   Features of Targeted Agents 179
9.2   One Targeted Agent 180
9.3   Combining Targeted and Cytotoxic Agents 186
9.4   Combining Two Molecularly Targeted Agents 195

9.1   Features of Targeted Agents

Recent accelerated development of novel molecularly targeted agents (MTAs) has challenged the conventional phase I $\rightarrow$ phase II paradigm, since the assumption that $\pi_T(x)$ and $\pi_E(x)$ increase with dose x may not hold. MTAs are developed to modulate specific aberrant pathways in cancer cells while sparing normal tissue. Examples include biospecimens targeting a specific tumor pathway, gene products aiming for DNA repair, and immunotherapies stimulating the immune system to attack a tumor.

Because of an MTA's working mechanism, rather than monotonically increasing, the dose-Efficacy curve $\pi_E(x)$ often plateaus at an intermediate dose, e.g., when the agent reaches a saturation level in the body, so further increasing x may not improve Efficacy. For example, the Efficacy of PTK/ZK, an orally active inhibitor of vascular endothelial growth factor receptor tyrosine kinases, does not change with higher dose once it reaches the plateau, of 1000 mg, which is below the MTD. Imatinib, a molecularly targeted agent heralded as a major advance in the treatment of chronic myeloid leukemia (CML) and gastrointestinal stromal tumors, demonstrates similar behavior. Analysis of responses in blood counts over time suggests that doses of 400 to 600 mg of imatinib are on the plateau of a dose-response curve (Druker, 2002). This was confirmed in a meta-analysis (Gafter-Gvili et al., 2011) of phase III randomized trials, in which no difference in outcome was found between imatinib using the 400 mg dose and higher doses.

In some cases, Efficacy of the MTA may even decrease at higher dose levels, showing an umbrella-shaped dose-Efficacy curve (Hoff and Ellis, 2007; Le Tourneau et al., 2009; Korn, 2004; Parulekar and Eisenhauer, 2004; LoRusso et al., 2010). For example, Postel-Vinay et al. (2008) investigated the dose-Efficacy relationship of monotherapy based on 135 patients enrolled in phase I trials at the Royal Marsden Hospital from 5 January 2005 to 6 June 2006. Patients were classified into three cohorts, A, B, and C according to the dose received as a percentage of the MTD (0-33%, 34-65%, >65%). The Efficacy endpoint was non-progression, i.e., complete/partial response or stable disease for at least 3 months. Monotherapy demonstrated a nonmonotonic dose-Efficacy relationship, with non-progression rates for the patients in cohorts A, B, and C of 21%, 50%, and 31%, respectively. That is, the median dose rather than the highest dose (i.e., cohort C) leads to the highest Efficacy.

For MTAs, the goal of a dose finding trial is to identify the *optimal biological dose* (OBD), defined as the lowest x having the highest $\pi_E(x)$, while also safeguarding patients against excessive Toxicity.

The shape of the Toxicity curve $\pi_T(x)$ depends on the particular MTA. In many cases, although it still is reasonable to assume that $\pi_T(x)$ increases with x, the Toxicity of an MTA is expected to be minimal within the therapeutic dose range. For example, FDA guidance points out that cancer vaccine trials using $3 + 3$ designs often fail to identify an MTD, since the $\pi_T(x)$ curve may be so flat that the highest dose that can be administered is limited by manufacturing or anatomic issues, rather than by Toxicity (Guidance for Industry: Clinical Considerations for Therapeutic Cancer Vaccines, U.S. Food and Drug Administration, 2011). For other MTAs, $\pi_T(x)$ may monotonically increase with the dose, similar to conventional cytotoxic agents, or increase at low dose levels and then approximately plateau at higher dose levels within the therapeutic dose range.

When designing dose-finding trials for MTAs, depending on the nature of the associated Toxicity, we distinguish two cases that require different strategies. In the first case, there is strong prior knowledge (e.g., based on preclinical data and biology) that the experimental agent has minimal Toxicity within the therapeutic dose range. Thus, Efficacy should be the main driving force for determining dose escalation. In this case, modeling $\pi_T(x)$ is not needed, and a simple safety monitoring rule can be used to safeguard patients from potentially toxic doses. This is analogous to safety monitoring in conventional phase II trials. The second case is that where there is no adequate prior evidence on the safety of the experimental agent, and it may cause substantial Toxicity. In this case, it is preferable to model $\pi_T(x)$ as well as $\pi_E(x)$ and use a phase I–II design. We will illustrate these approaches in following Sections.

9.2   One Targeted Agent

We first focus on the case where the MTA is expected to have minimal Toxicity, and dose finding is primarily driven by Efficacy. We describe a Toxicity monitoring rule, followed by two methods to find the OBD.

Let $x_1 < \cdots < x_J$ denote standardized doses with mean 0 and standard deviation 0.5, with $\pi_{T,j} = \Pr(Y_T = 1|x_j)$. Let n_j denote an interim sample size of patients assigned to dose x_j, with m_j experiencing Toxicity among the n_j, and o_j experiencing Efficacy. Toxicity of each dose level is modeled independently using a beta-binomial model

$$m_j \sim Binom(n_j, \pi_{T,j})$$
$$\pi_{T,j} \sim Beta(\zeta, \xi)$$

where ζ and ξ are hyperparameters. The posterior of $\pi_{T,j}$ follows a beta distribution

$$[\pi_{T,j}|n_j, m_j] \sim Beta(\zeta + m_j, \xi + n_j - m_j). \tag{9.1}$$

Let $\bar{\pi}_T$ denote the Toxicity upper bound, and define the posterior probability

$$\psi_j = \Pr(\pi_{T,j} > \bar{\pi}_T|n_j, m_j) = 1 - \mathcal{B}(\bar{\pi}_T; \zeta + m_j, \xi + n_j - m_j)$$

where $\mathcal{B}$ denotes the c.d.f. of the beta distribution.

To impose dose-Toxicity monotonicity and borrow information across dose levels, we apply isotonic regression to $\psi_1, \cdots, \psi_J$ using the pool adjacent violators algorithm (PAVA) (Barlow et al., 1972; Robertson et al., 1988), and denote the resulting isotonic estimates as $\{\tilde{\psi}_j\}$. The idea of PAVA is to replace adjacent monotonicity violators by their weighted average, and do this repeatedly until monotonic ordering is obtained. For example, denote the initial estimates $(\psi_1, \cdots, \psi_5) = (0.1, 0.3, 0.2, 0.4, 0.3)$ with equal weights 1. The PAVA algorithm scans $(\psi_1, \cdots, \psi_5)$, identifies the first pair of violators $(\psi_2, \psi_3) = (0.3, 0.2)$ and replaces them by their weighted average 0.25, and updates $(\psi_1, \cdots, \psi_5)$ to $(0.1, 0.25, 0.25, 0.4, 0.3)$. PAVA scans again and identifies the next pair of violators $(\psi_4, \psi_5) = (0.4, 0.3)$. After replacing these violators with their weighted average, PAVA yields the final isotonic estimates $(\tilde{\psi}_1, \cdots, \tilde{\psi}_5) = (0.1, 0.25, 0.25, 0.35, 0.35)$.

To monitor Toxicity, define the admissible dose set

$$\mathcal{A} = \{x_j : \tilde{\psi}_j < p_T, \ j = 1, \ldots, J\}, \tag{9.2}$$

where p_T is a prespecified toxicity probability cutoff. At the start of the trial, all investigational doses should be in $\mathcal{A}$. This can be ensured by choosing the hyperparameters ζ and ξ so that $\mathcal{B}(\bar{\pi}_T; \zeta, \xi) = 1 - p_T + \delta$, where δ is a small positive number, e.g., $\delta = 0.05$. That is, *a priori*, all doses must satisfy the safety rule given in (9.2). Since this single constraint is not enough to determine the values of ζ and ξ, one can add another constraint, such as $\zeta + \xi = 1$, to solve for ζ and ξ.

We now discuss how to find the OBD based on Efficacy, with dose assignments restricted to $\mathcal{A}$. We assume that $\pi_E(x)$ is unimodal in x, i.e., umbrella-shaped, or reaches a plateau within the therapeutic dose range. The methods described below also can handle a conventional monotonic dose-response curve. Although more complicated multimodal dose-Efficacy curves are possible, they rarely occur in practice within the therapeutic dose range and thus will not be considered here. Denote $\pi_{E,j} = \Pr(Y_E = 1|x_j)$. A straightforward approach is to assume a parametric dose-Efficacy model, such as,

$$\text{logit}\,(\pi_{E,j}) = \alpha + \beta x_j + \gamma x_j^2, \quad j = 1, \ldots, J.$$

At each interim decision, given the interim data $\mathcal{D}$, we fit the model, identify the dose that is safe and has highest estimated Efficacy, and then assign the new patient to that dose. This parametric design is simple, but is sensitive to model mis-specifications. See Zang et al. (2014) for details. For this reason, we will not discuss this approach further. Instead, in what follows, we describe two more robust approaches to find the OBD based on the isotonic regression and local regression, respectively.

Various isotonic regression-based designs have been proposed to find the MTD for conventional cytotoxic agents under the assumption that $\pi_T(x)$ increases with x. (Leung and Wang, 2001; Conaway et al., 2004; Yuan and Chappell, 2004). These isotonic designs cannot be used directly to find the OBD because the dose-response curve of MTAs may be non-monotonic. For the MTAs with unimodal or plateaued dose-Efficacy curves, the goal is to find the OBD, the dose level j^* such that

$$\pi_{E,1} \leq \cdots \leq \pi_{E,j^*} \geq \cdots \geq \pi_{E,J}. \tag{9.3}$$

The difficulty is that, before we identify the OBD, the order constraint (9.3) is unknown and thus standard isotonic regression methods (e.g., PAVA algorithm) cannot be applied to estimate $\{\pi_{E,j}\}$ and identify the OBD. One way to overcome this difficulty is to use double-sided isotonic regression (Turner and Wollan, 1997). In this approach, we first enumerate all J possible locations of j^*. Given each location, say $j^* = r$, the isotonic estimates $\{\tilde{\pi}_{E,j}^{(r)}\}$ can be obtained by fitting the following two separate standard isotonic regressions to the interim data:

(1) $\hat{\pi}_{E,1}, \ldots, \hat{\pi}_{E,j^*}$ with the known constraint $\pi_{E,1} \leq \cdots \leq \pi_{E,j^*}$,
(2) $\hat{\pi}_{E,j^*+1}, \ldots \hat{\pi}_{E,J}$ with the known constraint $\pi_{E,j^*+1} \geq \cdots \geq \pi_{E,J}$,

where $\hat{\pi}_{E,j} = o_j/n_j$ is observed efficacy rate. Each of these two isotonic regressions can be done using the PAVA algorithm. After applying this procedure to each of the J possible locations of j^*, we obtain J sets of possible isotonic estimates $\{\tilde{\pi}_{E,j}^{(r)}\}, r = 1, \ldots, J$. We select as the final isotonic estimates $\{\tilde{\pi}_{E,j}\} = \{\tilde{\pi}_{E,j}^{(r^*)}\}$, as that with smallest sum of square error, i.e.,

$$r^* = \text{argmin}_{r \in (1,\ldots,J)} \sum_{j=1}^{J} \left(\tilde{\pi}_{E,j}^{(r)} - \frac{o_j}{n_j}\right)^2.$$

The isotonic design is carried out as follows:

1. Treat the first cohort of patients at the lowest dose x_1, or at the physician-specified starting dose.

2. Determine the admissible set $\mathcal{A}$.

3. Identify the dose level j^* having largest $\tilde{\pi}_{E,j}$ among the tried doses in $\mathcal{A}$. If there are ties, select j^* as the lowest dose level among the ties. Let j denote the current dose level, and j^h denote the highest dose level tried thus far.

   (a) If $j^* > j$, escalate to $j + 1$;

   (b) if $j^* < j$, de-escalate to $j - 1$;

   (c) if $j^* = j = j^h$, escalate to $j + 1$ given that $j + 1$ is in $\mathcal{A}$;

   (d) otherwise, repeat dose level j.

4. Once the maximum sample size N is reached, select the lowest dose having the highest $\tilde{\pi}_{E,j}$ in $\mathcal{A}$ as the OBD.

One limitation of isotonic regression is that it cannot estimate the $\pi_{E,j}$'s for untried doses, at which no patients have been treated. Therefore, during trial conduct, when the dose with the highest estimate of Efficacy is the highest tried dose (i.e., $j^* = j = j^h$), there may be insufficient information to determine whether the maximum of the dose-Efficacy curve has been identified. To overcome this limitation, in the above dose-finding algorithm step 3(c), when $j^* = j = j^h$, we escalate the dose level to further explore the dose-Efficacy curve and search for the maximum, given that the next higher dose level is safe (i.e., within the admissible set $\mathcal{A}$).

The second approach to find the OBD is based on local regression. When the dose-response curve is umbrella-shaped or plateaus, finding the OBD is essentially the problem of finding the mode. This motivates the approach that uses the local gradient (or the first derivative) to guide dose escalation and de-escalation. Under the unimodal assumption, if the local gradient at the current dose is positive, it means that one should escalate to search for the mode. If the gradient at the current dose is negative, one should de-escalate. To do this, let $\mathcal{D}(j) = \{(o_{j'}, n_{j'}), j' = j - l + 1, \cdots, j\}$ denote "local" data collected from the current dose level j up to the previous $l - 1$ dose levels. Fit a local linear logistic model based on $\mathcal{D}(j)$,

$$\text{logit}(\pi_{E,j'}) = \alpha + \beta x_{j'}, \quad j' = j - l + 1, \ldots, j.$$

where $2 \leq l \leq j$. For practical use, we recommend $l = 2$ because increasing l yields similar or worse operating characteristics, based on simulation studies (Zang et al., 2014).

One may question the reliability of parameter estimates for the local logistic model, based on data from 2 doses. For dose finding, the goal is not to obtain precise estimates of model parameters, but rather to identify the local trend, i.e., whether the dose-response curve is increasing or decreasing, for directing dose escalation/de-escalation. As long as the estimates correctly identify the trend of the curve, i.e., the sign of the slope, they lead to appropriate dose escalation and de-escalation decisions. Simulation studies show that using two local doses yields good operating characteristics, suggesting that estimation using local data is adequately stable to identify the local trend of the dose-response curve. To complete the Bayesian model, following Gelman et al. (2008), we specify a Cauchy prior distribution with center 0 and scale 10 for α, i.e., $Cauchy(0, 10)$; and an independent Cauchy prior $Cauchy(0, 2.5)$ for β.

Given the interim data $\mathcal{D}(j)$, the decision of dose escalation/de-escalation is made based on the posterior probability $\Pr(\beta > 0|\mathcal{D}(j))$. Let p_{E1} and p_{E2} be pre-specified Efficacy cut-offs with $p_{E1} > p_{E2}$. If $\Pr(\beta > 0|\mathcal{D}(j)) > p_{E1}$ i.e., the current trend of the dose-Efficacy curve is increasing, we escalate the dose because the next higher dose level is expected to have higher Efficacy. In contrast, if $\Pr(\beta > 0|\mathcal{D}(j)) < p_{E2}$, which indicates a decreasing dose-Efficacy curve, we de-escalate the dose because the lower dose level is expected to have higher Efficacy. Otherwise, we repeat the current dose. The values of p_{E1} and p_{E2} can be calibrated by simulation to obtain good operating characteristics. Typically, p_{E1} should be larger than p_{E2} by a reasonable margin, such as 10% to 20%.

The local logistic design dose-finding algorithm is as follows:

1. Starting from the lowest l dose levels, treat one cohort of patients at each dose level. Alternatively, to be more conservative, the 3+3 dose escalation rule can be used to sequentially assign patients to the lowest l dose levels.

2. At the current dose level j, based on Toxicity, find the admissible set $\mathcal{A}$.

3. Based on the Efficacy outcomes in $\mathcal{D}(j)$ from the current and previous $l - 1$ dose levels, calculate $\Pr(\beta > 0|\mathcal{D}(j))$.

   (a) If $\Pr(\beta > 0|\mathcal{D}(j)) > p_{E1}$, escalate to $j + 1$ when $j + 1$ is in $\mathcal{A}$;
   (b) if $\Pr(\beta > 0|\mathcal{D}(j)) < p_{E2}$, de-escalate to $j - 1$;
   (c) otherwise, i.e., $p_{E2} \leq \Pr(\beta > 0|\mathcal{D}(j)) \leq p_{E1}$, dose level j is repeated.

4. Once the maximum sample size N is reached, based on the final data, carry out a double-sided isotonic regression and select the lowest dose that has the highest estimate of the Efficacy probability $\tilde{\pi}_{E,j}$ as the OBD.

A potential problem with the above algorithm is that the chosen dose may alternate between dose levels j and $j + 1$ if dose level j maximizes the dose-Efficacy curve. To avoid this problem, before conducting any dose escalation, we determine whether $\Pr(\beta > 0|\mathcal{D}(j+1)) < p_{E2}$ whenever the dose level $j+1$ has been used to treat any patients. If $\Pr(\beta > 0|\mathcal{D}(j + 1)) < p_{E2}$, indicating

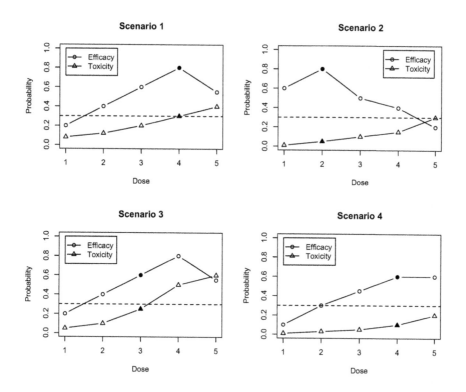

FIGURE 9.1: Simulation scenarios with filled symbols indicating the OBD.

that dose level j is the maximum point of the curve, we repeat the current dose level.

Operating characteristics of the isotonic and local regression designs are illustrated under four Efficacy and Toxicity scenarios shown in Figure 9.1. In the simulations, there were five dose levels, the trial started at the lowest dose, the Toxicity upper bound was $\bar{\pi}_T = 0.3$, with $p_T = 0.8$, maximum sample size $N = 30$, with cohorts of size 3. For the local regression design, the Efficacy cut-offs were $p_{E1} = 0.4$ and $p_{E2} = 0.3$, and two adjacent doses (i.e., $l = 2$) were used to fit the local logistic model. We compared the isotonic design and the local regression design with a design used in practice, in which the MTD is first identified by the 3+3 design, and then the remaining patients are randomized between the MTD and the dose one level lower than the MTD.

Table 9.1 shows the dose selection probabilities and the average percentages of patients treated at each dose level under the 3+3, isotonic, and local regression designs. In practice, besides the OBD, the other doses with high Efficacy and low Toxicity often are of interest to investigators. Therefore, Table 9.1 also reports the selection percentage of the OBD region, defined as the two doses having the highest response rates in $\mathcal{A}$. For example, in scenario 1, the OBD region is consisted of doses 3 and 4.

In Scenario 1, the dose-Efficacy curve is unimodal and the fourth dose level is the true OBD with the highest Efficacy rate and acceptable Toxicity. The 3+3 design yielded the lowest correct OBD selection percentage of 21.6%, The isotonic design had correct OBD selection percentage of 45.6%. The local regression design performed best and correctly selected the OBD 54.4% of the time. The isotonic and local regression designs also assigned higher percentages of patients to the OBD than the 3+3 design. In Scenario 2, the OBD is located at dose level 2, whereas the MTD is located at dose level 5. The 3+3 design incorrectly selected dose 4 as the OBD with percentage 40.0%, and correctly selected dose 2 as the OBD only 24.4% of the time. The isotonic and local regression designs correctly selected dose level 2 as the OBD with percentages of 78.6% and 77.0%, respectively. In Scenario 3, dose level 4 has the highest Efficacy, but is overly toxic, and dose level 3 is the OBD. The selection percentage of the OBD under the isotonic and local regression designs were about 20% higher than that of the 3+3 design. In Scenario 4, $\pi_{E,j}$ initially increases with dose and then plateaus. In this case, the true OBD is the lowest dose yielding the highest Efficacy, dose level 4, and the performances of three designs were comparable.

9.3 Combining Targeted and Cytotoxic Agents

Combining traditional cytotoxic agents with novel MTAs provides an important approach to treating cancer and achieving better patient outcomes. Since cytotoxic agents and MTAs work via different mechanisms, combining them can induce a synergistic treatment effect, target tumor cells with differing drug susceptibilities, and achieve a higher intensity of dose with non-overlapping toxicities. Because MTAs display different, potentially non-monotonic dose-Toxicity and dose-Efficacy profiles, the methods described in Chapter 8 for combinations of cytotoxic agents may not be suitable for combinations involving MTAs.

For trials combining a cytotoxic agent with an MTA, the goal is to find the biological optimal dose combination (ODC), defined as the dose pair with highest Efficacy and tolerable Toxicity, e.g., with Toxicity probability less than a prespecified upper bound $\bar{\pi}_T$. Under the assumption that the dose-Efficacy curve first increases and then plateaus, this is equivalent to finding the change point, i.e., the lowest dose where the dose-Efficacy curve first plateaus, given that the dose is tolerable.

Pishvaian et al. (2012) reported a phase I trial for the combination of imatinib and paclitaxel in patients with advanced solid tumors refractory to standard therapy. Imatinib is a tyrosine kinase inhibitor used in the treatment

TABLE 9.1: Dose selection percentages and average percentages of patients treated at each dose under the 3+3, isotonic, and local regression designs, with the OBD selection percentages in boldface, and the OBD regions in shade.

Design		Dose level					% OBD region
		1	2	3	4	5	
	Scenario 1						
	True Efficacy	0.2	0.4	0.6	0.8	0.55	
	True Toxicity	0.08	0.12	0.2	0.3	0.4	
3+3	Selection (%)	22.8	27.4	27.0	**21.6**	1.1	48.6
	Patients (%)	32.4	26.1	21.8	13.8	5.9	
Isotonic	Selection (%)	12.5	15.8	23.4	**45.6**	2.7	69.0
	Patients (%)	21.0	22.0	21.0	26.3	9.7	
Local reg	Selection (%)	6.8	10.0	24.9	**54.4**	3.9	79.3
	Patients (%)	16.7	19.3	20.3	28.0	15.7	
	Scenario 2						
	True Efficacy	0.6	0.8	0.5	0.4	0.2	
	True Toxicity	0.01	0.05	0.10	0.15	0.3	
3+3	Selection (%)	4.3	**24.4**	25.9	40.0	5.4	28.7
	Patients (%)	14.9	18.2	22.4	27.0	17.5	
Isotonic	Selection (%)	14.0	**78.6**	5.4	2.0	0.0	92.6
	Patients (%)	21.8	58.4	15.0	4.1	0.7	
Local reg	Selection (%)	11.4	**77.0**	9.1	2.5	0.0	88.4
	Patients (%)	14.9	49.3	22.4	9.8	3.8	
	Scenario 3						
	True Efficacy	0.2	0.4	0.6	0.8	0.55	
	True Toxicity	0.05	0.1	0.25	0.5	0.6	
3+3	Selection (%)	18.8	41.7	**30.4**	9.0	0.1	72.1
	Patients (%)	30.5	33.9	25.3	8.9	1.4	
Isotonic	Selection (%)	12.4	25.4	**49.5**	12.1	0.6	74.9
	Patients (%)	20.7	25.0	27.7	19.3	7.7	
Local reg	Selection (%)	5.8	21.4	**50.0**	21.7	1.1	71.4
	Patients (%)	15.3	23.3	29.7	21	10.7	
	Scenario 4						
	True Efficacy	0.1	0.3	0.45	0.6	0.6	
	True Toxicity	0.01	0.03	0.05	0.1	0.2	
3+3	Selection (%)	1.6	4.8	21.2	**42.7**	29.7	72.4
	Patients (%)	12.0	13.7	17.8	31.1	25.4	
Isotonic	Selection (%)	0.7	6.7	14.6	**45.5**	32.5	78.0
	Patients (%)	10.9	13.3	18.4	29.6	27.7	
Local reg	Selection (%)	0.6	4.9	20.1	**40.4**	34.0	74.4
	Patients (%)	10.5	11.6	14.0	23.5	40.4	

of multiple cancers, most notably chronic myelogenous leukemia (CML). Imatinib works by inhibiting the activity of the BCR-Abl tyrosine kinase enzyme that is necessary for cancer development, thus preventing the growth of cancer cells and leading to their death by apoptosis. Because the BCR-Abl tyrosine kinase enzyme exists only in cancer cells and not in healthy cells, imatinib works effectively as an MTA killing only cancer cells. The goal of the trial was to evaluate the safety of combining imatinib with the traditional cytotoxic chemotherapeutic agent paclitaxel, and to determine whether that combination improved the Efficacy of imatinib. In the trial, four doses, 300, 400, 600, 800 mg, of imatinib and three doses, 60, 80, 100 mg/m^2, of paclitaxel were investigated. Most of the grade 3 or 4 toxicities related to therapy were neutropenia, flu-like symptoms, or pain. Treatment response was evaluated using the RECIST criteria (Eisenhauer et al., 2009).

This phase I trial used a conventional 3+3 design, with only a subset of all 12 possible combinations of imatinib and paclitaxel investigated. As a result, the trial might completely miss the most desirable dose pair in the 4 × 3 dose combination space. The trial selectively investigated the 6 (paclitaxel, imatinib) dose combinations (60, 300), (60, 400), (80, 400), (80, 600), (100, 600), and (100, 800). The protocol specified daily oral administration of imatinib and weekly paclitaxel infusions. However, after treating patients at the first two dose pairs, the regimen resulted in an excessive number of Toxicities. The protocol thus was amended to investigate a less intensive schedule, with intermittent dosing of imatinib. A limitation of the 3+3 design is that it ignores Efficacy, but assumes implicitly that π_E increases with dose, which is not the case for imatinib. Druker (2002) pointed out that, for treating CML, any dose between 400 and 600 mg/day of imatinib reached the plateau of the dose-response curve. This result was confirmed in a meta-analysis (Gafter-Gvili et al., 2011) of phase III randomized trials, in which no treatment difference was found between 400 mg and higher doses of imatinib. This trial example demonstrates the need for a new dose-finding design to handle the clinical trials that combine an MTA with a traditional cytotoxic agent.

In general, consider a trial combining J doses of cytotoxic agent A, $d_{1,1} < \cdots < d_{1,J}$, with L doses of targeted agent B, $d_{2,1} < \cdots < d_{2,L}$. Let $(d_{1,j}, d_{2,l})$ denote the combination of the jth dose of agent A and the lth dose of agent B, Y_T denote the binary Toxicity outcome, and define $\pi_T(d_{1,j}, d_{2,l}) = \Pr(Y_{T,i} = 1 \mid d_{1,j}, d_{2,l})$, for $j = 1, \cdots, J$ and $l = 1, \cdots, L$. Toxicity is modeled as

$$\text{logit}(\pi_T(d_{1,j}, d_{2,l})) = \beta_0 + \beta_1 x_{1,j} + \beta_2 x_{2,l} \tag{9.4}$$

where β_0, β_1, and β_2 are unknown parameters, and $(x_{1,j}, x_{2,l})$ are "effective" or standardized doses ascribed to the raw doses $(d_{1,j}, d_{2,l})$ based on the prior estimates of the single-agent Toxicity probabilities for these two dose levels. The procedure of determining the values of $(x_{1,j}, x_{2,l})$ will be described below. We require $\beta_1 > 0$ and $\beta_2 > 0$, such that $\pi_T(d_{1,j}, d_{2,l})$ increases with the dose of the two agents.

In model (9.4), the interactive effect of the two agents, e.g., a term

$\beta_3 x_{1,j} x_{2,l}$, is not included because reliable estimation of β_3 would require a larger sample size than typically is available in early-phase trials. Recall that, for the purpose of dose finding, we do not seek to model the entire dose-Toxicity surface but aim to obtain an adequate local fit to facilitate dose escalation and de-escalation. A model may provide a poor global fit to the entire dose-Toxicity surface, but if the model provides a good local fit around the current dose, it will lead to reasonably reliable dose selection decisions. Numerical studies suggest that including the interaction term does not improve the performance of the design (Wang and Ivanova, 2005; Braun and Wang, 2010).

Unlike Toxicity, which often can be observed quickly, in some cases, Efficacy may require a longer follow-up time to be scored. In this case, the conventional approach of treating Efficacy as a binary outcome causes a serious logistic problem. When a new patient is enrolled and is waiting for dose assignment, some patients already treated might not be fully evaluated, and thus their Efficacy outcomes are not available for the adaptive dose assignment decision for the new patient. One way to overcome this difficulty is to model Efficacy as a time-to-event outcome. Thus, follow up time data on the incomplete Efficacy evaluations are incorporated into the dose assignment decision. Alternatively, the missing data approach, described in Chapter 5, can be used to handle the delayed Efficacy outcome.

Let t_E denote the time to Efficacy. In early phase trials, the typical way to evaluate Efficacy is to follow each patient for a fixed period of time T, e.g., 3 months, after the initiation of treatment. Within the assessment window (0, T], if the patient responds favorably, i.e., $t_E \le T$, it is scored as a response, otherwise nonresponse. Conceptually, one can think of $t_E = \infty$ for the patients who do not respond by T. A special feature of the trial combining an MTA with a cytotoxic agent is that the dose-Efficacy curve behaves differently with respect to the two agents: Efficacy is expected to increase monotonically with the dose of the cytotoxic agent, but not necessarily with the dose of the MTA. Let $\lambda_{jl}(t_E)$ denote the hazard function of t_E associated with combination $(d_{1,j}, d_{2,l})$, and $I(\mathcal{C}) = 1$ if $\mathcal{C}$ is true, 0 if not. The Efficacy endpoint t_E is modeled using a proportional hazards model, augmented with a plateau parameter τ, as follows,

$$\lambda_{jl}(t_E) = \lambda_0(t_E) \exp[\gamma_1 \tilde{x}_{1,j} + \gamma_2 \{\tilde{x}_{2,l} I(l < \tau) + \tilde{x}_{2,\tau} I(l \ge \tau)\}],$$

where $\lambda_0(t_E)$ is the baseline hazard, and $(\tilde{x}_{1,j}, \tilde{x}_{2,l})$ are "effective" or standardized doses ascribed to $(d_{1,j}, d_{2,l})$ based on the prior estimates of the single-agent Efficacy probabilities for these two doses, described below. We require that $\gamma_1 > 0$ and $\gamma_2 > 0$, so that Efficacy monotonically increases with the dose of the cytotoxic agent A, as well as the targeted agent B before the latter plateaus.

The plateau parameter τ is an integer between 1 and L, and indicates the dose level of agent B, i.e., the MTA, where Efficacy no longer increases with dose. When the dose level is lower than τ, Efficacy increases monotonically with the dose of the MTA, $\tilde{x}_{2,l}$, through the covariate effect $\gamma_2\{\tilde{x}_{2,l}I(l < \tau) + \tilde{x}_{2,\tau}I(l \geq \tau)\} = \gamma_2\tilde{x}_{2,l}$. When the dose level is equal to or higher than τ, the Efficacy plateaus (with respective to the dose level of agent B) with a constant dose effect $\gamma_2\tilde{x}_{2,\tau}$. This change-point model can also accommodate a monotonic dose-Efficacy relationship by taking $\tau = L$, i.e., the highest dose level of the MTA. One concern is that the dose-Efficacy curve may not be completely flat after reaching the plateau. This is not a problem here because the flat line is used to approximate where Efficacy does not change significantly after a certain dose level. Given the small sample size of early phase trials, with any model there is little statistical power to detect such small changes.

Assuming an exponential distribution for t_E with constant baseline hazard, i.e., $\lambda_0(t_E) = \lambda_0$, the survival function is

$$S_{jl}(t_E) = \exp[-\lambda_0 t_E \exp\{\gamma_1\tilde{x}_{1,j} + \gamma_2(\tilde{x}_{2,l}I(l < \tau) + \tilde{x}_{2,\tau}I(l \geq \tau))\}].$$

The Efficacy probability for combination $(d_{1,j}, d_{2,l})$ is

$$\pi_E(d_{1,j}, d_{2,l}) = \Pr(t_E \leq T \mid d_{1,j}, d_{2,l}) = 1 - S_{jl}(T), \tag{9.5}$$

which will be used for decision making.

We specify the effective doses, i.e., $(x_{1,j}, x_{2,l})$ in the Toxicity model, and $(\tilde{x}_{1,j}, \tilde{x}_{2,l})$ in the Efficacy model, based on the prior estimates of the single-agent Toxicity and Efficacy probabilities. Before two agents are combined, in most settings each has been studied individually. For example, prior to the solid tumor trial of combining imatinib with paclitaxel, (Pishvaian et al., 2012), many phase I and II trials had been conducted to study the single-agent Toxicity and Efficacy profiles for imatinib (Ramanathan et al., 2008; Gibbons et al., 2008; Lipton et al., 2010; van Oosterom et al., 2001) and paclitaxel (Kato et al., 2011; Tsimberidou et al., 2011; Takano et al., 2001; Lim et al., 2010; Horiguchi et al., 2009). Therefore, one often has prior estimates of the single-agent Toxicity and Efficacy probabilities. The purpose of defining and using effective doses is to obtain prior estimates of the single-agent Toxicity and Efficacy probabilities. This incorporates the available single-agent dose-Toxicity and -Efficacy information into the model and thus improves the efficiency of the design. This approach has been used previously for dose finding in single-agent trials (Chevret, 2006; Yin and Yuan, 2009b; Zohar et al., 2013) and drug-combination phase I trials (Yin and Yuan, 2010; Liu et al., 2013; Thall et al., 2003).

Let $\hat{\pi}_k(d_{1,j}, 0)$, $k = T, E$, denote the estimates of the single-agent Toxicity and Efficacy probabilities for agent A, and $\hat{\pi}_k(0, d_{2,l})$ for agent B. Under the Toxicity model (9.4), setting the dose of agent B (or A) to 0 gives the single-agent Toxicity models $\text{logit}(\pi_T(d_{1,j}, 0)) = \beta_0 + \beta_1 x_{1,j}$ for agent A and $\text{logit}(\pi_T(0, d_{2,l})) = \beta_0 + \beta_2 x_{2,l}$ for agent B. Therefore, based on the prior estimates $\hat{\pi}_T(d_{1,j}, 0)$ and $\hat{\pi}_T(0, d_{2,l})$, the "effective" doses $(x_{1,j}, x_{2,l})$ for Toxicity model are given by

$$x_{1,j} = \{\text{logit}(\hat{\pi}_T(d_{1,j}, 0)) - \hat{\beta}_0\}/\hat{\beta}_1$$
$$x_{2,l} = \{\text{logit}(\hat{\pi}_T(0, d_{2,l})) - \hat{\beta}_0\}/\hat{\beta}_2,$$

where $\hat{\beta}_0$ and $\hat{\beta}_1$ are prior means of β_0 and β_1. Similarly, setting $d_{1,j} = 0$ or $d_{2,l} = 0$ and $\hat{\tau} = L$ in the Efficacy model (9.5) gives the effective doses

$$\tilde{x}_{1,j} = \log[-\log\{1 - \hat{\pi}_E(d_{1,j}, 0)\}/(\hat{\lambda}_0 T)]/\hat{\gamma}_1$$
$$\tilde{x}_{2,l} = \log[-\log\{1 - \hat{\pi}_E(0, d_{2,l})\}/(\hat{\lambda}_0 T)]/\hat{\gamma}_2,$$

where $\hat{\lambda}_0, \hat{\gamma}_1, \hat{\gamma}_2$ are prior estimates.

To complete the prior specification for the Toxicity model, a vague normal prior $N(0, 100)$ is assumed for the intercept β_0, and, following Chevret (1993), the slopes β_1 and β_2 are given independent exponential distributions with rate parameter 1, i.e., $\beta_1, \beta_2 \overset{iid}{\sim} Exp(1)$. For the Efficacy model, vague priors $\lambda_0 \sim Exp(0.01)$ and $\gamma_1, \gamma_2 \sim Exp(0.1)$, are assumed, and τ is multinomial with probabilities $\varrho = (\varrho_1, ..., \varrho_L)$, where ϱ_l is the prior probability that the dose-Efficacy curve plateaus at dose level l of the MTA. When there is rich information on the location of τ, e.g., we know the saturation dosage of the MTA from pharmacokinetic and pharmacodynamic studies, we can choose a set of ϱ to reflect the likelihood of each dose level being the plateau point. When there is no good prior information regarding the location of τ, we recommend assigning τ an increasing sequence of prior probabilities, $\varrho_1 < \varrho_2 < ... < \varrho_L$, rather than a noninformative flat prior $\varrho_1 = \varrho_2 = ... = \varrho_L$. This recommendation is based on our experience with numerical studies, in which we found that using a noninformative prior often caused the dose selection to remain at low dose levels due to the sparsity of data. The prior with increasing ϱ_l's encourages the dose-finding algorithm to explore higher dose levels of agent B and actively learn the shape of the dose-Efficacy curve, thereby improving the ODC selection accuracy. In our simulation study, we took $\varrho = (0.14, 0.20, 0.28, 0.39)$, which led to good operating characteristics across various scenarios. Details for the likelihood and posterior sampling can be found in Riviere et al. (2015).

Dose finding is conducted in two stages. When no meaning is lost, the notation (j, l) is used for dose pair $(d_{1,j}, d_{2,l})$ $j = 1, \cdots, J$ and $l = 1, \cdots, L$. Stage I performs dose escalation using a rule similar to that proposed by Huang et al. (2007), which divides the dose combination matrix into a sequence of zones along the diagonal from low doses to high doses (Figure 9.2), and then conducts a 3+3 type dose escalation across the zones. The goal is to collect preliminary data to facilitate model fitting in stage II. Stage I starts by treating the first cohort of 3 patients at the lowest zone, i.e., the lowest combination $(1, 1)$, and then escalates the dose pair to higher dose zones until a zone in which all doses are "closed" is encountered. Given a dose pair, if > 1 patient experiences Toxicity out of the 3 or 6 patients given that dose,

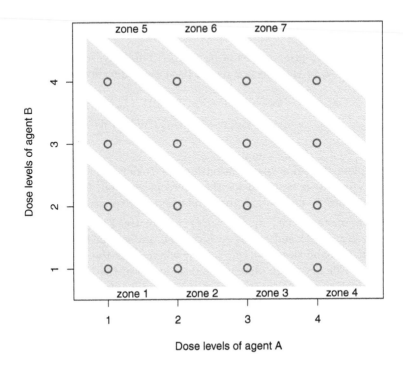

FIGURE 9.2: Illustration of zones for stage I dose escalation.

the dose is closed and all higher doses, i.e., any pair having a higher dose level of A or B or both, are closed and not eligible for use in treating future patients in the start-up phase. More precisely, if (j, l), is closed, then close all higher doses (j', l') for $j' \geq j$ and $l' \geq l$. Closed dose combinations can be reopened subsequently if the accumulating data indicate that they are safe. Dose escalation across zones is similar to 3+3 dose escalation rule: if 0/3 Toxicities are observed, escalate; if 3/3 Toxicities are observed, close the dose; and if 1/3 Toxicities are observed, treat 3 more patients at the current dose. In the latter case, if 0 or 1 out of the 6 patients experiences Toxicity, escalate; otherwise, close the dose. When escalating to a higher dose zone, if there are multiple combinations that are not closed in that zone, simultaneously assign patients to each of the combinations.

After the completion of stage I, we proceed to stage II for model-based dose finding. Let $\bar{\pi}_T$ and $\underline{\pi}_E$ denote the prespecified Toxicity upper bound and Efficacy lower bound, respectively. Let N denote the total sample size, and n denote the number of patients treated in the trial. A combination (j, l)

is *admissible* if

$$\Pr(\pi_T(d_{1,j}, d_{2,l}) < \bar{\pi}_T) > p_T \tag{9.6}$$

and

$$\Pr(\pi_E(d_{1,j}, d_{2,l}) > \underline{\pi}_E) \geq p_E I(n \geq N/2), \tag{9.7}$$

where p_T and p_E are probability cut-offs. The Efficacy requirement (9.7) takes effect when half of the patients have been enrolled, as controlled by the indicator function $I(n \geq N/2)$. Introducing the Efficacy condition too early causes a high frequency of misclassification of the admissible doses as inadmissible and thus results in the early termination of the trial. This can arise because, compared to evaluation of the Toxicity condition (9.6), reliable evaluation of the Efficacy condition (9.7) requires more data, since the Efficacy outcome is not immediately observable and the Efficacy model is relatively more complicated.

Let (j, l) denote the current dose, $\mathcal{Z}_n$ the set of combinations that have been used previously to treat patients, and $\mathcal{B} = \{(j', l'); j' \leq j + 1, l' \leq l + 1, \text{ and } (j', l') \neq (j + 1, l + 1)\}$ the set of combinations for which the doses are not two levels higher than the current dose pair (j, l). The dose-finding algorithm is as follows: After the start-up phase, assign the next cohort to the optimal combination that is *admissible* and has highest estimated Efficacy, $\hat{\pi}_E(d_{1,j}, d_{2,l})$, selected from the set $\mathcal{Z}_n \cup \mathcal{B}$. If several optimal combinations exist, e.g., Efficacy has reached a plateau with respect to the dose level of the MTA, select the optimal combination with lowest MTA dose level. At any time, if all combinations are not admissible, then terminate the trial. At the end of the trial, select the ODC as the admissible combination with highest estimated Efficacy and lowest estimated Toxicity.

For the solid tumor trial, cytotoxic agent A (paclitaxel) has 3 dose levels, and molecularly targeted agent B (imatinib) has 4 dose levels, giving 12 combinations. The prior single-agent Toxicity and Efficacy probabilities were $(0.2, 0.3, 0.4)$ and $(0.3, 0.4, 0.5)$, respectively, for agent A, and $(0.12, 0.2, 0.3, 0.4)$ and $(0.3, 0.4, 0.5, 0.59)$ for agent B. The Toxicity upper bound was $\bar{\pi}_T = 0.30$ and the Efficacy lower bound was $\underline{\pi}_E = 0.20$. The maximum sample size was 75, with cohort size 3.

Three simulation scenarios are given in Table 9.2. Table 9.3 gives the simulation results, including the ODC selection percentage, and average number of patients assigned to the ODC. In Scenario 1, the dose-Efficacy curve approximately plateaus at the lowest dose level of the targeted agent B, and the ODC is the combination $(3, 1)$, which yields the highest Efficacy with the lowest dose of the targeted agent. To mimic what may happen in practice, we designed the Scenarios to allow for some variation in Efficacy, even when it has reached the plateau. The design selected the ODC 75.6% of the time, and allocated on average 35.1 patients to the ODC. In Scenario 2, the dose-Efficacy curve plateaus after dose level 2 of agent B. The ODC selection percentage in that Scenario was 51.3%. Scenario 3 is a case where Efficacy monotonically increases with the dose of agent B, i.e., agent B does not reach a level of saturation within the range of the investigational doses. This is similar to what

TABLE 9.2: Three Toxicity and Efficacy scenarios for the combination of a cytotoxic agent (agent A) with an MTA (agent B). The ODCs are in bold, and the shaded areas indicate the Efficacy plateaus for the MTA

Agent	Agent A					
	1	2	3	1	2	3
B	Toxicity			Efficacy		
	Scenario 1					
4	0.45	0.50	0.65	0.27	0.42	0.56
3	0.30	0.45	0.55	0.26	0.41	0.56
2	0.15	0.30	0.45	0.25	0.41	0.55
1	0.10	0.15	**0.30**	0.25	0.40	**0.55**
	Scenario 2					
4	0.10	0.15	0.30	0.32	0.46	0.61
3	0.08	0.10	**0.15**	0.30	0.45	**0.60**
2	0.04	0.05	0.10	0.20	0.30	0.40
1	0.01	0.03	0.07	0.05	0.10	0.20
	Scenario 3					
4	0.10	0.15	**0.30**	0.40	0.55	**0.70**
3	0.07	0.10	0.15	0.25	0.40	0.55
2	0.05	0.08	0.10	0.15	0.30	0.40
1	0.01	0.05	0.07	0.05	0.10	0.30

may happen in conventional combination trials with two cytotoxic agents. The design performs well, with ODC selection percentage 66.4%, suggesting that the design also can be applied to combination trials of two cytotoxic agents.

Next, we retrospectively apply the design to the solid tumor trial. Recall that the trial selectively studied six dose combinations out of 12 possible combinations. Because the dosing schedule used in the original protocol resulted in too many toxicities, the protocol was amended to use a less intensive dose schedule. As a result, five dose combinations actually were used under the amended schedule. The window for assessing treatment response was set at $T = 13$ weeks. The trial did not report the time to response. Thus, we assumed that t_E was uniformly distributed on $(0, 13]$.

The trial started by treating the first cohort of 3 patients at the lowest dose combination (60, 400), at which one response and no dose-limiting Toxicity (DLT) was observed. Based on the data, our method identified the dose combination (100, 600) as the ODC, with estimated response rate 0.54, and thus recommended escalation to (80, 400) for the second cohort. Among the three patients treated at (80, 400), two responded to treatment and no Toxicities were observed. The method estimated the combination (100, 600) as the ODC, with an estimated response rate 0.56, and escalated to (80, 600) for the third cohort, among which 2/3 responded and 0/3 Toxicities were observed. The method escalated and assigned the fourth cohort to (100, 600), at which 2/3 responded and no Toxicites were observed, with estimated ODC (100, 600) and estimated response rate 0.45. Based on these results, the method

TABLE 9.3: ODC (in boldface) selection percentages and average numbers of patients treated at each combination

Scenario	Selection percentage			Average number of patients		
1	0.4	0.1	0.1	2.0	0.2	0.2
	0.9	1.0	0.0	4.0	1.3	1.3
	0.5	7.4	6.0	3.9	5.8	10.3
	0.1	7.9	**75.6**	4.0	6.9	**35.1**
2	0.0	0.8	32.5	3.5	3.3	16.3
	0.0	0.1	**51.3**	3.6	3.4	**18.1**
	0.0	0.0	13.9	3.4	3.3	9.4
	0.0	0.0	1.4	3.1	3.2	4.5
3	0.0	1.2	**66.4**	3.4	3.2	**23.1**
	0.0	0.0	19.8	3.5	3.2	13.1
	0.0	0.0	9.1	3.4	3.4	7.1
	0.0	0.0	3.5	3.1	3.4	5.1

would repeat the current dose and assign the remaining 6 patients to (100, 600), whereas the 3+3 design would escalate to (100, 800). At the end of the trial, the design selected (100, 600) as the ODC, while the 3+3 design selected (100, 800). According to the literature, a dose of 600mg of imatinib reaches the plateau of the dose-response curve and is the dose that has been administered widely to cancer patients in practice. The design successfully identified this, while the 3+3 design would have resulted in overdosing patients.

9.4 Combining Two Molecularly Targeted Agents

As more MTAs become available, it has become commonplace to combine multiple MTAs that target different elements of a genomic pathway or multiple pathways, to overcome treatment resistance and achieve synergistic treatment effects. As an example, a phase I–II trial at The University of Texas M.D. Anderson Cancer Center combined two novel MTAs to treat patients with relapsed lymphoma. The two agents target two different components in the PI3K/AKT/mTOR signaling pathway. Agent A is a PI3K kinase inhibitor and agent B is a downstream inhibitor of mTOR kinase within that pathway. Preclinical research suggested that some types of lymphomas are promoted and maintained by activation of the PI3K/AKT/mTOR pathway, making this pathway an important target for drug development (Smith et al., 2010). Combining these two agents may obtain a more complete inhibition of the PI3k/AKT/mTOR pathway, and thereby achieve better treatment responses.

The trial investigated the combinations of 4 dose levels of agent A with 4 dose levels of agent B, which results in 16 dose combinations. The goal was to find the ODC, defined as the dose combination with the highest Efficacy and tolerable Toxicity, specifically with $\bar{\pi}_T = .40$. The physicians expected the dose-Efficacy curve of the combination to be non-monotonic in either agent, so the dose of each agent in the combination having highest Efficacy may not be the highest dose of that agent. They also allowed the possibility that the Toxicity of the combinations may increase at low doses and become approximately flat within the dose range under investigation. Because of these new features, the design described in a previous section for the combination of a cytotoxic agent and an MTA cannot be used here. For this trial, Efficacy is quickly ascertainable, and (Y_T, Y_E) both are binary.

Let $x_{1,1} < \cdots < x_{1,J}$ denote J standardized doses for targeted agent A, and $x_{2,1} < \cdots < x_{2,L}$ denote L standardized doses of targeted agent B. As described previously, there are various ways to standardize the raw dose pairs $(d_{1,j}, d_{2,l})$. Here, $(x_{1,j}, x_{2,l})$ are given by $x_{1,j} = 0.5(d_{1,j} - \bar{d}_1)/\mathrm{sd}(d_1)$ and $x_{2,l} = 0.5(d_{2,l} - \bar{d}_2)/\mathrm{sd}(d_2)$, such that $\{x_{1,j}\}$ and $\{x_{2,l}\}$ have mean 0 and standard deviation 0.5.

To accommodate the possibility that the Toxicity of the combinations of MTAs may initially increase and then approximately plateau within the therapeutic dose range, we assume a change-point model given by

$$
\begin{aligned}
\mathrm{logit}(\pi_T(x_{1,j}, x_{2,l})) \;=\; & (\beta_0 + \beta_1 x_{1,j} + \beta_2 x_{2,l}) I(\beta_0 + \beta_1 x_{1,j} \\
& + \beta_2 x_{2,l} \le \omega) + \omega I(\beta_0 + \beta_1 x_{1,j} + \beta_2 x_{2,l} > \omega), \quad (9.8)
\end{aligned}
$$

where $I(\cdot)$ is the indicator function and $(\beta, \omega) = (\beta_0, \beta_1, \beta_2, \omega)$ are unknown parameters. Under this model, the dose-Toxicity surface initially is monotone in each dose but becomes flat once it passes the threshold defined by $\beta_0 + \beta_1 x_{1,j} + \beta_2 x_{2,l} = \omega$ (Figure 9.3). We require $\beta_1 > 0$ and $\beta_2 > 0$, so that the π_T initially increases with each dose before it plateaus at $e^\omega/(1 + e^\omega)$.

The change-point model is more flexible than the standard linear logistic model, such as (9.4), used in the previous section. It contains the standard monotonically increasing dose-Toxicity curve as a special case when the change point $\omega \ge \beta_0 + \beta_1 x_{1,J} + \beta_2 x_{2,L}$, so it also accommodates monotonic dose-Toxicity curves. A possible concern is that, under the change-point model, the dose-Toxicity curve is not smooth at the changing point ω. However, this is not problematic in our setting because the doses are discrete and sparse, and there are insufficient data to estimate the smoothness between two doses where the change point occurs. Cai et al. (2014b) found that the choice of the Toxicity model could be flexible as long as it accommodates a non-monotonic dose-Toxicity relationship. For example, an alternative model is $\pi_T(x_{1,j}, x_{2,l}) = \omega \mathrm{logit}^{-1}(\beta_0 + \beta_1 x_{1,j} + \beta_2 x_{2,l})$, which defines a smooth dose-Toxicity curve, yields a design with operating characteristics similar to those obtained under the change-point model.

For MTAs, the dose-Efficacy curve often is non-monotonic. For example,

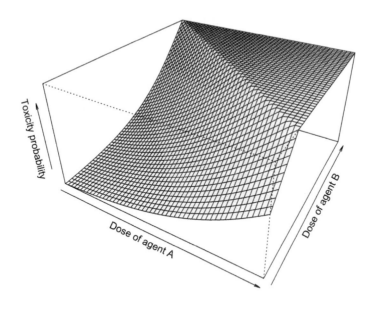

FIGURE 9.3: Toxicity probability surface for two-agent combination under the change-point model. The probability of Toxicity initially increases with each dose and plateaus after reaching the change line.

in immunotherapy trials, the dose-Efficacy relationship could be umbrella-shaped, so the most effective dose is in the middle of the therapeutic dose range. A simple model that incorporates such a non-monotonic pattern for the dose-Efficacy relationship is

$$\text{logit}\{\pi_E(x_{1,j}, x_{2,l})\} = \gamma_0 + \gamma_1 x_{1,j} + \gamma_2 x_{2,l} + \gamma_3 x_{1,j}^2 + \gamma_4 x_{2,l}^2, \quad (9.9)$$

where $\gamma = (\gamma_0, \cdots, \gamma_4)$ are unknown parameters. The quadratic terms render the model adequate flexibility to capture the non-monotonic shape of the dose-Efficacy surface. For the same reason described previously in Section 9.3, the interaction between $x_{1,j}$ and $x_{2,l}$ is not included in the Toxicity and Efficacy models.

For prior specification of the Efficacy model, we assign γ a weakly informative default prior proposed by Gelman et al. (2008) for logistic regression. To use this default prior, given the standardized doses with mean 0 and standard deviation 0.5, we assume the regression coefficients $\gamma_1, \cdots, \gamma_4$ are iid following a Cauchy prior with center 0 and scale 2.5, Cauchy(0, 2.5), and the intercept $\gamma_0 \sim$ Cauchy(0,10). Advantages of these weakly informative priors are that they are diffuse and provide reasonable coverages for plausible values of the parameters. For example, the Cauchy(0, 10) prior for γ_0 expects the Efficacy probability for an average case to be between 10^{-9} and $1 - 10^{-9}$. These priors also are appropriately regularized, so that a dramatic change in the Efficacy probability, e.g., from 0.01 to 0.5, is unlikely when a dose changes by one level. This stabilizes estimation while still being sufficiently vague to ensure that the data dominate the priors. For the Toxicity model, we use the Cauchy(0, 10) prior for the intercept β_0, and assign β_1 and β_2 a gamma prior with shape 0.5 and rate 0.5 to ensure monotonicity before the dose-Toxicity surface reaches the change line in model (9.8). For ω, we assume that the Toxicity probability at the plateau is between 0.2 and 0.8, which corresponds to a value of ω ranging from -1.39 to 1.39. Thus, we assign ω a $N(0, 4)$ prior, which provides sufficient coverage for all plausible Toxicity probabilities at the plateau, given by $e^\omega/(1 + e^\omega)$. Details on the likelihood and posterior can be found in Cai et al. (2014b).

The dose-finding design consists of two stages. Stage I is a run-in period, with the goal to explore the dose-combination space and collect preliminary data so that the proposed probability models can be estimated reliably in stage II. The algorithm is similar to that of Thall et al. (2003) used for a two-agent phase I design. Stage I begins with the first cohort treated at the lowest dose pair $(1, 1)$, and then escalates the dose pair along the diagonal of the dose pair matrix until a dose pair that violates the safety requirement

$$\Pr(\pi_T(x_{1,j}, x_{2,l}) > \bar{\pi}_T | \mathcal{D}) < p_T, \tag{9.10}$$

where $\bar{\pi}_T$ is the Toxicity probability upper limit and p_T is a prespecified cutoff. If the dose pair matrix is not square (i.e., $J > L$), the dose pair is escalated along the diagonal where $j = l$ until reaching (L, L), and thereafter escalated by fixing the dose level of B at L and increasing the dose level of A from (L, L) until reaching the highest dose combination (J, L). In stage I, only a small fraction of patients are enrolled and the observed data are sparse. Therefore, in this stage, we evaluate the safety requirement based on a simple beta-binomial model rather than the proposed dose-Toxicity models. Specifically, we assume that the number of toxicities m_{jl} follows a binomial distribution $Binom(n_{jl}, \pi_{T,jl})$, and that $\pi_{T,jl}$ follows a $Beta(\zeta, \xi)$ prior. To ensure that the data dominate the posterior distribution, we set ζ=0.1 and ξ=0.2. Under the beta-binomial model, $\Pr(\pi_T(x_{1,j}, x_{2,l}) > \bar{\pi}_T | \mathcal{D}) = 1 - \mathcal{B}(\bar{\pi}_T | \zeta + m_{jl}, \xi + n_{jl} - m_{jl})$. We also collect Efficacy data in stage 1, although these data are not used for decision making. If (j, l) violates the safety requirement, i.e., $\Pr(\pi_T(x_{1,j}, x_{2,l}) > \bar{\pi}_T | \mathcal{D}) \geq p_T$, or we reach (J, L), stage I is complete and the trial moves to stage II. Under this conservative stage I completion rule, the maximum number of patients allocated to the dose that violates the safety requirement will be no more than one cohort, which is comparable to the conventional 3+3 design.

Stage II uses the full Toxicity and Efficacy models for dose finding, and has two key features. First, the proposed algorithm encourages exploration of untried dose combinations to avoid the problem of becoming stuck at a suboptimal dose pair, which is of particular concern for combinations of MTAs. Due to possibly complex drug-drug interactions and non-monotonic dose-response patterns, the assumed (simple) dose-response model is not expected to estimate the dose-response surface well, especially early in the trial when only a few observations are available. The estimates of the $\pi_k(x_{1,j}, x_{2,l})$'s may deviate substantially from the truth, and the "optimal" dose identified based on these estimates may be suboptimal. Second, we introduce the concepts of *g-degree neighbor* and *g-degree admissible neighbor* to restrict dose escalation/de-escalation within a neighborhood of the current dose. This avoids dramatic dose changes and improves the reliability of the method.

Given the current dose combination (j, l), we define *g-degree neighbors* of (j, l), denoted by $\mathcal{N}_g$, as dose combinations $\{(j', l')\}$ whose dose levels are different from (j, l) no more than g levels, i.e., $\mathcal{N}_g = \{(j', l') : |j' - j| \le g \text{ and } |l' - l| \le g\}$. The dose set $\mathcal{N}_g$ includes the current dose combination. We define a *g-degree admissible dose set*

$$\mathcal{A}_g = \{(j', l') : (j', l') \in \mathcal{N}_g \text{ and } \Pr(\pi_T(x_{1,j'}, x_{2,l'}) > \bar{\pi}_T | \mathcal{D}) < p_T\},$$

which is a subset of the g-degree neighbors $\mathcal{N}_g$ satisfying the safety requirement $\Pr(\pi_T(x_{1,j'}, x_{2,l'}) > \bar{\pi}_T | \mathcal{D}) < p_T$. That is, $\mathcal{A}_g$ contains the safe g-degree neighbors of the dose combination (j, l).

Let N denote the maximum sample size, N_1 the number of patients in stage I, and $N_2 = N - N_1$ be the number of patients available for stage II. The algorithm for stage II is as follows:

1. Given the current data, determine the dose set $\mathcal{A}_{g^*}$, where $g^* = \min\{g : \mathcal{A}_g \ne \emptyset, g \ge 1\}$. That is, $\mathcal{A}_{g^*}$ is the nonempty admissible set with the smallest degree g^*. If $\mathcal{A}_{g^*}$ is empty, i.e., all dose pairs violate the safety requirement, terminate the trial.

2. Identify the combination (j^*, l^*) in $\mathcal{A}_{g^*}$ having largest posterior mean of Efficacy $\hat{\pi}_E(x_{1,j^*}, x_{2,l^*})$, subject to the safety constraint $(j^* - j) + (l^* - l) \le 1$, i.e., the total dose escalation for two agents cannot be more than one level.

3. If combination (j^*, l^*) has not been used to treat any patients thus far, or all doses in $\mathcal{A}_{g^*}$ have been used to treat patients, assign the next cohort to (j^*, l^*). If (j^*, l^*) has been used to treat patients and there are some untried doses in $\mathcal{A}_{g^*}$, assign the next cohort to (j^*, l^*) only if

$$\hat{\pi}_E(x_{1,j^*}, x_{2,l^*}) > \left(\frac{N_2 - n_2}{N_2}\right)^{\alpha}, \qquad (9.11)$$

where n_2 is the total number of patients that have been treated in stage II and α is a tuning parameter controlling how stringent the threshold is. Otherwise, exclude (j^*, l^*) from the admissible set $\mathcal{A}_{g^*}$ and return to step 2.

4. Repeat step 1-3 until the maximum sample size N_2 is reached or the trial is early terminated.

5. At the end of the trial, select as the ODC the dose combination with largest $\hat{\pi}_{E,jl}$ that satisfies the safety requirement $\Pr(\pi_T(x_{1,j}, x_{2,l}) > \bar{\pi}_T | \mathcal{D}) < p_T$.

The dose assignment rule (9.11) plays a key role by adaptively encouraging exploration of untried doses and avoiding the problem of becoming trapped at a suboptimal dose pair. Early in stage II, n_2 is small and thus the value of $\{(N_2 - n_2)/N_2\}^\alpha$ is close to 1. Consequently, rule (9.11) strongly encourages exploration of untried dose pairs. This is sensible because, at the beginning of stage II, estimates of the $\hat{\pi}_E(x_{1,j}, x_{2,l})$'s are highly variable, and high priority should be given to exploring new doses rather than placing too much faith in point estimates. Toward the end of the trial, when $n_2 \approx N_2$, the estimates of the $\hat{\pi}_E(x_{1,j}, x_{2,l})$'s are more precise. As $\{(N_2 - n_2)/N_2\}^\alpha$ approaches 0, the algorithm essentially assigns incoming patients to the dose combination with the highest $\hat{\pi}_E(x_{1,j}, x_{2,l})$ because rule (9.11) is almost always satisfied. In rule (9.11), the tuning parameter α controls how fast $\{(N_2 - n_2)/N_2\}^\alpha$ decays from 1 to 0, so α should be calibrated to obtain desirable operating characteristics.

This provides a pragmatic strategy to balance the two competing goals of achieving high statistical reliability and treating the patients in the trial ethically. This is the well-known "exploration versus exploitation" dilemma in sequential analysis and reinforcement learning (Sutton and Barto, 1998; Thall and Nguyen, 2012). On one hand, to achieve a high probability of identifying the true ODC, one should distribute patients evenly among dose combinations to learn about the Efficacy and Toxicity profiles of the entire dose pair domain. On the other hand, to conduct an ethical trial, one should concentrate patients at the dose pair having highest Efficacy and lowest Toxicity, if this dose pair can be identified reliably. The proposed adaptive rule balances these two goals. As described in Chapter 2, one approach to solving the exploration versus exploitation dilemma is use of AR. Compared to AR, the above approach provides higher priority to explore new doses, especially when the estimates of Efficacy for untried doses are low, and thus may be more effective to overcome stickiness for dose combination trials.

To demonstrate the importance of adaptively encouraging the exploration of dose space in two-dimensional dose finding, we compare the design to a "greedy" design that always assigns patients to the dose with the highest estimated Efficacy. The greedy design replaces the rule (9.11) with $\hat{\pi}_E(x_{1,j^*}, x_{2,l^*}) > 0$, so that the dose with the highest Efficacy among admissible dose set $\mathcal{A}_{g^*}$ is always selected.

The simulations considered trials combining two MTAs, A and B, each with 4 dose levels, maximum sample size 45, cohort size 3, and $\bar{\pi}_T = 0.3$. In the proposed design, we set the safety decision cut-off $p_T = 0.6$ and the tuning parameter $\alpha = 2$. Table 9.4 gives the scenarios. In Scenario 1, the dose-Toxicity surface initially increases with the doses of both agents and then plateaus at

TABLE 9.4: Two dose-Toxicity and dose-Efficacy scenarios for the simulation studies. The target ODCs are bolded, and shaded areas indicate plateaus of Toxicity.

	Agent A							
Agent	Toxicity probability				Efficacy probability			
B	1	2	3	4	1	2	3	4
	Scenario 1							
4	.14	**.25**	.25	.25	.42	**.60**	.38	.32
3	.09	.15	.18	.25	.19	.44	.20	.18
2	.04	.08	.13	.18	.12	.29	.15	.10
1	.02	.04	.07	.12	.05	.22	.10	.08
	Scenario 2							
4	.23	.42	.43	.44	.05	.08	.15	.10
3	.15	.23	.42	.43	.10	.14	.24	.18
2	.10	.15	.23	.42	.20	.28	.37	.26
1	.05	.10	**.18**	.25	.30	.40	**.60**	.37

higher doses of the dose pairs with Toxicity probability 0.25. The dose-Efficacy curve increases with $x_{1,j}$ but not with $x_{2,l}$. In Scenario 2, the dose-Toxicity surface becomes flat at high dose levels that are overly toxic.

The simulation results are summarized in Table 9.5. In Scenario 1, the target ODC is $(2, 4)$. The "adaptively encouraging" design outperformed the greedy design with 12.1% higher selection percentage of the ODC and 7.1% more patients allocated to the ODC. The greedy dose assignment rule often caused the design to become trapped at suboptimal doses, such as $(4, 4)$. This demonstrates that the dose assignment rule that adaptively encourages new dose exploration is useful to avoid trapping in suboptimal doses and improve the overall performance of the trial design. Similar results are seen in Scenario 2, where the greedy design was trapped in the lowest dose $(1, 1)$, and had a low selection percentage of the ODC.

TABLE 9.5: Dose pair selection percentages, and percentage of patients treated at each dose pair, under the "adaptively encouraging" (AdptEnc) and greedy designs. The target ODCs are bolded. Shaded areas indicate where the greedy design was trapped at suboptimal dose pairs.

Sc.	Design	Selection percentage				Percentage of patients			
1	AdptEnc	26.0	**36.2**	12.2	8.1	15.3	**17.3**	9.8	8.7
		1.5	5.0	1.8	1.8	2.4	6.0	7.6	5.3
		0.8	1.6	0.7	0.9	1.3	7.6	3.8	2.7
		0.8	1.5	0.7	0.4	6.9	1.8	1.6	2.0
	Greedy	20.0	**24.1**	6.0	27.1	10.0	**10.2**	5.3	31.3
		1.8	4.5	1.3	2.8	1.3	2.7	10.4	3.6
		0.4	3.9	0.7	1.0	0.9	10.0	1.3	1.8
		0.7	2.5	0.9	2.1	7.6	1.6	1.1	0.9
2	AdptEnc	0.8	0.8	0.2	0.4	1.6	1.6	2.5	4.2
		0.4	0.8	0.9	0.2	2.5	4.2	6.9	2.8
		2.2	1.9	3.0	1.8	5.1	8.3	5.1	2.5
		11.6	15.0	**36.1**	19.4	13.9	11.3	**16.4**	11.1
	Greedy	2.0	0.9	0.4	0.4	1.4	1.4	1.6	5.5
		0.6	0.9	1.1	0.5	1.6	2.5	10.3	1.6
		1.9	3.1	4.3	2.2	2.5	12.8	3.7	2.5
		22.1	7.1	**29.8**	18.9	26.5	4.8	**11.4**	10.0

10

Optimizing Doses in Two Cycles

CONTENTS

10.1   The Two-Cycle Problem 203
10.2   A Two-Cycle Model 205
10.3   Decision Criteria 209
10.4   Illustration 212
10.5   Simulation Study 215

"The right thing at the wrong time is the wrong thing."

Joshua Harris

10.1   The Two-Cycle Problem

The designs discussed in the previous chapters dealt with medical settings where a treatment regime, ρ, consisted of either a single dose or a pair of doses of two agents, and administration of the regime is followed by a clinical outcome, Y, that is observed once. Actual medical practice often is more complex than choosing a single ρ and observing Y, however, since a patient's therapy may involve multiple cycles. In this common setting, the physician chooses the patient's treatment in each cycle adaptively based on the patient's history of treatments and clinical outcomes in previous cycles. In such settings, a patient's regime is not one treatment, but rather is a sequence of treatments, with each chosen using a sequentially adaptive decision algorithm. The within-patient regime used by a physician might be described generally as "Observe $\rightarrow$ Act $\rightarrow$ Observe $\rightarrow$ Act $\rightarrow$ $\cdots$" and so on. Here, the first "Observe" means to examine the patient's baseline diagnostic information and prognostic covariates. At each cycle thereafter, observation includes the patient's accumulated history, from all previous cycles, of treatments given, clinical outcomes, and possibly updated baseline covariates. "Act" may mean choose a treatment from a set of alternatives, choose a dose or schedule of a given treatment, suspend therapy to see whether an observed Toxicity is resolved within a given time period, or stop treatment because therapeutic success has been achieved, excessive Toxicity has been observed, or it is considered futile to continue. For each cycle, the treatment given to the patient or other action taken by the physician depends on the particular disease. In oncology, the treatment in each cycle may be a chemical or biological agent, radiation therapy, surgery, cellular therapy, immunotherapy, or some combination of these. Other medical areas where DTRs are applied include chronic diseases such as behavioral or psychological disorders (Collins et al., 2005; Almirall et al., 2010) and drug or alcohol addiction (Murphy et al., 2007). In these settings, the interventions typically include some form of behavior modification or psychotropic drugs to alleviate depression, reduce anxiety, or mitigate psychotic behavior. This paradigm is known variously as a dynamic treatment regime (DTR) (Murphy et al., 2001; Lavori and Dawson, 2004; Murphy, 2003; Moodie et al., 2007), multi-stage treatment strategy (Thall et al., 2000, 2002) or treatment policy (Lunceford et al., 2002; Wahed and Tsiatis, 2004). This DTR paradigm also is used in many areas other than medicine, including control theory, computing, education, and marketing.

Statistical methods for DTRs have seen limited application in actual clinical trials (Rush et al., 2003; Thall et al., 2007; Wang et al., 2012). This is remarkable, since multi-cycle decision-making is an inherent part of routine medical practice. Recently, there has been extensive methodological research to develop or optimize DTRs in medicine. Some examples are semiparametric methods (Wahed and Tsiatis, 2006) and reinforcement learning (Zhao et al., 2011). The general aim is to do a better job of reflecting the intrinsically multi-stage, adaptive structure of what physicians actually do, in both trial design and analysis of observational data, and to construct or identify optimal regimes. This statistical methodology had its origins in research to define and estimate causal parameters in complex longitudinal data, pioneered by Robins (1986, 1993, 1997, 1998) and applied to the analysis of AIDS data (Hernan et al., 2000; Robins et al., 2000) More recently, there has been intensive research activity in sequential, multiple assignment, randomized trial (SMART) designs, which randomize each patient repeatedly at successive stages of their regime (Murphy and Bingham, 2009; Kosorok and Moodie, 2015).

In actual conduct of phase I–II trials, the patient's attending physician often uses a DTR to make multi-cycle decisions. Depending on the patient's history of doses and outcomes, the dose given in each cycle may be above, below, or the same as the dose given in the previous cycle, or the patient's therapy may be terminated due to excessive Toxicity or poor Efficacy. Because the designs we have discussed so far ignore such within-patient multi-cycle decision making, the optimal dose that they choose at the end of the trial actually pertains only to the first cycle of therapy, or possibly may be based on 2 or 3 cycles of therapy while ignoring any between-cycle adaptive decision rules.

In this chapter, we will discuss the problem of adaptively optimizing each patient's dose in each of two cycles of therapy in a phase I–II trial based on binary Efficacy and binary Toxicity. The model and method that we will present are given by Lee et al. (2015). This is the simplest case of the general multi-cycle phase I–II trial design problem, which may be formulated using ordinal or time-to-event outcomes and an arbitrary number of cycles. As the development in this chapter will show, while generalizing dose-finding to two cycles may seem relatively simple, the problem actually is much more complicated than the one-cycle case. This complexity will be seen in the dose-outcome model, which includes a Bayesian hierarchical latent variable structure, and in the methodology used to define and derive optimal two-cycle regimes.

Following Lee et al. (2015), we refer to the methodology as DTM2, an acronym for "Decision-Theoretic Method for 2-cycles." The DTM2 regime consists of two decisions, one for each cycle, with the cycle 1 decision a dose, and the cycle 2 decision depending on the patient's cycle 1 dose and outcomes, including the possibility that the cycle 2 decision is to not treat the patient. A model-based Bayesian objective function is used, defined in terms of utilities for bivariate binary Y of the form $U(y)$ for $y \in \{0,1\}^2$. The action in each cycle is chosen to maximize the posterior expected mean of a Bayesian objective function that is structurally similar to that used in reinforcement learning (Sutton and Barto, 1998) or Q-learning functions (Watkins, 1989). The optimization algorithm is a modified version of the recursive Bellman equation (1957) that makes the usual assumption, when deriving the optimal decision in cycle 1, that the optimal decision will be made in cycle 2. At the end of the trial, the method does not recommend two optimal doses, one for each cycle. Rather, it provides an optimal two-stage regime consisting of an optimal cycle 1 dose, and an optimal function of the patient's cycle 1 dose and outcomes that either chooses a cycle 2 dose or says to not treat the patient in cycle 2. The optimal regime may recommend different cycle 2 doses for two different patients, depending on their cycle 1 data. Because the objective function uses posterior estimates computed using data from other patients in the trial as well as each patient's own cycle 1 data for his/her cycle 2 decision, the decision algorithm is adaptive both between and within patients. This methodology may be considered a hybrid of a utility-based phase I–II design, and a design to optimize a two-cycle DTR.

10.2   A Two-Cycle Model

Denote the number of patients accrued and given at least one cycle of treatment up to trial time t by $n(t)$ and index patients by $i = 1, ..., n(t)$. The dose-outcome model does not depend on numerical dose values. Since we must keep track of patients, outcomes, and cycles, to avoid triple indexing we denote the outcomes as follows. For patient i and treatment cycle $c = 1, 2$, denote dose by $d_{i,c}$, outcome indicators $Y_{i,c}$ for Toxicity and $Z_{i,c}$

for Efficacy. Denote the 2-cycle vectors $d_i = (d_{i,1}, d_{i,2})$, $Y_i = (Y_{i,1}, Y_{i,2})$, and $Z_i = (Z_{i,1}, Z_{i,2})$, and the observed data from all patients at trial time t by $\mathcal{D}_{n(t)} = \{(Y_i, Z_i, d_i) : i = 1, ..., n(t)\}$. Each $d_{i,c}$ is an action that may be either a dose or the decision to not treat the patient in that cycle, is indexed by $d_{i,c} = 0$, so the set of possible actions in each cycle is $\mathcal{R} = \{0, 1, \cdots, m\}$. Denoting the optimal pair chosen by the end of the trial (d_1^{opt}, d_2^{opt}), while d_1^{opt} simply chooses an element from $\mathcal{R}$, $d_2^{opt} = d_2^{opt}(d_1^{opt}, Y_{i,1}, Z_{i,1})$ uses the patient's cycle 1 dose and outcomes to decide what action to take in cycle 2. If $d_1^{opt} = 0$, this corresponds to a case where, after considering the data on actions and outcomes in two cycles of therapy, the recommended action is to not treat the patient with the agent.

A very important point is that optimizing (d_1, d_2) together, "globally," may give a different answer compared to what would be obtained if each cycle were optimized by itself, "myopically." That is, if d_1 where optimized based on the cycle 1 dose and outcomes alone without any consideration of treatment and outcomes in cycle 2, then the optimal dose or action would not necessarily be the same as the first component of the globally optimal two-cycle regime $d^{opt} = (d_1^{opt}, d_2^{opt})$. This is true in general with optimization of any DTR. A common example in cancer chemotherapy is that a high dose of an agent may maximize the response rate in cycle 1, but if it fails to achieve a response then the patient's immune system and organs are so damaged that only a low dose, if any, is possible in cycle 2, so it is very unlikely that a cycle 2 response will be achieved. As a numerical illustration, ignoring Toxicity for simplicity, suppose that the goal is to achieve a response in 1 or 2 cycles of therapy. Suppose that the cycle 1 response probability with $d_1 = 400$ is .60, but if a response is not achieved then a second cycle of chemotherapy is not possible. Suppose that the cycle 1 response probability with $d_1 = 200$ is .50, and if a response is not achieved in cycle 1 then a second cycle using $d_2 = 200$ is given, and the response probability is .40. Thus, while $d_1 = 400$ has a higher cycle response probability than $d_1 = 200$, the overall 2-cycle response probability starting with $d_1 = 400$ is .60, compared to $.50 + (1-.50) \times .40 = .70$ with the two-cycle strategy (200, 200). This illustrates the general fact that making the best decision based only on consideration of the most immediate outcome may be a very bad idea.

The model underlying DTM2 exploits the idea, first introduced by Ashford and Sowden (1970), of generating a multivariate probit model for a vector of binary variables from a corresponding vector of unobserved, correlated, latent multivariate normal variables. This is done by defining each observed variable as the indicator that its corresponding latent variable is greater than 0. Since the multivariate distribution of the vector of observed binary variables is induced by the distribution of the latent normal variables, this construction induces association among the binary variables.

In the present setting, the four observable binary outcome variables of the ith patient are $(Y_i, Z_i) = (Y_{i,1}, Y_{i,2}, Z_{i,1}, Z_{i,2})$. The joint distribution of $[Y_i, Z_i \mid d_i]$ is constructed by defining the binary outcomes in terms of four real-valued latent variables, $\xi_i = (\xi_{i,1}, \xi_{i,2})$ for Y_i and $\eta_i = (\eta_{i,1}, \eta_{i,2})$ for Z_i, with (ξ_i, η_i) following a multivariate normal distribution having means that vary with d_i. This multivariate probit model is elaborated by including hierarchical structures, and it provides a computationally feasible basis for deriving optimal two-cycle regimes for a phase I–II trial. Denoting the indicator of event A by $\mathrm{I}(A)$, the assumptions are $Y_{i,c} = \mathrm{I}(\xi_{i,c} > 0)$ and $Z_{i,c} = \mathrm{I}(\eta_{i,c} > 0)$, so the distribution of $[Y_i, Z_i \mid d_i]$ is induced by that of $[\xi_i, \eta_i \mid d_i]$.

To use this structure to construct the model, a conditional likelihood first is defined for the cycle-specific pairs of latent variables, $[\xi_{i,c}, \eta_{i,c} \mid d_{i,c}]$, for $c = 1, 2$. This is done by using patient-specific random effects (u_i, v_i) to characterize association among the four observed outcomes between and within cycles. Denote a univariate normal distribution with mean μ and variance σ^2 by $N(\mu, \sigma^2)$, and denote its pdf by $\phi(\cdot \mid , \mu, \sigma^2)$. The construction assumes the following Level 1 and Level 2 priors, i.e., priors and hyperpriors:

Level 1 Priors on the Latent Variables. For patient i treated with dose $d_{i,c} = d$ in cycle c,

$$\xi_{i,c} \mid u_i, \bar{\xi}_{c,d}, \sigma_\xi^2 \sim \mathrm{N}(\bar{\xi}_{c,d} + u_i, \ \sigma_\xi^2) \quad \text{and} \quad \eta_{i,c} \mid v_i, \bar{\eta}_{c,d}, \sigma_\eta^2 \sim \mathrm{N}(\bar{\eta}_{c,d} + v_i, \ \sigma_\eta^2),$$
$$(10.1)$$

with ξ_i and η_i conditionally independent given (u_i, v_i) and fixed variances, σ_ξ^2 and σ_η^2.

Level 2 priors of the patient effects, (u_i, v_i), and mean cycle-specific dose effects, $(\bar{\xi}_{c,d}, \bar{\eta}_{c,d})$, are as follows. Let MVN_k denote a k-variate normal distribution, and let $\Sigma_{u,v}$ denote the 2×2 matrix with all diagonal elements τ^2 and all off-diagonal elements $\rho\tau^2$.

Level 2 Priors on the Random Patient Effects. For patient $i = 1, \cdots, n$,

$$u_i, v_i \mid \rho, \ \tau^2 \ \overset{iid}{\sim} \ \mathrm{MVN}_2((0,0), \Sigma_{u,v}). \tag{10.2}$$

The prior hyperparameters, $-1 \leq \rho \leq 1$ and $\tau^2 > 0$, are fixed. This Level 2 prior induces association, parameterized by (ρ, τ^2), among the mean parameters $(\xi_{i,1}, \eta_{i,1}, \xi_{i,2}, \eta_{i,2})$ via the latent variable model (10.1), and thus among the corresponding observed Toxicity and Efficacy outcomes, (Y_i, Z_i).

Denote the vectors of mean dose effects by $\bar{\xi}_c = (\bar{\xi}_{c,1}, \cdots, \bar{\xi}_{c,m})$ and $\bar{\eta}_c = (\bar{\eta}_{c,1}, \cdots, \bar{\eta}_{c,m})$. Let $\bar{\xi}_{c,-d}$ denote the vector $\bar{\xi}_c$ with $\bar{\xi}_{c,d}$ deleted, and similarly let $\bar{\eta}_{c,-d}$ denote $\bar{\eta}_c$ with $\bar{\eta}_{c,d}$ deleted.

Level 2 Priors on the Mean Dose Effects $(\bar{\xi}_{c,d}, \bar{\eta}_{c,d})$. The following Level 2 prior induces association among the elements of the Level 1 prior hyperparameters $\bar{\xi}_{c,d}$ and $\bar{\eta}_{c,d}$, for each dose d :

$$p(\bar{\xi}_{c,d} \mid \bar{\xi}_{c,-d}) \ \propto \ \phi(\bar{\xi}_{c,d} \mid \xi_{c,0}, \sigma_{\bar{\xi}_{c,0}}^2) 1(\bar{\xi}_{c,d-1} < \bar{\xi}_{c,d} < \bar{\xi}_{c,d+1})$$
$$p(\bar{\eta}_{c,d} \mid \bar{\eta}_{c,-d}) \ \propto \ \phi(\bar{\eta}_{c,d} \mid \eta_{c,0}, \sigma_{\eta_{c,0}}^2) 1(\bar{\eta}_{c,d-1} < \bar{\eta}_{c,d} < \bar{\eta}_{c,d+1}). \quad (10.3)$$

The order constraints ensure that $\xi_{i,c}$ and $\eta_{i,c}$ each increases stochastically in dose, which implies that the per-cycle probabilities of Toxicity and Efficacy increase with dose. In settings where this assumption is not appropriate, such as trials of biologic agents, these constraints should be dropped.

Collecting terms from (10.1), (10.2), and (10.3), the 12 fixed hyperparameters that determine all Level 1 and Level 2 priors are

$$\tilde{\theta} = (\xi_0, \eta_0, \sigma^2_{\xi_0}, \sigma^2_{\eta_0}, \sigma^2_\xi, \sigma^2_\eta, \tau^2, \rho)$$

where $\xi_0 = (\xi_{1,0}, \xi_{2,0})$, $\eta_0 = (\eta_{1,0}, \eta_{2,0})$, $\sigma^2_{\xi_0} = (\sigma^2_{\xi_{1,0}}, \sigma^2_{\xi_{2,0}})$ and $\sigma^2_{\eta_0} = (\sigma^2_{\eta_{1,0}}, \sigma^2_{\eta_{2,0}})$. Denote the parameter vectors $\bar{\xi} = (\bar{\xi}_1, \bar{\xi}_2)$, $\bar{\eta} = (\bar{\eta}_1, \bar{\eta}_2)$, and $\mu_{d_i} = (\bar{\xi}_{1,d_{i,1}}, \bar{\xi}_{2,d_{i,2}}, \bar{\eta}_{1,d_{i,1}}, \bar{\eta}_{2,d_{i,2}})$, and the covariance matrix

$$\Sigma_{\xi,\eta} = \begin{bmatrix} \sigma^2_\xi + \tau^2 & \tau^2 & \rho\tau^2 & \rho\tau^2 \\ & \sigma^2_\xi + \tau^2 & \rho\tau^2 & \rho\tau^2 \\ & & \sigma^2_\eta + \tau^2 & \tau^2 \\ & & & \sigma^2_\eta + \tau^2 \end{bmatrix}.$$

The joint distribution of $[\xi_i, \eta_i \mid d_i, \bar{\xi}, \bar{\eta}, \tilde{\theta}]$ is computed by integrating over (u_i, v_i), yielding

$$\xi_i, \eta_i \mid d_i, \bar{\xi}, \bar{\eta}, \tilde{\theta} \overset{iid}{\sim} \text{MVN}_4\left(\mu_{d_i}, \Sigma_{\xi,\eta}\right). \tag{10.4}$$

The mean vector μ_{d_i} is a function of the dose levels, and it does not depend on numerical dose values. The hyperparameters, τ^2 and ρ, induce associations between Efficacy outcomes and Toxicity outcomes both between and within cycles. If $-1 < \rho < 0$, this model implies that Efficacy and Toxicity are negatively associated, that is, higher Toxicity is associated with lower Efficacy. If $0 < \rho < 1$, then Efficacy and Toxicity are positively associated, and lower Toxicity is associated with lower Efficacy.

For either cycle, denote the pair of possible observed Toxicity outcomes by $y = (y_1, y_2) \in \{0, 1\}^2$ and Efficacy outcomes by $z = (z_1, z_2) \in \{0, 1\}^2$. Denote $\theta = (\bar{\xi}, \bar{\eta})$. Integrating over (u_i, v_i) and suppressing $\tilde{\theta}$ and patient index i, the joint likelihood for the observables of a patient is given by

$$
\begin{aligned}
p(y, z \mid d, \theta) &= \Pr(Y_1 = y_1, Y_2 = y_2, Z_1 = z_1, Z_2 = z_2 \mid d, \theta) \\
&= \Pr(\gamma_{1,y_1} \leq \xi_1 < \gamma_{1,y_1+1}, \gamma_{1,y_2} \leq \xi_2 < \gamma_{1,y_2+1}, \\
&\qquad \gamma_{2,z_1} \leq \eta_1 < \gamma_{2,z_1+1}, \gamma_{2,y_2} \leq \eta_2 < \gamma_{2,z_2+1} \mid d, \theta)
\end{aligned}
$$

$$= \int_{\gamma_{1,y_1}}^{\gamma_{1,y_1+1}} \int_{\gamma_{1,y_2}}^{\gamma_{1,y_2+1}} \int_{\gamma_{2,z_1}}^{\gamma_{2,z_1+1}} \int_{\gamma_{2,z_2}}^{\gamma_{2,z_2+1}} \phi(\xi, \eta \mid \mu_d, \Sigma_{\xi,\eta}) d\eta_2 d\eta_1 d\xi_2 d\xi_1,$$

where the cut-off vectors $(\gamma_{10}, \gamma_{11}, \gamma_{12})$ for Y_c and $(\gamma_{20}, \gamma_{21}, \gamma_{22})$ for Z_c both are $(-\infty, 0, \infty)$, for $c = 1, 2$. The conditional distribution of the cycle 2 outcomes (Y_2, Z_2) given the cycle 1 outcomes $(Y_1 = y_1, Z_1 = z_1)$ is

$$p(y_2, z_2 \mid y_1, z_1, d, \theta) = \Pr(Y_2 = y_2, Z_2 = z_2 \mid Y_1 = y_1, Z_1 = z_1, d)$$

$$= \frac{p(y, z \mid d, \theta)}{p(y_1, z_1 \mid d_1, \theta)},$$

where the cycle 1 bivariate marginal is computed as the double integral

$$p(y_1, z_1 \mid d_1, \theta) = \int_{\gamma_{1y_1}}^{\gamma_{1,y_1+1}} \int_{\gamma_{2z_1}}^{\gamma_{2,z_1+1}} \phi([\xi_1, \eta_1] \mid \mu_{d_1}^1, \Sigma_{\xi,\eta}^1) d\eta_1 d\xi_1 \quad (10.5)$$

with

$$\mu_{d_1}^1 = \begin{bmatrix} \bar{\xi}_{1,d_1} \\ \bar{\eta}_{1,d_1} \end{bmatrix} \text{ and } \Sigma_{\xi,\eta}^1 = \begin{bmatrix} \sigma_\xi^2 + \tau^2 & \rho\tau^2 \\ \rho\tau^2 & \sigma_\eta^2 + \tau^2 \end{bmatrix}.$$

The structure of this hierarchical model in the two cycle setting is similar to the non-hierarchical model for multiple toxicities in one cycle of therapy used by Bekele and Thall (2004). Posterior computation relies on the MCMC methods for latent variable models given by Albert and Chib (1993) and extended by Chib and Greenberg (1998) to use Gibbs sampling.

10.3 Decision Criteria

Recall that the action in each cycle either chooses a dose from the set $\{1, \cdots, m\}$ or makes the decision to not treat the patient, indexed by 0. If the optimal cycle 1 action is $d_1^{opt} = 0$ at any point in the trial then the study is terminated. Otherwise, the patient receives d_1^{opt} for cycle 1 and $d_2^{opt} \in \mathcal{R}$ for cycle 2, where d_2^{opt} is a function of the cycle 1 dose and outcomes, (d_1^{opt}, Y_1, Z_1), and the current data, $\mathcal{D}_{n(t)}$, from all $n(t)$ patients. The optimal actions (d_1^{opt}, d_2^{opt}) change throughout the course of the trial as patients are treated, their outcomes are observed, and thus $\mathcal{D}_{n(t)}$ expands.

For example, if the cycle 1 dose $d_{i,1}^{opt} = d_1$ given to patient i produced Toxicity, $Y_{i,1} = 1$, then one possible optimal cycle 2 action is $d_{i,2}^{opt}(d_1, 1, 1, \mathcal{D}_{n(t)}) = d_1 - 1$ if $Z_{i,1} = 1$, and $d_{i,2}^{opt}(d_1, 1, 0, \mathcal{D}_{n(t)}) = 0$ if $Z_{i,1} = 0$. Similarly, if $d_{i,1}^{opt} = 1$, the lowest dose level, and $Y_{i,1} = 1$ was observed, then it may be that $d_{i,2}^{opt}(d_1, 1, Z_1, \mathcal{D}_{n(t)}) = 0$ regardless of whether $Z_{i,1} = 0$ or 1. In general, a two-cycle regime is far more general than a dose pair chosen from $\mathcal{D}_{n(t)} \times \mathcal{D}_{n(t)}$, and a regime for which $d_{i,2}^{opt}$ ignores the patient's cycle 1 dose and outcomes, $(d_{i,1}, Y_{i,1}, Z_{i,1})$, is unlikely to be optimal. In the DTR literature, $(d_{i,1}^{opt}, Y_{i,1}, Z_{i,1})$ would be called "tailoring variables."

To optimize (d_1, d_2), an objective function is constructed by exploiting the basic ideas of Bellman (1957), starting in cycle 2 and working backwards. A point of departure from conventional DTR methodology is that DTM2 uses per-cycle utilities $U(y, z)$ to quantify the desirability of outcome $(Y_c, Z_c) = (y, z)$ in cycle $c = 1$ or 2.

Depending on the levels of marginalization and aggregation over cycles and patients, many different variations of the objective function defined below may be obtained. We will refer to any of these generically as a "utility" or "objective function" when we want to highlight that a particular expected utility is a function only of known quantities and the action taken, and thus can be used to select the optimal action. We fix $U(0,1) = 100$ and $U(1,0) = 0$, with the intermediate values $U(0,0)$ and $U(1,1)$ elicited from the physicians. In the simulations given below, the numerical utilities $U(0,0) = 35$ and $U(1,1) = 65$ are used.

In the language of Q-learning (Watkins, 1989; Murphy, 2005; Zhao et al., 2011), the cycle c "action" is d_c, the "reward" is $U(Y_c, Z_c)$, and the "state" prior to taking action d_2 in cycle 2 is (d_1, Y_1, Z_1). Ideally, baseline covariates such as age, disease severity, or performance status also would be included in the patient's state for $c = 1$. This is an important extension of the methodology presented here.

Suppress patient index i and trial time t to simplify notation. Given a patient's cycle 1 data (d_1, Y_1, Z_1), the *mean utility of action d_2 in cycle 2* is

$$
\begin{aligned}
Q_2(d_2, d_1, Y_1, Z_1, \theta) &= E\{U(Y_2, Z_2) \mid d_2, d_1, Y_1, Z_1, \theta\} \\
&= \sum_{y_2=0}^{1} \sum_{z_2=0}^{1} U(y_2, z_2) p(y_2, z_2 \mid d_2, d_1, Y_1, Z_1, \theta).
\end{aligned}
$$

A cycle 2 objective function is obtained by computing the posterior mean of Q_2 given $\mathcal{D}_{n(t)}$,

$$
q_2(d_2, d_1, Y_1, Z_1, calD_t) = E\{Q_2(d_2, d_1, Y_1, Z_1, \theta) \mid d_2, d_1, Y_1, Z_1, \mathcal{D}_{n(t)}\}.
$$

Given (d_1, Y_1, Z_1) and the current data $\mathcal{D}$, the optimal cycle 2 action is

$$
d_2^{opt}(d_1, Y_1, Z_1, \mathcal{D}_{n(t)}) = \underset{d_2}{\operatorname{argmax}} \ \{q_2(d_2, d_1, Y_1, Z_1, \mathcal{D}_{n(t)})\},
$$

subject to acceptability rules for d_2.

If $d_2 = 0$, i.e., no treatment is given in cycle 2, then

$$
p(Y_2 = 0, Z_2 = 0 \mid d_2 = 0, d_1, Y_1, Z_1, \theta) = 1
$$

and consequently the cycle 2 payoff is

$$
q_2(d_2 = 0, d_1, Y_1, Z_1, \mathcal{D}_{n(t)}) = U(0,0),
$$

the utility of having neither Toxicity nor Efficacy. The fact that $U(0,0)$ is what is achieved by not treating the patient plays a key role in constructing optimal rules. If $d_2 \neq 0$, then $q_2(d_2, d_1, Y_1, Z_1, \mathcal{D})$ is the posterior expected utility of giving dose d_2 in cycle 2 given (d_1, Y_1, Z_1). This underscores the importance of requiring $U(0,0) > U(1,0)$, namely, that it must be more desirable to have neither Toxicity nor Efficacy than to have Toxicity and no Efficacy.

Next, the procedure moves backward to the cycle 1 optimization under the Bellman assumption that $q_2(d_2^{opt}, d_1, Y_1, Z_1, \mathcal{D})$ has been computed for all $(d_1, Y_1, Z_1, \mathcal{D})$. The expected utility of administering dose d_1 given θ is

$$Q_1(d_1, \theta) = E\{U(Y_1, Z_1) \mid d_1, \theta\} = \sum_{y_1=0}^{1} \sum_{z_1=0}^{1} U(y_1, z_1) p(y_1, z_1 | d_1, \theta).$$

To define the overall objective function, the cycle 2 payoff is discounted using the fixed parameter $0 < \lambda < 1$, as is done traditionally in Q-learning. The expected entire future utility of administering dose d_1 in cycle 1, assuming that d_2^{opt} will be taken in cycle 2, is

$$
\begin{aligned}
q_1(d_1, \mathcal{D}_{n(t)}) &= E\Big[E\{U(Y_1, Z_1) \\
&\quad + \lambda\, q_2(d_2^{opt}(d_1, Y_1, Z_1, \mathcal{D}), d_1, Y_1, Z_1, \mathcal{D}_{n(t)}) | \theta, d_1\} | d_1, \mathcal{D}_{n(t)} \Big] \\
&= E\{Q_1(d_1, \theta) | d_1, \mathcal{D}_{n(t)}\} \\
&\quad + \lambda \sum_{y_1=0}^{1} \sum_{z_1=0}^{1} q_2(d_2^{opt}(d_1, y_1, z_1, \mathcal{D}_{n(t)}), d_1, y_1, z_1, \mathcal{D}) \\
&\quad \times\ p(y_1, z_1 | d_1, \mathcal{D}_{n(t)}),
\end{aligned}
$$

where $p(y_1, z_1 | d_1, \mathcal{D})$ is the posterior expected density for (Y_1, Z_1). The optimal cycle 1 action is

$$d_1^{opt} = \underset{d_1}{\arg\max}\ q_1(d_1, \mathcal{D}_{n(t)}),$$

subject to dose acceptability rules for d_1.

The maximizations in q_1 and q_2 yield the optimal pair of actions $d^{opt} = (d_1^{opt}, d_2^{opt})$, where d_1^{opt} is either a dose or 0, d_2^{opt} is applicable only when $d_1^{opt} \neq 0$, d_2^{opt} is a function of (d_1^{opt}, Y_1, Z_1), and both are functions of $\mathcal{D}_{n(t)}$. These maximizations include the possibilities of selecting $d_c = 0$ by comparing the expected utility to that of no treatment. Thus, while a given dose or dose pair may be optimal in the sense that they maximize q_1 and q_2 over the doses $1, \cdots, m$, it still is possible that their expected utilities may be smaller than those of $d = \{0, 0\}$ or $d_2 = 0$. This is an ethical constraint on the method. If new data from other patients are obtained between administration of d_1^{opt} and optimization of $q_2(d_2(d_1), \mathcal{D}_{n(t)})$, then $\mathcal{D}_{n(t)}$ changes while waiting to evaluate the patient's cycle 1 outcomes (Y_1, Z_1). In this case, the posterior and hence the patient's optimal cycle 2 action d_2^{opt} might change.

As in the single cycle cases, the method includes dose acceptability gatekeeper criteria. The first constraint is the usual one that an untried dose level may not be skipped when escalating. Let d_1^M denote the highest dose among those that have been tried in cycle 1 and d_2^M the highest dose among those that have been tried in either cycle. The search for optimal actions is constrained so that $1 \le d_1 \le \min(d_1^M + 1, m)$ and $1 \le d_2 \le \min(d_2^M + 1, m)$. The second constraint does not allow escalating a patient's dose in cycle 2 if Toxicity was observed in cycle 1, $Y_1 = 1$. While this may seem obvious clinically, it is possible that the formal method without this constraint might recommend that one should escalate in cycle 2 after observing $Y_1 = 1$, say if $Z_1 = 1$ and $U(1, 1)$ is sufficiently large. The third criterion, defined in terms of expected utility, is included to avoid giving undesirable dose pairs.

For cycle 2, *action d_2 is unacceptable* if it violates the do-not-skip rule, escalates after $Y_1 = 1$, or

$$q_2(d_2, d_1, Y_1, Z_1, \mathcal{D}_{n(t)}) < U(0, 0),$$

that is, if the posterior expected utility of treating the patient with d_2 given $(d_1, Y_1, Z_1, \mathcal{D}_{n(t)})$ is smaller than what one would expect to obtain by not treating the patient at all. We denote the set of acceptable cycle 2 doses for a patient with cycle 1 data (d_1, Y_1, Z_1) by $\mathcal{A}_2(d_1, Y_1, Z_1, \mathcal{D}_{n(t)})$. Note that a given d_2 may be acceptable for some (d_1, Y_1, Z_1) but not acceptable for others.

We require that $d_2^{opt}(d_1, Y_1, Z_1, \mathcal{D}_{n(t)})$ is chosen from $\mathcal{A}_2(d_1, Y_1, Z_1, \mathcal{D}_{n(t)})$. For cycle 1, we say that *action d_1 is unacceptable* if it violates the do-not-skip rule or satisfies the utility-based criterion, similar to that for cycle 2,

$$q_1(d_1, \mathcal{D}_{n(t)}) < U(0, 0) + \lambda U(0, 0).$$

This says that d_1 is unacceptable in cycle 1 if it yields a smaller posterior expected utility than not treating the patient. We denote the set of acceptable cycle 1 doses by $\mathcal{A}_1 \subset \mathcal{D}_{n(t)}$. Note that, while $\mathcal{A}_1$ is adaptive between patients since it is a function of other patients' data, $\mathcal{A}_2(d_1, Y_1, Z_1, \mathcal{D}_{n(t)})$ is adaptive both between and within patients.

10.4   Illustration

Table 10.1 illustrates true expected cycle 2 utilities of d_2 conditional on (d_1, Y_1, Z_1) using simulation Scenario 4, given below. For example, the true values of $Q_2(d_2, d_1 = 3, Y_1 = 0, Z_1 = 0, \theta^{true})$ given in the first row of the third box from the top are (35.98, 39.49, 39.70, 36.30, 27.17) for $d_2 = (1, 2, 3, 4, 5)$, respectively. Since $Q_2(5, 3, 0, 0, \theta^{true}) < U(0, 0)$, the payoff for treating the patient at $d = 5$ is less than the payoff for not treating the patient at all in cycle 2. Thus, $d_2 = 5$ is not acceptable. The other dose levels are acceptable, so $\mathcal{A}_2(3, 0, 0, \theta^{true}) = \{1, 2, 3, 4\}$, with $d_2^{opt}(d_1 = 3, Y_1 = 0, Z_1 = 0, \theta^{true}) = 3$. When $(d_1, Y_1, Z_1) = (3, 1, 0)$, no d_2 has expected utility $> U(0, 0)$, and moreover $d_2 = 3, 4, 5$ are not allowed due to the no-escalation-after-Toxicity rule. Thus, $\mathcal{A}_2(3, 0, 0, \theta^{true})$ is the empty set and $d_2^{opt}(d_1 = 3, Y_1 = 1, Z_1 = 0, \theta^{true}) = 0$. The last column of the table gives $d_2^{opt}(d_1, Y_1, Z_1, \theta^{true})$ for all combinations of (d_1, Y_1, Z_1).

TABLE 10.1: True expected utilities $Q_2(d_2, d_1, Y_1, Z_1, \theta^{true})$ in simulation scenario 4

d_1	true $q_1(d_1, \theta)$	(Y_1, Z_1)	d_2 1	2	3	4	5	d_2^{opt}
1	66.2	(0,0)	37.3	41.4	41.9	38.5	*29.7*	3
		(0,1)	48.2	55.1	56.8	54.0	45.0	3
		(1,0)	30.6	33.6	33.1	29.6	23.3	NT
		(1,1)	41.2	47.2	48.0	44.8	38.2	NT
2	73.4	(0,0)	36.5	40.3	40.7	37.3	*28.4*	3
		(0,1)	45.1	51.4	52.9	50.1	41.2	3
		(1,0)	*30.1*	32.9	32.3	28.7	22.3	NT
		(1,1)	38.4	43.7	44.3	41.1	34.5	1
3	80.6	(0,0)	36.0	39.5	39.7	36.3	*27.2*	3
		(0,1)	43.3	49.2	50.6	47.7	38.7	3
		(1,0)	*30.3*	*32.8*	32.1	28.4	21.5	NT
		(1,1)	37.3	42.3	42.8	39.5	32.5	2
4	69.7	(0,0)	37.2	40.9	41.4	38.2	*28.7*	3
		(0,1)	44.4	50.5	52.1	49.5	40.1	3
		(1,0)	*32.1*	*34.9*	*34.4*	30.7	22.9	NT
		(1,1)	39.2	44.3	45.0	41.7	33.9	3
5	68.2	(0,0)	38.1	42.0	42.8	39.8	*30.1*	3
		(0,1)	45.3	51.5	53.5	51.0	41.5	3
		(1,0)	*33.0*	35.9	35.5	*31.9*	23.7	2
		(1,1)	40.1	45.3	46.2	43.0	34.8	3

The expected utilities given in gray boxes are those for d_2 violating the do-not-escalate-after-$Y_1 = 1$ rule. The expected utilities given in italics are those for d_2 unacceptable.

Recall that AR can be very useful to reduce stickiness. This also is the case in the two-cycle setting. While d^{opt} yields the best clinical outcomes on average, the reliability of the methodology over the course of the trial can be improved by including AR among the d having objective function values near the maximum at d^{opt}. Thus, AR is included as part of DTM2.

To implement AR in the 2-cycle setting, first define ϵ_i to be a function decreasing in patient index i, and denote $\epsilon = (\epsilon_1, \cdots, \epsilon_n)$. The set $\mathcal{R}_{i,1}$ of ϵ_i-*optimal doses for cycle 1* is defined as all $d_1 \in \mathcal{A}_{i,1}(\mathcal{D}_{n(t)})$ such that

$$\left| q_1(d_{1,i}^{opt}, \mathcal{D}_{n(t)}) - q_1(d_1, \mathcal{D}_{n(t)}) \right| < \epsilon_i.$$

That is, $\mathcal{R}_{i,1}$ contains acceptable d_1 having posterior mean utility within ϵ_i of the maximum posterior mean utility. Similarly, $\mathcal{R}_{i,2}$ of $(\epsilon_i/2)$-optimal doses for cycle 2 given $(d_{i,1}, Y_{i,1}, Z_{i,1})$ is defined as the $d_2 \in \mathcal{A}_{i,2}(d_{i,1}, Y_{i,1}, Z_{i,1}, \mathcal{D}_{n(t)})$ satisfying

$$\left| q_2(d_{i,2}^{opt}, d_{i,1}, Y_{i,1}, Z_{i,1}, \mathcal{D}_{n(t)}) - q_2(d_2, d_{i,1}, Y_{i,1}, Z_{i,1}, \mathcal{D}_{n(t)}) \right| < \epsilon_i/2,$$

keeping in mind that $d_{i,2}^{opt}$ is a function of $(d_{i,1}, Y_{i,1}, Z_{i,1})$. The value $\epsilon_i/2$ is used for cycle 2 because $q_2(d_2, d_1, Y_1, Z_1, \mathcal{D}_{n(t)})$ is the posterior expected utility for cycle 2 only, whereas q_1 is the total payoff for both cycles. For each cycle $c = 1, 2$, patient i is randomized fairly among the doses in $\mathcal{D}_{i,c}$. This is called AR(ϵ). The numerical values of ϵ_i depend on the numerical range of $U(y, z)$, and must be determined by preliminary trial simulations.

The trial studied in the simulations is constructed to mimic a typical phase I–II chemotherapy trial with five dose levels, but accounting for two cycles of therapy rather than one. The maximum sample size is $N = 60$ patients with a cohort size 2. Based on preliminary simulations, the values $\epsilon_i = 20$ are used for the first 10 patients, $\epsilon_i = 15$ for the next 10 patients, and $\epsilon_i = 10$ for the remaining 40 patients. An initial cohort of 2 patients is treated at the lowest dose in cycle 1, their cycle 1 Toxicity and Efficacy outcomes are observed, the posterior of θ is computed, and actions are taken for cycle 2 of patients in the initial cohort. If $\mathcal{R}_{i,2} = \{0\}$ then patient i does not receive a second cycle of treatment. If $\mathcal{R}_{i,2} \neq \{0\}$, then AR($\epsilon$) is used to choose an action from $\mathcal{R}_{i,2}$ for cycle 2. When $(Y_{i,2}, Z_{i,2})$ are observed from cycle 2, the posterior of θ is updated. The second cohort is not enrolled until the cycle 1 outcomes of the first cohort have been evaluated.

For all subsequent cohorts, the posterior is updated after the outcomes of all previous cohorts are observed, and the posterior expected utility, $q_{i,1}(d_1, \mathcal{D}_{n(t)})$, is computed using $\lambda = 0.8$. If $\mathcal{R}_{i,1}(\mathcal{D}_{n(t)}) = \emptyset$ for any interim $\mathcal{X}$, then $d_{i,1}(\mathcal{D}) = 0$, and the trial is terminated with no d selected. If $\mathcal{R}_{i,1} \neq \emptyset$, then a cycle 1 dose is chosen from $\mathcal{D}_{i,1}$ using AR(ϵ). Once the outcomes in cycle 1 are observed, the posterior is updated. Given $(d_{i,1}, Y_{i,1}, Z_{i,1}, \mathcal{D}_{n(t)})$ and ϵ_i, the set $\mathcal{R}_{i,2}$ of cycle 2 actions is searched. If $\mathcal{R}_{i,2} = \{0\}$, then $d_{i,2} = 0$

and a cycle 2 dose is not given to patient i. Otherwise, $d_{i,2}$ is selected from $\mathcal{R}_{i,2}(d_{i,1}, Y_{i,1}, Z_{i,1}, \mathcal{D}_{n(t)})$ using AR(ϵ). All adaptive decisions are made based on the most recent data $\mathcal{D}$. In particular, a new d_{select} may be chosen utilizing partial data from recent patients for whom $(Y_{i,1}, Z_{i,1})$ but not $(Y_{i,2}, Z_{i,2})$ have been evaluated. These steps are repeated until either the trial has been stopped early or $N = 60$ has been reached, in which case a final optimal two-cycle regime d_{select} is chosen. The aim is that the chosen pair d_{select} should be the true $d_1^{opt} \in \{1, \cdots, m\}$ and $d_2^{opt}(d_1^{opt}, y_1, z_1) \in \mathcal{R}$. Note that the final recommendation for phase III is d_{select}, rather than a single "optimal" dose as is done conventionally.

10.5 Simulation Study

The simulations compare DTM2 with four other designs. These are two-cycle extensions of the CRM, a Bayesian phase I–II method using toxicity and efficacy odds ratios (TEOR, Yin et al., 2006), and the 3+3a and 3+3b methods discussed in Chapter 1. Each of these one-cycle methods was extended to include additional decision rules for a second cycle. For both 3+3 methods, the deterministic rule was used in cycle 2 that if $Y_1 = 1$ then the dose is lowered by 1 level ($d_2 = d_1 - 1$) and if $Y_1 = 0$ then the first dose is repeated ($d_2 = d_1$). The 3+3a method, with this deterministic rule for cycle 2, is used very commonly in actual phase I trials.

For cycle 1 of the extended CRM, called the ECRM, the usual model was assumed with $\Pr(Y_1 = 1|d_1) = p_{d_1}^{\exp(\alpha)}$ and $\alpha \sim N(0, 2)$ with skeleton $(p_1, \cdots, p_5)$. The skeleton was calibrated using the "getprior" subroutine in the package "dfcrm," with target toxicity probability $\pi_T^* = 0.30$, the prior guess that the MTD is level 4, and the desired halfwidth of the indifference intervals equal to 0.05 (Cheung, 2011). This produced the skeleton $(p_1, \cdots, p_5) = (0.063, 0.123, 0.204, 0.300, 0.402)$. With this model, each patient's cycle 1 dose is chosen to have posterior mean toxicity probability closest to 0.30. This was implemented using the R function, "crm" in dfcrm, while imposing the do-not-skip rule for cycle 1. To determine a cycle 2 dose, the same deterministic rule as for the extended (3+3) methods was used, with one more safety requirement. For ECRM, a cycle 2 dose was not given if $\Pr\{\Pr(Y_1 = 1 \text{ or } Y_2 = 1) > p_T|\mathcal{D}_{n(t)}, d\} > \psi_T$, with $p_T = 0.5$ and $\psi_T = 0.9$, assuming independence of $P(Y_1 = 1)$ and $P(Y_2 = 1)$ for simplicity. For example, following the deterministic rule, a patient treated in cycle 1 at d_1 may be treated at $d_2 \in \{d_1 - 1, d_1\}$ depending on the cycle 1 Toxicity outcome. This, d_1 is repeated in cycle 2 if $Y_1 = 0$. If (d_1, d_1) does not satisfy the safety requirement, then the cycle 2 treatment is not given to a patient with $Y_1 = 0$. If the cycle 2 treatment is not allowed for any d_1 regardless of Y_1, that is, if no (d_1, d_2) with $d_2 \in \{d_1 - 1, d_1\}$ satisfies the safety rule, then d_1 is lowered until the cycle 2 treatment is safe for either of $Y_1 = 0$ or $Y_1 = 1$.

TEOR was extended to 2-cycles similarly to ECRM, and this was called ETEOR. For ETEOR, the patient was not treated in cycle 2 if Toxicity in both cycles or Efficacy in neither cycle was likely. Formally, $d_2 = 0$ if $\Pr\{\Pr(Y_1 = 1 \text{ or } Y_2 = 1) > p_T | \mathcal{D}_{n(t)}, d\} > \psi_T$ or $\Pr\{\Pr(Z_1 = 0 \text{ and } Z_2 = 0) > p_E | \mathcal{D}_{n(t)}, d\} > \psi_E$ with $p_T = 0.6$, $p_E = 0.8$, and $\psi_T = \psi_E = 0.9$, assuming the two cycles are independent for simplicity. The priors of Yin et al.(2006) were calibrated using prior ESS, which gave their hyperparameters as $\sigma_\phi^2 = 20$, $\sigma_\psi^2 = 5$ and $\sigma_\theta^2 = 10$. We set $\bar{\pi}_T = 0.35$, $\underline{\pi}_E = 0.5$, $p^{escl} = 0.5$, $p^\star = 0.25$ and $q^\star = 0.1$, and used $w_d^{(3)}$ to select a dose for the next patient. The trials were simulated under each of eight scenarios using each of the five designs: DTM2, the extended 3+3a and 3+3b algorithms, ECRM, and ETEOR.

For the simulations, 2-cycle scenarios were determined by specifying joint distributions $p(y_1, z_1 \mid d_1)$ for each d_1 and $p(y_2, z_2 \mid d_1, d_2, y_1, z_1)$ for each (d_1, d_2, y_1, z_1). The first seven scenarios were constructed using the model that underlies DTM2, and Scenario 8 was obtained using a very different model to study robustness, but using the same marginal probabilities as Scenario 5. The data were simulated assuming $\sigma_\xi^{2,true} = \sigma_\eta^{2,true} = 0.5^2$, $\tau^{2,true} = 0.3^2$ and $\rho^{true} = -0.2$. The true marginals $\pi_{T,c}(d_j)$ and $\pi_{E,c}(d_j)$ for Scenarios 1–7 are given in Table 10.2, with these identical for Scenarios 5 and 8. Values of $\bar{\xi}^{true}$ and $\bar{\eta}^{true}$ were determined by matching

$$\Pr(Y_c < 0) = \Phi(0 \mid \bar{\xi}_{d_c}^{true}, \sigma_\xi^{2,true} + \tau^{2,true})$$

and

$$\Pr(Z_c < 0) = \Phi(0 \mid \bar{\eta}_{d_c}^{true}, \sigma_\eta^{2,true} + \tau^{2,true}).$$

To study robustness in Scenario 8, outcomes were simulated using the following logistic regression model. The marginal cycle 1 Toxicity and Efficacy probabilities $(p_T(d_1), p_E(d_1))$ are the same as those of Scenario 5, with outcomes generated using true probabilities

$$\Pr(Y_1 = 1 \mid d_1) = p_T(d_1)$$

$$\Pr(Z_1 = 1 \mid d_1, Y_1) = \text{logit}^{-1}\{\text{logit}(p_E(d_1)) - 0.34(Y_1 - 0.5)\}$$

$$\Pr(Y_2 = 1 \mid d_1, d_2, Y_1, Z_1)$$

$$= \text{logit}^{-1}\{\text{logit}(p_T(d_1)) + 0.33 d_2 + 0.4(Y_1 - 0.5) - 0.3(Z_1 - 0.5)\},$$

and

$$\Pr(Z_2 = 1 \mid d_1, d_2, Y_1, Z_1, Y_2)$$

$$= \text{logit}^{-1}\{\text{logit}(p_E(d_1)) + 0.76 d_2 - 0.22(Y_1 - 0.5) + 2.4(Z_1 - 0.5) - 1.8(Y_2 - 0.5)\}.$$

TABLE 10.2: True marginal probabilities $(p_T, p_E)^{true}$ for each cycle under each scenario used in the simulation studies

	Dose Levels				
	1	2	3	4	5
Cycle			Scenario 1		
1	(0.10, 0.02)	(0.15, 0.03)	(0.30, 0.05)	(0.45, 0.08)	(0.55, 0.10)
2	(0.13, 0.01)	(0.18, 0.02)	(0.33, 0.04)	(0.48, 0.07)	(0.58, 0.09)
			Scenario 2		
1	(0.30, 0.50)	(0.32, 0.60)	(0.35, 0.70)	(0.38, 0.80)	(0.40, 0.90)
2	(0.33, 0.45)	(0.35, 0.55)	(0.38, 0.65)	(0.41, 0.75)	(0.43, 0.85)
			Scenario 3		
1	(0.05, 0.10)	(0.18, 0.13)	(0.20, 0.25)	(0.40, 0.26)	(0.50, 0.27)
2	(0.30, 0.20)	(0.31, 0.35)	(0.32, 0.45)	(0.45, 0.65)	(0.65, 0.70)
			Scenario 4		
1	(0.13, 0.06)	(0.15, 0.18)	(0.25, 0.35)	(0.55, 0.38)	(0.75, 0.40)
2	(0.20, 0.14)	(0.25, 0.23)	(0.35, 0.29)	(0.50, 0.32)	(0.80, 0.35)
			Scenario 5		
1	(0.52, 0.01)	(0.61, 0.15)	(0.71, 0.20)	(0.82, 0.25)	(0.90, 0.30)
2	(0.53, 0.04)	(0.55, 0.20)	(0.62, 0.25)	(0.85, 0.27)	(0.95, 0.33)
			Scenario 6		
1	(0.25, 0.10)	(0.28, 0.13)	(0.30, 0.25)	(0.40, 0.35)	(0.50, 0.45)
2	(0.30, 0.20)	(0.31, 0.35)	(0.32, 0.45)	(0.43, 0.65)	(0.56, 0.70)
			Scenario 7		
1	(0.25, 0.10)	(0.28, 0.13)	(0.30, 0.25)	(0.40, 0.38)	(0.65, 0.40)
2	(0.30, 0.20)	(0.31, 0.35)	(0.32, 0.45)	(0.43, 0.65)	(0.66, 0.67)

TABLE 10.3: Optimal actions under the eight simulation scenarios using the simulation truth, θ^{true}. The last four columns give cycle 1 outcomes (y_1, z_1).

Scenario	d_1^{opt}	$d_2^{opt}(y_1, z_1)$			
		(0,0)	(0, 1)	(1,0)	(1,1)
1	0	0	0	0	0
2	5	5	5	4	4
3	3	4	4	2	2
4	3	3	3	0	0
5	0	0	0	0	0
6	5	4	4	4	4
7	4	4	4	3	3
8	5	5	3	4	4

To apply DTM2, the hyperparameters, $\tilde{\theta}$, were calibrated using ESS, by first simulating 1,000 pseudo samples of θ, setting $\sigma_{\xi_{c0}}^2 = \sigma_{\eta_{c0}}^2 = 6^2$, and computing the probabilities of interest, such as $P(Y_c = 0|d_c)$ and $P(Z_c = 0|d_c)$, based on the pseudo samples, then setting $\sigma_\xi^2 = \sigma_\eta^2 = 2^2$, $\tau^2 = 1$ and $\rho = -0.5$. The values of $\tilde{\theta}$ were determined to give $0.5 \leq ESS \leq 2$ for the quantities of interest, and this $\tilde{\theta}$ was used to determine the prior for all simulations.

Table 10.3 gives the optimal actions, d_1^{opt} and $d_2^{opt}(d_1^{opt}, Y_1, Z_1)$, under each scenario. For example, in Scenario 3, the optimal cycle 1 action is $d_1^{opt} = 3$, and the optimal cycle 2 action is $d_2^{opt}(d_1 = 3, Y_1 = 0, Z_1) = 4$ and $d_2^{opt}(d_1 = 3, Y_1 = 1, Z_1) = 2$, regardless of the cycle 1 Efficacy outcome Z_1.

The following summary statistics are used to evaluate each method's performance. The outcomes of the n patients in a given trial who received at least one cycle of therapy are $\{(Y_{i,1}, Z_{i,1}), (Y_{i,2}, Z_{i,2}), i = 1, ..., n\}$. Note that $n < 60$ if the trial was stopped early. The empirical mean total utility for the n patients is

$$\bar{U} = \frac{1}{n} \sum_{i=1}^n \{U(Y_{i,1}, Z_{i,1}) + U(Y_{i,2}, Z_{i,2})\},$$

where $U(Y_{i,2}, Z_{i,2}) = U(0,0)$ for patients who did not receive a second cycle of therapy. Indexing the simulated replications of the trial by $r = 1, ..., N$, the empirical mean total payoff for all patents in a given trial is

$$\bar{\bar{U}} = N^{-1} \sum_{r=1}^N \bar{U}^{(r)}.$$

This may be thought of as an index of the ethical desirability of the method, given the utility $U(y, z)$.

To evaluate design performance in terms of benefit to future patients, the expected payoff in cycle 1 of the selected dose level d_1^{sel} for a future patient is

$$Q_1^{sel}(d_1^{sel}) = E\{U(Y_1, Z_1) \mid d_1^{sel}, \theta^{true}\},$$

for $d_1^{sel} \neq 0$. This expectation is computed under the distribution of (Y_1, Z_1) conditional on d_1^{sel} and θ^{true}, so it may be written more generally as $E^{true}\{U(Y_1, Z_1) \mid d_1^{sel}\}$. For rule d_2^{sel}, denoting $d^{sel} = (d_1^{sel}, d_2^{sel})$, the expected cycle 2 payoff is

$$Q_2^{sel}(d_2^{sel}) = \sum_{y_1=0}^{1} \sum_{z_1=0}^{1} E\{U(Y_2, Z_2) \mid d^{sel}, y_1, z_1, \theta^{true}\} \times p(y_1, z_1 \mid d_1^{sel}, \theta^{true}),$$

where

$$E\{U(Y_2, Z_2) \mid d^{sel}, y_1, z_1, \theta^{true}\} = U(0, 0)$$

if $d_2^{sel}(y_1, z_1) = 0$. The total expected payoff for a future patient treated using the selected regime d^{sel} is

$$Q^{sel}(d^{sel}) = Q_1^{sel}(d_1^{sel}) + \lambda Q_2^{sel}(d_2^{sel}).$$

Empirical Toxicity and Efficacy rates were defined as follows. Define $\delta_{i,2} = 1$ if patient i was treated in cycle 2. For each simulated trial with each method, for patients who received at least one cycle of therapy, the empirical rates were

$$\Pr(\text{Tox}) = \frac{1}{n} \sum_{i=1}^{n} \frac{1(Y_{i,1} = 1) + \delta_{i,2} 1(Y_{i,2} = 1)}{1 + \delta_{i,2}}$$

and

$$\Pr(\text{Eff}) = \frac{1}{n} \sum_{i=1}^{n} \frac{1(Z_{i,1} = 1) + \delta_{i,2} 1(Z_{i,2} = 1)}{1 + \delta_{i,2}}.$$

For each of the five designs studied under each scenario, a total of $1,000$ trials were simulated. The simulation results are summarized in Table 10.4. In Scenario 1, Table 10.2 shows that doses $d = 1,2,3$, are safe, $d = 4,5$ are too toxic, and all doses have very low Efficacy. In this case there is little benefit from giving any dose. The value $\bar{\bar{U}} = 66.48$ for DTM2 in Table 10.4 is close to the utility $U(0, 0) + 0.8U(0, 0) = 66$ of $(d_1 = 0, d_2 = 0)$, and the utility-based stopping rule of DTM2 correctly stops the trial early 97.7% of the time, while ETEOR stops the trial early 95.6% of the time. In contrast, the extended 3+3 and CRM designs are very likely to run the trial to completion, because they ignore Efficacy. This provides a striking illustration of the fact that there is little benefit in exploring the safety of an agent if it is inefficacious. Methods that ignore Efficacy are very likely to make this mistake. This actually has very little to do with the 2-cycle structure, since it also can be seen when comparing one-cycle phase I–II to phase I methods. Thus, in Scenario 1, DTM2 and ETEOR are the only reasonable designs, and in this case DTM2 is superior to ETEOR in terms of both $\bar{\bar{U}}$ and Q^{sel}.

In Scenario 2, Table 10.2 shows that Toxicity probabilities increase with dose from 0.30 to 0.40 in cycle 1 and from 0.33 to 0.43 in cycle 2, while Efficacy probabilities are very high in both cycles, increasing with dose from 0.50 to 0.90 in cycle 1 and from 0.45 to 0.85 in cycle 2. If $\pi_{T,c}(d_j)$ values around 0.40

are considered acceptable trade-offs for such high $\pi_{E,c}(d_j)$ values, then there is a payoff for escalating to higher doses. The utility function reflects this, with the optimal action $d_1^{opt} = 5$ and $d_2^{opt}(5, Y_1, Z_1) = 4$ or 5 (Table 10.3). DTM2 obtains larger values of $\bar{\bar{U}}$ and Q^{sel} due to much larger $\pi_{E,c}(d_j)$ and slightly larger $\pi_{ETc}(d_j)$, compared to all other methods.

In Scenario 3, $d_1^{opt} = 3$, with $d_2^{opt} = 4$ if $Y_1 = 0$ in cycle 1 and $d_2^{opt} = 2$ if $Y_1 = 1$ (Table 10.3). This illustrates the within-patient adaptation of DTM2. The $(3+3)$a, $(3+3)$b, and ECRM methods select $d_1^{opt} = 3$ often since the toxicity probability of $d_1 = 3$ is close to 0.30, but they never select $d_2^{opt} = 2$ for patients with $(d_1, Y_1) = (3, 0)$ because their deterministic rules ignore Z_1 and do not allow escalation in cycle 2 even with $Y_1 = 0$. DTM2 again achieves the largest $\bar{\bar{U}}$, Q^{sel}, and Pr(Eff), with slightly larger Pr(Tox).

Scenario 4 is challenging for DTM2 and favorable for the other four designs. In Scenario 4, $d_1^{opt} = 3$ since its toxicity probability 0.25 is closest to 0.30. In addition, $d_2^{opt}(d_1^{opt}, Y_1, Z_1)$ is exactly the same as the cycle 2 dose levels chosen by the deterministic rules of $(3+3)$a, $(3+3)$b and ECRM, except for $(Y_1, Z_1) = (0, 1)$, which occurs about 5% of the time. From Table 10.1, the true expected utility of $d_2 = 2$ given $(d_1, Y_1, Z_1) = (3, 0, 1)$ is 32.82, very close to $U(0, 0)$. The three methods, $(3+3)$a, $(3+3)$b, and ECRM thus are likely to select d_1^{opt} by considering only Toxicity and select d_2^{opt} following their deterministic rules. CRM thus selects $d_1^{opt} = 3$ most of time, leading to the largest $\bar{\bar{U}}$ and Q^{sel}. Similar performance is seen for ETEOR because d_1^{opt} is considered optimal by ETEOR, and it uses the same deterministic rule for cycle 2. The smaller values of $\bar{\bar{U}}$ and Q^{sel} for DTM2 are due to the fact that it does a stochastic search to determine the optimal actions, using much more general criteria than the other methods. Table 10.1 shows that, for $(d_1, Y_1) = (3, 1)$, the expected cycle 2 utilities are smaller than or very close to $U(0, 0)$ for all the cycle 2 doses, so all cycle 2 doses are barely acceptable or not acceptable. However, $d_1 = 5$ is acceptable and, given $d_1 = 5$, many cycle 2 doses are acceptable, so DTM2 often explores higher doses in cycle 1 than d_1^{opt}. This scenario illustrates the price that must be paid for using more of the available information to explore the dose domain more extensively using an Efficacy–Toxicity utility-based objective function.

In Scenario 5, the lowest dose $d_1 = 1$ is too toxic and thus unacceptable. All methods terminate the trial early most of time, with DTM2 stopping trials due to the low posterior expected utilities caused by the high toxicity at d_1. Scenarios 6 and 7 have identical true Toxicity and Efficacy for doses 1, 2, and 3, while for doses 4 and 5, Scenario 7 has higher Toxicity and lower Efficacy, so that its d_1^{opt} is lower than d_1^{opt} of Scenario 6. In these two scenarios, since dose 3 has a π_T closest to 0.3, the other four methods perform very similarly, but DTM2 again has much higher $\bar{\bar{U}}$ and Q^{sel}.

For Scenario 8, which is included to evaluate robustness, DTM2 has greatly superior performance compared to all four other methods, in terms of both $\bar{\bar{U}}$ and Q^{sel}. This is because DTM2 allows a higher rate of Toxicity as a trade-off for much higher Efficacy, while the phase I methods $(3+3)$a, $(3+3)$b,

TABLE 10.4: Simulation results for DTM2 and 2-cycle extensions of 3+3a, 3+3b, the CRM, and TEOR

Scenarios	Criterion	DTM2	(3+3)a	(3+3)b	ECRM	ETEOR
1	$\bar{U}$	66.48	59.27	58.81	56.56	61.90
	Q^{sel}	57.77	54.36	52.30	51.75	52.43
	Pr(Tox)	0.25	0.22	0.23	0.27	0.25
	Pr(Eff)	0.07	0.03	0.03	0.05	0.07
	% completed trials	2.3	88.6	96.5	99.6	4.4
2	$\bar{U}$	136.35	124.36	118.32	115.86	122.13
	Q^{sel}	135.76	103.85	104.48	102.43	108.47
	Pr(Tox)	0.39	0.30	0.33	0.36	0.35
	Pr(Eff)	0.72	0.58	0.55	0.56	0.60
	% completed trials	99.4	39.2	64.7	95.6	78.2
3	$\bar{U}$	94.23	85.95	85.75	89.93	88.04
	Q^{sel}	84.39	77.98	80.14	78.43	78.47
	Pr(Tox)	0.38	0.27	0.27	0.30	0.26
	Pr(Eff)	0.38	0.27	0.27	0.33	0.28
	% completed trials	79.4	96.6	99.2	100.0	78.50
4	$\bar{U}$	75.84	81.81	80.12	85.40	84.94
	Q^{sel}	69.49	74.92	75.76	78.67	78.87
	Pr(Tox)	0.51	0.25	0.26	0.29	0.28
	Pr(Eff)	0.29	0.22	0.21	0.29	0.27
	% completed trials	96.7	83.2	94.7	99.4	81.7
5	$\bar{U}$	66.65	52.87	52.72	50.41	NA
	Q^{sel}	50.64	40.66	40.70	40.61	NA
	Pr(Tox)	0.84	0.43	0.44	0.53	NA
	Pr(Eff)	0.35	0.08	0.04	0.03	NA
	% completed trials	0.4	6.8	20.0	9.0	0.0
6	$\bar{U}$	96.43	82.82	79.27	81.50	86.14
	Q^{sel}	92.78	70.30	71.28	71.29	76.24
	Pr(Tox)	0.45	0.28	0.32	0.32	0.32
	Pr(Eff)	0.41	0.24	0.23	0.25	0.29
	% completed trials	90.9	51.5	74.7	97.6	58.3
7	$\bar{U}$	91.88	82.66	79.31	80.99	86.32
	Q^{sel}	84.91	70.28	71.27	71.16	76.34
	Pr(Tox)	0.47	0.28	0.32	0.32	0.32
	Pr(Eff)	0.38	0.24	0.22	0.25	0.29
	% completed trials	90.3	51.4	73.6	97.5	58.7
8	$\bar{U}$	95.92	80.24	76.09	79.83	80.75
	Q^{sel}	93.22	68.23	69.26	69.28	70.73
	Pr(Tox)	0.54	0.34	0.36	0.37	0.34
	Pr(Eff)	0.45	0.25	0.22	0.27	0.27
	% completed trials	84.7	49.4	73.2	97.6	57.9

and ECRM all ignore efficacy, and the other phase I–II method, ETEOR, terminates the trial early much more frequently. It also appears that DTM2 is robust to the actual probability mechanism that generates the outcomes. The superior performance of DMT2 in Scenario 8 may be attributed to its use of a 2-cycle utility function to account for Efficacy–Toxicity trade-offs as a basis for early stopping, as well as the robustness of the underlying probability dose-outcome model.

11

Optimizing Dose and Schedule

CONTENTS

11.1   Schedule-Dependent Effects 223
11.2   Trinary Outcomes 224
11.3   Event Times Outcomes 231

11.1   Schedule-Dependent Effects

So far, we have discussed phase I–II designs with the goal to optimize a dose, the dose pair of a two-agent combination, or the doses of an agent given in two successive cycles. However, it is well known that many agents have highly schedule-dependent effects. An example is given by Thall et al. (2013), who describe a nucleoside analog used to treat solid tumors that has three different MTDs, depending on the schedule of administration. For a 30-minute infusion, the MTD is 2100 mg/m^2 if it is given as a single bolus, 1000 mg/m^2 if it is administered weekly for three weeks with total dose 3000 mg/m^2 over 21 days, and 300 mg/m^2 if it is administered twice in each of weeks 1, 3, and 5 for total dose 1800 mg/m^2 over 35 days.

In many clinical settings, what may appear to be small or trivial changes in schedule may have unexpected effects on clinical outcome, including substantially increased rates of Toxicity. An example of such a schedule effect was encountered in a phase I allogeneic stem cell transplantation (allosct) trial described by Thall (2010, Section 1.1). In allosct, the patient's bone marrow first is intentionally ablated (destroyed) by a preparative regimen, either high-dose chemotherapy or radiation. At this point in the therapeutic process, the patient has no blood cell production (hematopoiesis) and no immune system, so is susceptible to infection. Ablating the bone marrow is motivated by the idea that the cancer cells originate there. Next, blood cells obtained from a human leukocyte antigen (HLA) matched donor are infused into the patient, with the goal that the donor cells will repopulate the patient's bone marrow (engraft), and provide a new, cancer-free hematopoietic process. The preparative regimen for the trial consisted of the standard agents intravenous busulfan and melphalan, (Andersson et al., 2002; Nieto et al., 2012), with the addition of gemcitabine. These three agents were given according to fixed schedules on days -10 to -1 prior to allosct on day 0. The doses and schedules of the standard agents were fixed, with the goal to find an optimal dose of gemcitabine. Toxicity was defined as any regimen-related grade 4 or 5 adverse event, occurring within 30 days post transplant, that affected a vital organ, excluding adverse events that occur routinely in allosct. Given 10 specified gemcitabine doses in the range 225 to 3675 mg/m^2, the CRM was used with $\pi_T^* = .10$. For each total dose d of gemcitabine, $d/2$ administered on each of days -8 and -3. No Toxicities were observed in the first 24 patients enrolled in the trial. Given this, and motivated by the desire to improve Efficacy without changing Toxicity, the PI decided to change the gemcitabine schedule from $(d/2, d/2)$ on days (-8, -3) to $(d/3, d/3, d/3)$ on days (-8, -6, -3). Unexpectedly, this resulted in severe skin toxicities in the first two patients treated with the new schedule, causing the investigators to shut down the trial. The trial was re-designed using the initial 2-day gemcitabine schedule, but also expanding the set of gemcitabine doses, broadening the definition of Toxicity to include severe mucositis and skin Toxicity, and changing π_T^* from .10 to .15.

Although it is generally true that $\pi_T(d)$ increases monotonically with dose of a cytotoxic agent, this is not necessarily true for $\pi_E(d)$. If schedule also is varied, the joint effects of dose and schedule on outcomes may be quite complicated. For some agents, given the same total dose, a more frequent administration schedule may be associated with lower Toxicity. For example, in treating metastatic breast cancer, Blomqvist et al. (1993) found that the Toxicity of the combination of fluorouracil, epirubicin, and cyclophosphamide (FEC) was reduced when the conventional every-4-week dosing regimen was divided into four weekly doses. The same pattern was observed for doxorubicin in treating the same patient population (Blomqvist et al., 1993). Similarly, when treating metastatic renal cell cancer with sunitinib, Gyergyay et al. (2009) showed that a 2-week on and 1-week off schedule is more tolerable than a 4-week on and 2-week off schedule. However, for dasatinib, a prolonged schedule can lead to higher Toxicity in treating CP-CML patients (Shah et al., 2008). The effect of schedule on Efficacy is similarly complex. Clark et al. (1994) suggested that for treating small-cell lung cancer, a prolonged exposure to low concentrations of etoposide may improve the therapeutic ratio of this drug, whereas Blomqvist et al. (1993) showed that for treating metastatic breast cancer with FEC, a prolonged schedule was associated with lower Efficacy.

11.2   Trinary Outcomes

Consider a (dose, schedule)-finding trial with J doses of an investigational drug, and schedules $m = 1, \cdots, M$, where schedule refers to the method, frequency, or timing of administration, for a given total dose during a treatment cycle. For example, given a 21-day treatment cycle, a total dose of $d_j = 210$

mg drug can be administered according to different schedules, e.g., continuous 3-day administration with a 4-day rest, or a continuous 7-day administration with a 14-day rest. We assume that dose has been standardized so that all doses fall in the range of $(0, 1]$. Let (j, m) denote a (dose, schedule) combination with dose d_j administered under schedule m. The possible treatment regimes may be represented by a $J \times M$ (dose, schedule) matrix.

The following phase I–II design for jointly optimizing a (dose, schedule) regime $\rho = (j, m)$ among $J \times M$ possible combinations is given by Guo et al. (2016). Let Y denote a trinary outcome in a setting where Efficacy and Toxicity are disjoint, as in the EffTox design with trinary outcomes described in Chapter 4. Let $Y = 0$, 1, or 2 with 0 indexing $N = $ [no Efficacy and no Toxicity], 1 indexing $E = $ [Efficacy and no Toxicity], and 2 indexing $T = $ [Toxicity and no Efficacy]. Let $\pi_{y,j,m} = \Pr(Y = y \mid (j, m))$ for $y = 0, 1, 2$. Because $\pi_{0,j,m} + \pi_{1,j,m} + \pi_{2,j,m} = 1$, we only model two of the three probabilities for each (j, m). We do this by assuming the transformation

$$\alpha_{j,m} = g(\pi_{2,j,m}),$$
$$\beta_{j,m} = g(\pi_{1,j,m} + \pi_{2,j,m}),$$

where $g(\cdot)$ is a link function, such as the logit or probit.

The following Bayesian dynamic model provides a flexible representation of possible (dose, schedule) effects on Y. Letting x_j denote a standardized d_j, the model assumes

$$\alpha_{j,m} \mid \alpha_{j-1,m}, \gamma \quad \sim \quad N\left(\alpha_{j-1,m} + \gamma(x_j - x_{j-1}), \sigma^2\right) \qquad (11.1)$$
$$\alpha_{1,m} \quad \sim \quad N(\alpha_{0,m}, \sigma_0^2) \qquad (11.2)$$

for $j = 2, \cdots, J$ and $m = 1, \cdots, M$, where $\gamma > 0$ represents the dose effect, σ^2 is a fixed variance, and $\alpha_{0,m}$ and σ_0^2 are hyperparameters. This model is flexible in the sense that it specifies a treatment effect for each (dose, schedule) combination as $\alpha_{j,m}$ without making overly restrictive assumptions on the ordering pattern of the schedule effects.

The model also borrows strength across (dose, schedule) combinations by centering the parameter in the outcome distribution associated with each (j, m) on that of the next lower dose with the same schedule, plus the dose effect, while allowing random variation via σ^2. It is difficult to estimate σ^2 because of the small sample size of typical phase I–II trials, and thus appropriate to use σ^2 as a tuning parameter and calibrate its value by simulation. The magnitude of any dose-schedule interaction is controlled by σ^2. This is desirable, especially when the compound has slow clearance or a long half-life (Simon et al., 1997; Legedza and Ibrahim, 2000). By tuning σ^2, the model can be formulated to borrow strength at a predetermined level, and thus obtain desirable design operating characteristics. The hyperparameters $\alpha_{0,m}$ and σ_0^2 can be determined similarly. Since $\alpha_{1,m} = g(\pi_{2,1,m})$, where $\pi_{2,1,m}$ is the probability of Toxicity at the lowest dose level of schedule m, and $\alpha_{0,m}$ is the prior mean of $\alpha_{1,m}$, one can choose $\alpha_{0,m}$ based on the investigators' best guess of the Toxicity probability at the lowest dose of each schedule, while σ_0^2 quantifies the uncertainty of this prior guess.

Similarly to the proportional odds model, we assume

$$\beta_{j,m} = \delta + \alpha_{j,m}$$

with $\delta > 0$. Since by definition

$$\beta_{j,m} = g(\pi_{1,j,m} + \pi_{2,j,m}) = g\left\{\Pr(Y > 0 \mid (j,m))\right\},$$

if g is the logit link, the above model is the proportional odds model. From a computational perspective, the probit link may be preferable because of its connection to latent normal variables that facilitate sampling posteriors using the Gibbs sampler (Albert and Chib, 1993).

Suppose that n patients have been treated, with the ith patient being treated at (dose, schedule) (j_i, m_i), $i = 1, \cdots, n$, yielding data $\mathcal{D}_n = \{y_1, (j_1, m_1), \cdots, y_n, (j_n, m_n)\}$. Let $\alpha = \{\alpha_{j,m}; j = 1, \cdots, J, m = 1, \cdots, M\}$. The likelihood is

$$
\begin{aligned}
\mathcal{L}(\mathcal{D}_n \mid \alpha, \delta) &= \prod_{i=1}^{n} \left[1 - \Phi(\delta + \alpha_{j_i, m_i})\right]^{I(y_i=0)} \\
&\times \left[\Phi(\delta + \alpha_{j_i, m_i}) - \Phi(\alpha_{j_i, m_i})\right]^{I(y_i=1)} \\
&\times \left[n\Phi(\alpha_{j_i, m_i})\right]^{1(y_i=2)}
\end{aligned}
\tag{11.3}
$$

Let $f(\delta)$ and $f(\gamma)$ denote the priors of δ and γ, respectively. For example, $\delta \sim Uniform(0, U_\delta)$ and $\gamma \sim Uniform(0, U_\gamma)$, where U_δ and U_γ are hyperparameters. The posterior of $\theta = (\alpha, \delta, \gamma)$ is

$$
\begin{aligned}
f(\theta \mid \mathcal{D}_n) &= \mathcal{L}(\mathcal{D}_n \mid \alpha, \delta) \\
&\times \prod_{m=1}^{M} \left(\phi(\alpha_{1,m}; \alpha_{0,m}, \sigma_0^2) \prod_{j=2}^{J} \phi(\alpha_{j,m}; \alpha_{j-1,m} + \gamma(x_j - x_{j-1}), \sigma^2)\right) \\
&\times f(\delta) \times f(\gamma)
\end{aligned}
$$

where $\phi(x; \mu, \sigma^2)$ represents the density of the normal distribution with mean μ and variance σ^2. Details on sampling the posterior using the Gibbs sampler can be found in Guo et al. (2016).

Let $\underline{\pi}_E$ denote the lower limit for Efficacy and $\bar{\pi}_T$ the upper limit for Toxicity. A (dose, schedule) combination (j, m) has acceptable Efficacy if

$$\psi_E(j, m) \equiv \Pr(\pi_{1,j,m} \geq \underline{\pi}_E \mid \mathcal{D}_n) > p_E(n), \tag{11.4}$$

and acceptable Toxicity if

$$\psi_T(j, m) \equiv \Pr(\pi_{2,j,m} \leq \bar{\pi}_T \mid \mathcal{D}_n) > p_T(n), \tag{11.5}$$

where probability cut-offs $p_E(n)$ and $p_T(n)$ are functions of n. The target (dose, schedule) combination is defined as the (j, m) with highest Efficacy probability $\pi_{1,j,m}$ among combinations with acceptable Efficacy and acceptable Toxicity.

As usual, only a small amount of data are available early in the trial and the posterior distribution of $\pi_{y,j,m}$ is disperse, but becomes more informative as data accumulate during the trial. This motivates allowing the cut-offs that define Toxicity and Efficacy acceptability to change adaptively with sample size n, with the criteria liberal at the beginning of the trial and becoming more stringent as n increases (Wathen and Thall, 2008; Cai et al., 2014b; Riviere et al., 2015; Guo and Li, 2014; Hobbs et al., 2016). Let N denote the maximum sample size for the trial, N_0 denote the minimal sample size at which the criteria (11.4) and (11.5) are first applied, and n denote the current sample size. The adaptive cut-offs are given by

$$p_k(n) = p_{k,a} + \frac{n - N_0}{N - N_0}(p_{k,b} - p_{k,a}), \qquad k = E, T$$

which increases linearly from $p_{k,a}$ to $p_{k,b}$ as n increases from N_0 to N, where $0 < p_{k,a} < p_{k,b} < 1$.

Let $\mathcal{A}_n$ denote the set of all admissible (dose, schedule) combinations based on $\mathcal{D}_n$. The adaptive (dose, schedule)-finding algorithm is as follows:

1. During the trial, regardless of schedule an untried dose is never skipped when escalating.

2. For each schedule $m = 1, \cdots, M$, treat one cohort at the lowest dose of the (dose, schedule) combination, $(1, m)$.

3. Let $h_m, m = 1, \cdots, M$, denote the highest tried dose under schedule m.

   (a) If all $h_m = J$ or have unacceptable Toxicity (i.e., dose escalation has reached the highest dose level J or overly toxic dose under each of the M schedules), then the next cohort is treated at the (dose, schedule) combination in $\mathcal{A}_n$ with largest $\psi_E(j, m)$.

   (b) The trial is terminated with no (j, m) chosen if $\mathcal{A}_n$ is empty.

   (c) If some $h_m < J$, the next cohort of patients is randomized to combination $(h_m + 1, m)$ with probability

   $$\psi_E(h_m + 1, m) / \sum_{m \in \mathcal{B}} \psi_E(h_m + 1, m),$$

   where $m \in \mathcal{B}$ and $\mathcal{B} = \{m : h_m < J$ and has acceptable Toxicity$\}$ denotes the set of schedules where the highest tried dose is safe and has not reached the highest dose.

   The last rule says that, if there is any schedule for which the highest tried dose is safe and is not the highest dose, then escalate the dose for that schedule. The algorithm thus gives high priority to exploring the dose space within each schedule, to avoid getting stuck at a suboptimal dose. AR is used to ensure that patients have a higher chance to be assigned to effective doses, while mitigating stickiness.

4. The trial is terminated when the maximum sample size N is reached. The (dose, schedule) combination in $\mathcal{A}_n$ with the maximum $\psi_E(j, m)$ is selected as the recommended combination.

As an illustration, consider a phase I–II trial to study a γ-secretase inhibitor as a single agent in patients with refractory metastatic or locally advanced solid tumors. The investigators were interested in identifying an optimal (dose, schedule) combination. The four doses were 210, 273, 336, and 395 mg, the total dose given during a 21-day treatment cycle. The three schedules were a continuous 3-day administration with a 4-day rest, a continuous 7-day administration with a 14-day rest, and a continuous daily administration. Toxicity was defined as grade 3 or 4 non-hematologic Toxicity, grade 4 neutropenia lasting ≥ 7 days, febrile neutropenia and/or documented infection with absolute neutrophil count (ANC) $< 1.0 \times 10^9$/L, or thrombocytopenia grade 4 or any thrombocytopenia requiring platelet transfusion. Efficacy was defined as CR or PR per RECIST criteria. The acceptability limits were $\bar{\pi}_E = 0.3$ and $\underline{\pi}_T = 0.2$.

Operating characteristics of the design are given in Table 11.1. In all scenarios, given the schedule, the Toxicity probability, denoted as "Pr(Tox)," increases with dose, and the probability of Efficacy without Toxicity, denoted as "Pr(Eff and no Tox)," either increases or first increases and then decreases with dose. The maximum sample size is 40 and patients are treated in cohort size of 2. Uniform priors $\delta \sim Uniform(0, U_\delta)$ and $\gamma \sim Uniform(0, U_\gamma)$ are used with $U_\delta = 4$ such that a reasonable range of $\beta_{j,m}$ (or equivalently, $\Pr(Y = 1 \mid (j, m)) + \Pr(Y = 2 \mid (j, m))$) that may be encountered in practice is covered. For example, when the Toxicity probability $\Pr(Y = 2 \mid (j, m)) = 0.1$, the support for $\Pr(Y = 1 \mid (j, m)) + \Pr(Y = 2 \mid (j, m))$ is $(0.1, 0.99)$ under this prior. Similarly, U_γ is set as $U_\gamma = 8$ to reflect a reasonable range of Toxicity probability increase between adjacent doses. Based on the physicians' prior knowledge, we set $\alpha_{0,1} = \alpha_{0,2} = \alpha_{0,3} = -1$ so that the prior average Toxicity probability at the lowest dose level of each schedule was about 0.15, and set $\sigma_0^2 = 4$ to reflect prior uncertainty. The variance $\sigma^2 = 0.5$ and cut-off probabilities $p_{k,a} = 0.05$ and $p_{k,b} = 0.18$ for $k = E, T$ were tuned to obtain desirable operating characteristics.

Scenarios 1 and 2 have one optimal (dose, schedule) combination, and Scenarios 3 and 4 have two optimal (dose, schedule) combinations. In all scenarios, the percent of inconclusive trials using the proposed design is $< 3\%$. The combination at which the highest average number of patients have been treated is always an optimal combination. In the first two scenarios, the optimal combinations are $(3, 1)$ and $(4, 3)$, respectively, with selection percentages 48.3% and 63.6%, and average sample sizes 8.2 and 10.8. In Scenario 3, the

TABLE 11.1: True probabilities of (1) Efficacy and no Toxicity and (2) Toxicity at each (dose, schedule) combination. The numbers in boldface correspond to optimal combinations

	Dose							
	True Pr(Eff and no Tox)				True Pr(Tox)			
Schedule	1	2	3	4	1	2	3	4
				Scenario 1				
1	0.3	0.32	**0.53**	0.43	0.02	0.06	**0.1**	0.5
2	0.28	0.3	0.31	0.32	0.01	0.08	0.1	0.15
3	0.29	0.31	0.46	0.43	0.02	0.13	0.46	0.5
				Scenario 2				
1	0.18	0.23	0.24	0.27	0.01	0.01	0.02	0.02
2	0.24	0.27	0.33	0.4	0.01	0.01	0.02	0.03
3	0.33	0.4	0.44	**0.6**	0.01	0.02	0.03	**0.1**
				Scenario 3				
1	0.28	0.3	0.32	**0.52**	0.02	0.03	0.04	**0.12**
2	0.28	0.34	0.35	0.43	0.02	0.05	0.08	0.4
3	0.31	0.32	**0.52**	0.43	0.02	0.03	**0.12**	0.4
				Scenario 4				
1	0.3	0.33	**0.56**	0.54	0.01	0.02	**0.1**	0.4
2	0.3	**0.56**	0.5	0.49	0.02	**0.1**	0.42	0.46
3	0.48	0.49	0.46	0.42	0.45	0.46	0.5	0.54

selection percentages of the two optimal combinations $(4,1)$ and $(3,3)$ are 17.1% and 44.1%, respectively, and mean sample sizes 4 and 8.1. In Scenario 4, the selection percentages of the two optimal combinations $(3,1)$ and $(2,2)$ are 39.1% and 45%, with sum 84.1%, and sample sizes 8.4 and 9.1.

TABLE 11.2: Selection percentage and average number of patients treated at each (dose, schedule) combination, with the target (dose, schedule) combinations in boldface

| | Selection percentage | | | | Number of patients | | | |
| | Dose | | | | Dose | | | |
Schedule	1	2	3	4	1	2	3	4
				Scenario 1				
1	0.3	4.6	**48.3**	3.2	2	2	**8.2**	2.8
2	0	1.5	4.3	8.7	2	2.2	2.9	3.1
3	0.9	19.2	5.3	0.5	2.2	5.2	4.4	1.7
				Scenario 2				
1	0.2	0.3	0.6	1	2.1	2.1	2.2	2.5
2	0.9	0.9	1.2	10.7	2.2	2.2	2.4	4
3	2.9	5.1	11.8	**63.6**	2.5	2.8	4.2	**10.8**
				Scenario 3				
1	0.1	0.3	3	**17.1**	2	2.1	2.6	**4**
2	0.1	1.1	16.6	7.9	2	2.3	4.5	3.8
3	0.1	1.9	**44.1**	6.8	2	2.6	**8.1**	3.7
				Scenario 4				
1	0	1.4	**39.1**	3.6	2	2.4	**8.4**	2.8
2	0.4	**45**	5.6	0.1	2.2	**9.1**	5	1.6
3	2.9	1.4	0.2	0.1	3	2.4	0.9	0.3

11.3 Event Times Outcomes

The following phase I–II design, given by Thall et al. (2013), jointly optimizes (dose, schedule) of an experimental agent based on Y_E = time to Efficacy and Y_T = time to Toxicity. Sequentially adaptive decisions are made based on a joint utility of the two event times. The design has two versions, to accommodate the possibilities that the schedules are nested, or differ qualitatively and thus may or may not be nested.

The design was motivated by an autologous stem cell transplantation (auto-SCT) trial in multiple myeloma (MM). In auto-SCT, the patient's own blood stem cells first are collected and cryopreserved, a preparative regimen then is given to ablate the patient's bone marrow and thus kill the cancer cells, and the stem cells are infused. As in allo-SCT, the goal is that the infused cells will re-populate the patient's bone marrow and restore normal blood cell production and immune function. An advantage of auto-SCT is that, because the patient's own cryopreserved cells are used rather than cells from a matched donor, there is no risk of graft-versus-host disease. Melphalan is an alkalating agent commonly used as part of the preparative regimen for auto-SCT trials in MM. The goal of the trial was to determine the best (dose, schedule) combination of melphalan in older patients. To address this, a phase I–II trial was designed to evaluate total melphalan doses $d = 140$, 180, or 200 mg/m^2, given either as a single 30-minute bolus d infused on day -2 before SCT, or with the dose split into two equal boluses $d/2$ infused on days -3 and -2. Toxicity was defined as severe (grade 3 or 4) gastrointestinal Toxicity or diarrhea, graft failure, or regimen-related death. Efficacy in MM is defined to have the following three requirements, based on urine and serum analyzed by immunofixation electrophoresis: (1) normal bone marrow ($< 5\%$ myeloma cells), (2) no new lytic lesions on bone X-ray, and (3) absence of β_2 microglobulin, a monoclonal protein characterizing MM in two consecutive tests. Efficacy was evaluated at 1, 3, 6, 9, and 12 months post transplant, so Y_E was interval censored while Y_T was observed continuously.

Denoting the treatment regime $\rho = (j, m)$, first transforming pre-transplant administration days (-3, -2) to (0, 1) for convenience, transplant was on day 3 after the first administration, and the six regimes were $\rho_1 = \{140, 1\}$, $\rho_2 = \{180, 1\}$, $\rho_3 = \{200, 1\}$, $\rho_4 = \{140, (0, 1)\}$, $\rho_5 = \{180, (0, 1)\}$, $\rho_6 = \{200, (0, 1)\}$. Each of the subsets $\mathcal{R}_1 = \{\rho_1, \rho_2, \rho_3\}$ of one-day schedules and $\mathcal{R}_2 = \{\rho_4, \rho_5, \rho_6\}$ of two-day schedules has a natural ordering, since the probabilities of Toxicity and Efficacy each increase with d within each schedule. In contrast, for either Efficacy or Toxicity, there is no obvious ordering among all six regimes in $\mathcal{R} = \mathcal{R}_1 \cup \mathcal{R}_2$. For example, although ρ_1 and ρ_4 deliver the same total dose, it is not clear whether a 1-day or 2-day schedule is more toxic or has a higher Efficacy rate. Similarly, while ρ_5 delivers a larger total dose than ρ_1, due to possible schedule effects either of these regimes may be either more or less toxic, or more or less efficacious. The terms "escalate" or "de-escalate" thus are meaningful only when assigning doses within $\mathcal{R}_1$ or $\mathcal{R}_2$, but not for assigning regimes within the entire set of regimes $\mathcal{R}$.

Following the general utility-based approach in Chapter 7, the criterion for choosing each cohort's treatment regime was the posterior mean utility $u(\rho, \mathcal{D}_n) = E_\theta[\bar{U}(\rho, \theta) \mid \mathcal{D}_n]$, where $\bar{U}(\rho, \theta) = E\{U(Y) \mid \rho, \theta\}$. The problem of establishing a utility function $U(y)$ for the two-dimensional continuous outcome in this case may be solved as follows.

Step 1. Identify a finite rectangle in $[0, \infty)^2$ where Y pairs are likely to occur. This is done by eliciting a maximum follow up time $\bar{t}_{E,max}$ for observing Y_E and a maximum follow up time $\bar{t}_{T,max}$ for observing Y_T.

Step 2. Given these upper limits, ask the physician(s) to partition the interval $[0, \bar{t}_{E,max}]$ for observing Y_E into subintervals, and similarly partition the interval $[0, \bar{t}_{T,max}]$ for observing Y_T into subintervals. These two sets of subintervals determine a grid of subrectangles that partition the rectangle $[0, \bar{t}_{E,max}] \times [0, \bar{t}_{T,max}]$ where all (y_E, y_T) may be observed.

Step 3. For each subrectangle in the partition, elicit a numerical utility, $U^{(e)}$, subject to the constraint that the utilities must decrease as y_E gets larger and increase as y_T gets larger.

Step 4. Formulate a regression model for $U(y)$ as a function of y.

Step 5. Treat the midpoints of the subrectangles as predictors and the corresponding elicited utilities $U^{(e)}$ as outcomes in the regression model, and fit the model to obtain estimates $\hat{U}(y)$ for all $y \in [0, \bar{t}_{E,max}] \times [0, \bar{t}_{T,max}]$. Use these estimates as the utilities for the trial design.

The partition obtained from the subintervals of $[0, \bar{t}_{E,max}]$ and $[0, \bar{t}_{T,max}]$ should be sufficiently refined to provide a reasonable discretization of Y in terms of the anticipated joint probability distribution that is realistic based on clinical experience, but sufficiently coarse that the elicitation is feasible. To facilitate refinement of the elicited utilities or the grid, it is useful to show the physician a plot of the fitted utility surface, and iterate this process until an acceptable utility surface is obtained. It may be most practical to carry out both the utility elicitation and prior elicitation during the same sessions with the physician(s). Step 3 reflects the belief that both smaller Y_E (quicker Efficacy) and larger Y_T (later Toxicity) are more desirable. Given the subrectangles of the outcome domain $[0, \bar{t}_{E,max}] \times [0, \bar{t}_{T,max}]$, this approach mimics the previous utility structure used for two-dimensional tables of discrete outcomes, and it provides a utility for any realization (y_E, y_T) of (Y_E, Y_T).

The design presented here obtains a utility surface by assuming the para-

TABLE 11.3: Utilities for subrectangles of the times to response and Toxicity in the multiple myeloma auto-SCT trial. For each rectangle, the two tabled values are the elicited $U^{(e)}$ and model based estimate $\hat{U}$.

Months	Months to Response				
to Toxicity	[0, 1)	[1, 3)	[3, 6)	[6, 9)	[9, 12)
[9, 12)	95, 93.9	88, 86.0	74, 74.5	64, 62.8	54, 53.1
[6, 9)	85, 85.3	76, 77.4	63, 65.8	53, 54.0	43, 44.3
[3, 6)	75, 73.5	64, 65.5	52, 53.8	42, 41.9	32, 32.1
[1, 3)	62, 60.2	52, 52.1	41, 40.3	31, 28.3	21, 18.4
[0, 1)	50, 50.3	40, 42.2	30, 30.2	20, 18.1	10, 8.1

metric function

$$U(y \mid b_1, b_2, c_1, c_2) = 100 \, \frac{b_1 \, e^{-c_1 y_E} + b_2 \, e^{-c_2 y_T} + b_3 \, e^{-c_1 y_E - c_2 y_T} - U_{min}}{U_{max} - U_{min}}.$$

(11.6)

The inequalities $c_1, c_2 > 0$, $b_2 < 0 < b_1$, and $b_2 < -b_3 < b_1$ ensure monotonicity of $U(y_E, y_T \mid b_1, b_2, c_1, c_2)$ in each argument. To obtain $0 \leq U(y_E, y_T) \leq 100$ with 0 corresponding to the worst and 100 to the best possible outcomes, one may use the norming constants $U_{max} = U^o(y_{R,min}, y_{T,max})$ and $U_{min} = U^o(y_{R,max}, y_{T,min})$, denoting

$$U^o(y_E, y_T) = b_1 \, e^{-c_1 y_E} + b_2 \, e^{-c_2 y_T} + b_3 \, e^{-c_1 y_E - c_2 y_T}.$$

This utility function may be used quite generally as a basis for decision making with any type of treatment regime, since this functional form is not limited to the particular (dose, schedule) optimization design discussed here.

For the auto-SCT MM trial, $\bar{t}_{E,max} = \bar{t}_{T,max} = 12$ months. Table 11.3 gives the intervals for each outcome that determined the subrectangles. The numerical values of obtained estimates in a nonlinear least squares fit were $(\hat{c}_1, \hat{c}_2, \hat{b}_1, \hat{b}_2, \hat{b}_3) = (0.0631, 0.1088, 9.3557, -7.8677, 0.5301)$. Table 11.3 gives both the elicited utility $U^{(e)}$ and fitted utility $\hat{U} = U(y_{mid} \mid \hat{c}_1, \hat{c}_2, \hat{b}_1, \hat{b}_1, \hat{b}_3)$ for each of the 25 subrectangles, where y_{mid} denotes the subrectangle midpoint. For example, the rectangle defined by the two intervals $1 < y_E < 3$ and $3 < y_T < 6$ has midpoint $y_{mid} = (2, 4.5)$, elicited utility $U^{(e)} = 64$, and $\hat{U} = 65.5$. The surface $\hat{U}(y)$ is illustrated by Figure 11.1. This utility function is the basis for the auto-SCT MM trial design.

The modeling strategy is to first construct marginals for Y_E and Y_T that are functions of dose and schedule, and then use a copula to obtain a joint distribution. For each outcome $k = E, T$, denote $Y_k^o = $ time to the event or right-censoring and $\delta_k = I(Y_k = Y_k^o)$, with $Y^o = (Y_E^o, Y_T^o)$, and $\delta = (\delta_E, \delta_T)$. Denote the pdf, cdf, and survivor function of Y_k at time $y > 0$ by $f_k(y \mid \rho, \theta_k)$, $F_k(y \mid \rho, \theta_k) = \Pr(Y_k \leq y \mid \rho, \theta_k)$ and $\bar{F}_k(y \mid \rho, \theta_k) = 1 - F_k(y \mid \rho, \theta_k)$, where θ_k is the marginal model parameter vector. The hazard function is $\lambda_k(t \mid \rho, \theta_k)$

Estimated Utilities of Parametric Model

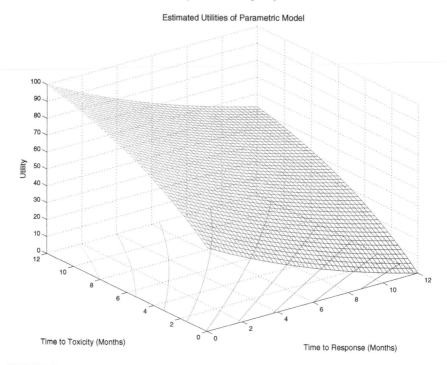

FIGURE 11.1: Fitted utility surface for the times to response and Toxicity in the multiple myeloma auto-SCT trial.

$= f_k(t \mid \rho, \theta_k)/\bar{F}_k(t \mid \rho, \theta_k)$ and the cumulative hazard is $\Lambda_k(t \mid \rho, \theta_k) = \int_0^t \lambda_k(u \mid \rho, \theta_k) du = -\log\{\bar{F}_k(t \mid \rho, \theta_k)\}$. The joint model parameter vector is $\theta = (\theta_E, \theta_T, \zeta)$, where ζ is the copula's association parameter.

Index doses by $j = 1, \cdots, J$ and schedules by $m = 1, \cdots, M$, with (dose, schedule) regime $\rho = (j, m)$. The design is based on the assumption that, given schedule, larger d_j is associated with stochastically smaller Y_E and smaller Y_T, equivalently, higher rates of both Efficacy and Toxicity. This assumption says that, at any follow-up time y, the probability of Efficacy, $F_E(y \mid (j, m), \theta_E)$, and the probability of Toxicity, $F_T(y \mid (j, m), \theta_T)$ by y both increase in d for any s. The conflict between increasing both Toxicity and Efficacy as the treatment regime is intensified is a central issue when optimizing $\rho = (j, m)$. The marginals are formulated so that these probabilities may either vary qualitatively with schedule or have monotone schedule effects. The utility function addresses the conflict between the goals to choose ρ to make $F_E(y_E \mid \rho, \theta_E)$ large while not allowing $F_T(y_T \mid \rho, \theta_T)$ to become unacceptably large, by quantifying the desirability of each possible (y_E, y_T) pair.

A practical difficulty when using $u((j, m), \mathcal{D}_n)$ for decision making based on bivariate time-to-event outcomes is that simply assuming $F_E(t \mid (j, m), \theta_E)$ and $F_T(t \mid (j, m), \theta_T)$ both are monotone in d_j may not distinguish adequately between different values of $u((j, m), \mathcal{D}_n)$ for doses d_j near the optimum, in the case $d_1 < d_j < d_J$, i.e., where d_j is an intermediate dose. Because a given change in an intermediate d_j to either d_{j+1} or d_{j-1} may produce changes of very different magnitudes in $F_E(t \mid (j, m), \theta_E)$, $F_T(t \mid (j, m), \theta_T)$, it may be difficult to identify a middle dose for which (j, m) has true maximum posterior mean utility, $u((j, m), \mathcal{D}_n)$. To address this problem in the context of optimizing (j, m), as in the model for the combination agent trial discussed in Chapter 8, outcome-specific *parametrically standardized doses* are used. Denoting $\bar{d} = (d_1 + \cdots + d_J)/J$, these are are defined as

$$d_{k,j}^\lambda = \frac{d_1}{\bar{d}} + \left(\frac{d_j - d_1}{d_J - d_1} \right)^{\lambda_k} \left(\frac{d_J - d_1}{\bar{d}} \right), \qquad (11.7)$$

for $k = E, T$ and $j = 1, ..., J$. With the formulation 11.7, the parameter λ_k controls the relative effects on the distribution of Y_k of doses that are between d_1 and d_J, since $d_{k,1}^\lambda = d_1/\bar{d}$ and $d_{k,J}^\lambda = d_J/\bar{d}$ do not depend on λ_k.

The following generalized gamma regression model provides a robust parametric form for the marginal event time distributions. It was chosen based on preliminary simulations exploring various parameterizations of the lognormal, Weibull, and gamma distributions across an array of regime-outcome scenarios and true event time distributions. The formulation generalizes a conventional gamma regression model in that both the scale and shape parameters have linear terms that vary with schedule and dose, rather than only assuming this structure for the scale parameter, as usually is done. For each outcome $k = E, T$, the marginal gamma pdf is

$$f_k(t \mid \rho, \theta_k) = \frac{t^{\phi_{k,1}-1} e^{-t/\phi_{k,2}}}{\Gamma(\phi_{k,1}) \phi_{k,2}^{\phi_{k,1}}},$$

where $\Gamma(\cdot)$ denotes the gamma function. In the generalized gamma regression model, the shape parameter $\phi_{k,1}$ and the scale parameter $\phi_{k,2}$ as functions of dose and schedule and are given by

$$\phi_{k,1}\{(j, m), \theta_k\} = \beta_{k,1}(\gamma_{k,m} d_{k,j}^\lambda)^{-\alpha_{k,1}} \qquad (11.8)$$

and

$$\log\{\phi_{k,2}\{(j, m), \theta_k\} + 1\} = \beta_{k,2}(\gamma_{k,m} d_{k,j}^\lambda)^{-\alpha_{k,2}}, \qquad (11.9)$$

denoting $\theta_k = (\beta_{k,1}, \beta_{k,2}, \alpha_{k,1}, \alpha_{k,2}, \gamma_{k,1}, \cdots, \gamma_{k,M})$. The model requires $\alpha_{k,1}$, $\alpha_{k,2}$, $\beta_{k,1}$, $\beta_{k,2} > 0$. To ensure numerical stability, it is assumed that the schedule effects, $\gamma_{k,1}, \cdots, \gamma_{k,M}$, have support $[0, 2]$. Different transformations are used to define $\phi_{k,1}(j, m)$ and $\phi_{k,2}(j, m)$ because the shape and scale parameters play very different roles in determining the form of the gamma distribution. In the models (11.8) for shape and (11.9) for scale, the $\gamma_{k,m}$'s are schedule-specific dose coefficients. The parametrically standardized doses $d_{E,j}^\lambda$ and $d_{T,j}^\lambda$ do a better job than the common form $d_j/\bar{d}$ of reflecting actual dose effects on the posterior mean utility, $u\{(j,m), \mathcal{D}_n\}$. In this model, $\beta_{k,1}$ may be thought of as the usual shape and $\beta_{k,2}$ as the usual scale parameter of the gamma, but with each modified by the effects of schedule and dose.

To formulate the likelihood function at study time t^*, for patient $i = 1, \cdots, n(t^*)$, denote the entry time $e_i < t^*$, treatment regime $\rho_{[i]}$, outcome vectors $Y^o_{i,t^*} = (Y^o_{i,E,t^*}, Y^o_{i,T,t^*})$ and $\delta_{i,t^*} = (\delta_{i,E,t^*}, \delta_{i,T,t^*})$. Since the outcomes are event times, each patient's outcome data may change over time, starting at $Y_{i,t^*} = Y^o_{i,t^*} = (0,0)$ and $\delta_{i,t^*} = (0,0)$ at accrual. Thereafter, each $Y^o_{i,m,t^*} = t^* - e_i$ as long as $\delta_{i,m,t^*} = 0$, and Y^o_{i,m,t^*} achieves the final value $Y_{i,m}$ that no longer changes with t^*, if and when the patient experiences event m, at which time δ_{i,m,t^*} jumps from 0 to 1. One may think of each $(Y^o_{i,t^*}, \delta_{i,t^*})$ as a bivariate sample path of two step functions, each jumping from 0 to 1 at their respective event times, subject to administrative right-censoring, from the time of the patient's accrual to the most recent follow-up time. Posterior quantities required for making outcome-adaptive interim decisions at any study time t^* are based on the most recent the trial data. The interim data at trial time t^* are

$$\mathcal{D}^* = \{(e_i, \rho_{[i]}, Y^o_{i,t^*}, \delta_{i,t^*}) : \ i = 1, \cdots, n(t^*)\}.$$

When both Y_E and Y_T are observed continuously, the likelihood for patient i at study time t^* is

$$
\begin{aligned}
\mathcal{L}(Y^o_{i,t^*}, \delta_{i,t^*} \mid \rho_{[i]}, \theta) \ &= \ \left\{ f_{E,T}(Y^o_{i,E,t^*}, Y^o_{i,T,t^*} \mid \rho_{[i]}, \theta) \right\}^{\delta_{i,E,t^*} \delta_{i,T,t^*}} \\
&\times \ \left\{ \int_{v=Y^o_{i,T,t^*}}^{\infty} f_{E,T}(Y^o_{i,E,t^*}, v \mid \rho_{[i]}, \theta) dv \right\}^{\delta_{i,E,t^*}(1-\delta_{i,T,t^*})} \\
&\times \ \left\{ \int_{u=Y^o_{i,E,t^*}}^{\infty} f_{E,T}(u, Y^o_{i,T,t^*} \mid \rho_{[i]}, \theta) du \right\}^{(1-\delta_{i,E,t^*})\delta_{i,T,t^*}} \\
&\times \ \left\{ \bar{F}_{E,T}(Y^o_{i,E,t^*}, Y^o_{i,T,t^*} \mid \rho_{[i]}, \theta) \right\}^{(1-\delta_{i,E,t^*})(1-\delta_{i,T,t^*})} \quad (11.10)
\end{aligned}
$$

Once the marginals have been specified, a joint distribution for $Y = (Y_E, Y_T)$ may be defined using a bivariate FGM copula. Hereafter, t^*, i, $\rho_{[i]}$, and θ will be suppressed for brevity when no meaning is lost. Denote the joint cdf of $[Y \mid \rho]$ by

$$F_{E,T}(y \mid \rho, \theta) \ = \ \mathrm{Pr}(Y_E \le y_E, Y_T \le y_T \mid \rho, \theta),$$

and the joint survivor function by

$$\bar{F}_{E,T}(y \mid \rho, \theta) \ = \ \mathrm{Pr}(Y_E > y_E, Y_T > y_T \mid \rho, \theta).$$

Temporarily suppressing ρ for brevity, the FGM copula for continuous variables is given in terms of the marginals and one association parameter $\zeta \in [-1, 1]$ by

$$F_{E,T}(y_E, y_T \mid \zeta) = F_E(y_E)F_T(y_T)\{1 + \zeta \, \bar{F}_E(y_E)\bar{F}_T(y_T)\}. \quad (11.11)$$

To obtain the terms in (11.10) under the FGM copula, for $(\delta_E, \delta_T) = (1,1)$ the joint pdf is

$$f_{E,T}(y_E, y_T \mid \zeta) = f_E(y_E)f_T(y_T)\Big[1 + \zeta\,\{1 - 2F_E(y_E)\}\{1 - 2F_T(y_T)\}\Big],$$

and

$$\bar{F}_{E,T}(y_E, y_T) = F_{E,T}(y_E, y_T) + \bar{F}_E(y_E) + \bar{F}_T(y_T) - 1.$$

For $(\delta_E, \delta_T) = (0,1)$ and $a > 0$,

$$\int_a^\infty f_{E,T}(y, y_T)dy = \bar{F}_E(a)f_T(y_T)\Big[1 - \zeta F_E(a)\{1 - 2F_T(y_T)\}\Big],$$

and the term for $(\delta_E, \delta_T) = (1,0)$ is obtained by symmetry. All likelihood contributions thus are determined by ζ and the marginal generalized gamma regression model pdfs, with F_E and F_T and terms corresponding to administratively censored event times computed by numerical integration.

In practice, the outcomes may be interval censored, for example, if each patient's disease status is evaluated every six weeks or the database is updated at the end of each month. To account for interval censoring when Efficacy is evaluated at successive times $0 = a_0 < a_1 < \cdots < a_{L-1} < a_L = \infty$, rather than continuously, denote the lth subinterval by $A_l = (a_{l-1}, a_l]$. Thus, Y_E is evaluated at each successive a_k until Efficacy is observed. If Efficacy does not occur by a_{l-1} but occurs by a_l, then $Y_E \in A_l$. Let $\delta_{1,l}$ denote this event. Given the partition $\{A_1, \cdots, A_L\}$ of $[0, \infty)$, the pair $(Y_{i,E}^o, \delta_{i,E})$ for continuously observed $Y_{i,E}$ are replaced by the vector of indicators $\delta_{i,E} = (\delta_{i,E,1}, \cdots, \delta_{i,E,L})$, which has one entry $= 1$ and all other entries $= 0$. At study time t^*, the observed outcome data of the ith patient are $\{\delta_{i,E}(t^*), Y_{i,T,t^*}^o, \delta_{i,T,t^*}\}$. If $Y_{i,T}^o = Y_{i,T}$ has been observed by study time t^*, so that $\delta_{i,T,t^*} = 1$, the ith patient's contribution to the likelihood is

$$\mathcal{L}(\delta_{i,E}(t^*), Y_{i,T,t^*}^o, 1 \mid \rho_{[i]}, \theta) = \prod_{l=1}^L \left\{ P_{E,T}^{(1)}(A_l, Y_{i,T,t^*}^o \mid \rho_{[i]}, \theta) \right\}^{\delta_{i,E,l}(t^*)},$$

where we denote the joint probability $P_{E,T}^{(1)}(A_l, Y_T^o) = \int_{A_l} f_{E,T}(y, Y_T^o)dy$. Under the assumed copula model (11.11), this takes the form

$$\begin{aligned}
P_{E,T}^{(1)}(A_l, Y_T^o) &= f_T(Y_T^o)\{F_E(a_l) - F_E(a_{l-1})\} \\
&\times [1 + \zeta\{2F_T(Y_T^o) - 1\}\{F_E(a_l) + F_E(a_{l-1}) - 1\}].
\end{aligned}$$

If patient i has not yet experienced Toxicity, so that $\delta_{i,T,t^*} = 0$ and $Y_{i,T}$ is censored at study time t^*, the likelihood contribution is

$$\mathcal{L}(\delta_{i,E}(t^*), Y_{i,T,t^*}^o, 0 \mid \rho_{[i]}, \theta) = \prod_{l=1}^L \left\{ P_{E,T}^{(2)}(A_l, Y_{i,T}^o(t^*) \mid \rho_{[i]}, \theta) \right\}^{\delta_{i,l}(t^*)},$$

denoting the joint probability

$$P_{E,T}^{(2)}(A_l, Y_T^o) = \int_{Y_T^o}^{\infty} \int_{A_l} f_{E,T}(y, w) \, dy \, dw.$$

Under the copula model, this takes the form

$$\begin{aligned} P_{E,T}^{(2)}(A_l, Y_T^o) &= \bar{F}_T(Y_T^o)\{F_E(a_l) - F_E(a_{l-1})\} \\ &\times \left[1 + \zeta F_T(Y_T^o)\{F_E(a_l) + F_E(a_{l-1}) - 1\}\right]. \end{aligned}$$

Combining all of the above terms, if Y_E is interval censored, then the likelihood of patient i at trial time t^* is

$$\begin{aligned} \mathcal{L}(Y_{i,T,t^*}^o, \delta_i(t^*) \mid \rho_{[i]}, \theta) = \prod_{l=1}^{L} &\left[P_{E,T}^{(1)}(A_l, Y_{i,T}^0(t^*) \mid \rho_{[i]}, \theta)^{\delta_{i,T,t^*}} \right. \\ &\left. \times P_{E,T}^{(2)}(A_l, Y_{i,T}^0(t^*) \mid \rho_{[i]}, \theta)^{1-\delta_{i,T,t^*}} \right]^{\delta_{i,l}(t^*)}. \end{aligned}$$

For each outcome $k = E, T$, let t_k^{ref} be a reference time from the start of therapy for evaluation of Y_k. The regime acceptability rule will specify a limit on the probability $F_k(t_k^{ref} \mid \rho, \theta)$ that the event will occur by t_k^{ref}. In some settings, it may be reasonable to set $t_E^{ref} = t_T^{ref}$. Let $\bar{\pi}_T$ be a fixed upper limit on $F_T(t_T^{ref} \mid \rho, \theta)$ and $\underline{\pi}_E$ be a fixed lower limit on $F_E(t_E^{ref} \mid \rho, \theta)$, both specified by the physician. Given upper probability cut-offs p_T and p_E, a regime ρ is *unacceptable* based on the data at trial time t^* if it is too toxic,

$$\Pr\{F_T(t_T^{ref} \mid \rho, \theta) > \bar{\pi}_T \mid \mathcal{D}^*\} > p_T$$

or if it is inefficacious,

$$\Pr\{F_E(t_E^{ref} \mid \rho, \theta) < \underline{\pi}_E \mid \mathcal{D}_{n(t^*)}\} > p_E.$$

The set of acceptable regimes at t^* is denoted by $\mathcal{A}^*$.

The methodology for the case where the schedules are not nested is called Design 1. The underlying idea for this design is to first learn about the behavior of regimes (j, m) while requiring a minimal sample size for each schedule $m = 1, \cdots, M$ in a first stage. In stage 1 of Design 1, patients are distributed evenly among the schedules, while optimizing dose within each schedule. Once enough has been learned about all schedules, the design then optimizes (j, m) globally in stage 2.

Denote the regime maximizing $u(\rho, \mathcal{D}^*)$ among all $\rho \in \mathcal{A}^*$ by

$$\rho^{opt} = \operatorname*{argmax}_{\rho \in \mathcal{A}} \ u(\rho, \mathcal{D}^*).$$

Denote the index of the optimal dose among acceptable regimes having schedule m by

$$j^{opt}(m) = \underset{1 \leq j \leq J, \ (j,m) \in \mathcal{A}^*}{\operatorname{argmax}} u((j,m), \mathcal{D}^*).$$

As before, because the posterior mean utility $u(\rho, \mathcal{D}^*)$ is highly variable throughout much of the trial, the design uses AR among regimes with $u(\rho, \mathcal{D}^*)$ $= u((j,m), \mathcal{D}^*)$ close to ρ^{opt}, to reduce the risk of getting stuck at a suboptimal regime. Since only $\rho \in \mathcal{A}^*$ may be chosen, as usual if $\mathcal{A}^*$ is empty then the trial is stopped and no ρ is selected. If $\mathcal{A}^*$ is not empty, then Design 1 proceeds as follows. Let N_1 denote the maximum stage 1 sample size. Patients are treated in cohorts of size c, so N_1 should be chosen to be a multiple of Jc that is reasonably close to $N/2$. This ensures that at least one cohort of size c will be treated at some dose for each schedule. For example, if the maximum trial sample size is $N = 72$, $M = 3$ schedules, and $c = 3$, then $Mc = 9$, so $N_1 = 36$ gives exactly $36/9 = 4$ cohorts for each schedule in Stage 1. Denote $n(j,m) = $ number of patients treated with regime $\rho = (j,m)$, that is, with dose j and schedule m.

Stage 1 of Design 1. Randomize M cohorts of size c fairly among the schedules, restricted so that each schedule is assigned to exactly c patients. Within schedule m, starting at the lowest dose and not skipping an untried dose when escalating, treat the next patient at dose $j^{opt}(m)$, unless

$$n(j^{opt}(m), m) \geq \underset{j}{max}\{n(j,m): \ j \neq j^{opt}(m), \ (j,m) \in \mathcal{A}^*\} + \Delta_1 c, \quad (11.12)$$

where Δ_1 is a small positive integer. If (11.12) holds, then within schedule m, choose an acceptable dose using AR with probability proportional to $u((j,m), \mathcal{D}^*)$. Repeat this until N_1 patients have been treated.

The underlying idea for Stage 1 is that the design is greedy, i.e., uses the optimal dose within schedule m based on the posterior mean utilities, until a large enough number of patients have been treated at the optimal dose for schedule m, which is $j^{opt}(m)$, and then proceeds to use AR. The inequality (11.12) in Stage 1 says that, to use AR within schedule m, the current sample size at the best acceptable dose within schedule m must be at least $\Delta_1 c$ larger than the current sample size at any other acceptable dose with that schedule.

Stage 2 allows the optimization to be done globally, rather than choosing an optimal dose within each schedule.

Stage 2 of Design 1. For $N - N_1$ more patients, choose (j,m) to maximize $u(j,m,\mathcal{D}^*) \in \mathcal{A}^*$ among all JM regimes, unless

$$n(j^{opt}(m^{opt}), m^{opt}) \geq$$

$$\underset{m}{max}\{n(j^{opt}(m), m): \ m \neq m^{opt}, \ (j^{opt}(m), m) \in \mathcal{A}^*\} + \Delta_2 c, \quad (11.13)$$

where Δ_2 is a small positive integer. If (11.13) holds, choose a schedule using AR with probability proportional to $u((j^{opt}(m), m), \mathcal{D}^*)$.

Practical values of Δ_1 and Δ_2 are small integers such as 1, 2, or 3, chosen depending on c and possibly N, to control the amount of sample size imbalance between regimes. The AR probabilities among doses within schedule m in stage 1 at t^* are

$$r_1(j, m) = \frac{u((j, m), \mathcal{D}^*) \, I((j, m) \in \mathcal{A}^*)}{\sum_{j'=1}^{J} u((j', m), \mathcal{D}^*) \, I((j', m) \in \mathcal{A}^*)} \quad j = 1, \cdots, J.$$

Similarly, the inequality (11.13) says that, to use AR, the current sample size at the best acceptable regime must be at least $\Delta_2 \, c$ larger than the current sample size at any other acceptable regime. The AR probabilities among schedules in stage 2 at t^* are

$$r_2(m) = \frac{u((j^{opt}(m), m), \mathcal{D}^*) \, I((j^{opt}(m), m) \in \mathcal{A}^*)}{\sum_{m'=1}^{M} u((j^{opt}(m'), m'), \mathcal{D}^*) \, I((j^{opt}(m'), m') \in \mathcal{A}^*)}, \quad m = 1, \cdots, M.$$

Design 2 for non-nested schedules is a greedy design, and is much simpler than Design 1. Design 2 chooses $\rho \in \mathcal{A}^*$ by simply maximizing $u((j, m), \mathcal{D}^*)$, subject to acceptability and the constraint that an untried dose may not be skipped when escalating within any schedule. With Design 2, schedules are chosen by fair randomization without replacement, as in Design 1, but this is done throughout the trial, and within schedule m the best current dose $j^{opt}(m)$ is chosen.

The problem is very different if schedules are nested. In this case, $\gamma_{k,1} < \gamma_{k,2} < \cdots < \gamma_{k,M}$ for each outcome $k = E, T$. Consequently, both Y_E and Y_T are stochastically increasing in schedule m as well as dose j, so the regime-finding algorithm may take advantage of this. In this case, the word "escalate" pertains to both dose and schedule, i.e., to both j and m, and the trial may be conducted by choosing (j, m) to globally maximize $u\{(j, m), \mathcal{D}^*\}$, subject to the two regime acceptability criteria and the usual two-dimensional "do-not-skip" rule similar to that used by Braun et al. (2007). Escalation from (j, m) to optimize $u\{\rho, \mathcal{D}^*\}$ is restricted to the three adjacent untried combinations $(j+1, m)$, $(j, m+1)$, or $(j+1, m+1)$. For example, while moving from (j, m) to either untried $(j + 1, m - 1)$ or untried $(j - 1, m + 1)$ is not strictly an "escalation," one could not skip from (j, m) to $(j + 2, m - 1)$ if $(j + 1, m - 1)$ were untried. This could be elaborated, as in Design 1, to include AR among nearly optimal regimes based on $u\{(j, m), \mathcal{D}^*\}$.

In some settings one may wish to account for death during follow-up, or discontinuation of follow-up due to Toxicity, possibly because the regime was changed at Y_T, or the possibility that the patient's follow-up may be terminated at the time of non-fatal Toxicity. The model and utility may be modified to account for this by using the following semi-competing risks model. First, call either death or discontinuation of follow up at Y_T "fatal" Toxicity, indicated by δ_{TD}, in which case Y_T censors Y_E. Define δ_{TA} to indicate "non-fatal" Toxicity that allows follow-up to continue after Y_T to possibly observe Y_E. Thus, $\delta_{TD} + \delta_{TA} = \delta_T$, and the pair $(\delta_{TD}, \delta_{TA})$ has the two possible values (1,0) or (0,1) if $\delta_T = 1$ and (0,0) if $\delta_T = 0$. If $\delta_{TD} = 1$ and $Y_T < Y_E$ then Efficacy cannot be observed. In this case, a device to account for this is to define $Y_E = +\infty$ and $\delta_E = 1$, and extend the domain of (Y_E, Y_T) from $R_2 = [0, \infty)^2$ to its one point compactification $R_2^+ = R_2 \cup [\{+\infty\} \times [0, \infty)]$. It is not assumed that Y_E censors Y_T, that is, each patient is followed after Efficacy with (Y_T^o, δ_T) observed, up to $\bar{t}_{T,max}$. Suppressing ρ and θ, define an extended distribution $f_{E,T,D}^+(Y_E, Y_T, \delta_{TD})$ in terms of $\pi_{TD} = \Pr(\delta_{TD} = 1)$ and the conditional probabilities

$$f_{E,T|D}^+(y_E, y_T \mid \delta_{TD} = 0) = f_{E,T}(y_E, y_T)$$

and

$$f_{E,T|D}^+(y_E, y_T \mid \delta_{TD} = 1) = f_{E,T}(y_E, y_T)I(y_E < y_T) + f_T(y_T)\pi_{NE}I(y_E > y_T),$$

where $\pi_{NE} = \Pr(Y_E > Y_T)$ is the probability of death before Efficacy if $\delta_{TD} = 1$. It follows that $f_{E,T,D}^+$ is a probability distribution on R_2^+, since

$$\int_{R_2^+} \sum_{a=0}^{1} f_{E,T|D}^+(y_E, y_T \mid \delta_{TD} = a)\Pr(\delta_{TD} = a)dy_E dy_T = 1.$$

To extend the likelihood (11.10) to this case, first note that lines 2 and 4 of (11.10) are unchanged since in these cases Y_T is right-censored. The first line of (11.10) becomes

$$\left[\{f_{E,T}(Y_E^o, Y_T^o)\}^{I(Y_E^o < +\infty)} \{f_T(Y_T^o)\pi_{NE}\}^{I(Y_E^o = +\infty)} \pi_{TD}^{\delta_{TD}}(1 - \pi_{TD})^{\delta_{TA}}\right]^{\delta_E \delta_T}.$$

For line 3 of (11.10), if Y_E is censored at the time of fatal Toxicity, then $\delta_{TD} = 1$ and $Y_E = +\infty$, a case already accounted for by line 1. If Y_E is censored at the time of non-fatal Toxicity, this is accounted for simply by replacing δ_T with δ_{TA} in line 3.

The utility may be modified to accommodate death by considering the scaled original utility, $U(y_E, y_T)/100$, as a multiplicative discount factor for survival time on the follow-up interval $[0, \bar{t}_{T,max}]$ for Y_T. A utility function that reflects this is

$$U^+(y_E, y_T) = \bar{t}_{T,max} U(y_E, y_T)/100 \quad \text{if} \quad \delta_{TA} = 1$$

and

$$U^+(y_E, y_T) = y_{TD} U(y_E, y_T)/100 \quad \text{if} \quad \delta_{TD} = 1.$$

This definition ensures that, for subjects i and i' with $y_{E,i} = y_{E,i'} = y_E$ and $y_{T,i} = y_{T,i'} = y_T$ but $\delta_{TD,i} = 1$ and $\delta_{TA,i'} = 1$, it must be the case that $U^+(y_{E,i}, y_{T,i}) < U^+(y_{E,i'}, y_{T,i'})$. That is, non-fatal toxicity at y_T has a higher utility than death at y_T. The trial is conducted as described above. The model may be extended similarly if follow-up is stopped at Y_E, although this

TABLE 11.4: Elicited prior means of $F_E(t \mid \rho)$ and $F_T(t \mid \rho)$ for the auto-SCT trial. For each total dose, prior means for the regimes $\rho = (-2, d)$ and $((-3, -2), d)$ were identical

Days of Follow up	Prior Mean $F_E(t \mid \rho)$ Melphalan Dose			Prior Mean $F_T(t \mid \rho)$ Melphalan Dose		
	140	180	200	140	180	200
1	–	–	–	.01	.02	.03
3	–	–	–	.05	.07	.09
6	–	–	–	.15	.18	.20
10	–	–	–	.25	.30	.32
14	–	–	–	.30	.35	.40
28	–	–	–	.33	.38	.43
30	.05	.08	.10	–	–	–
90	.09	.11	.15	–	–	–
180	.13	.16	.19	.34	.39	.44
270	.16	.19	.24	–	–	–
360	.20	.25	.30	.35	.40	.45

is not commonly done if Toxicity occurring during follow-up period $[0, \bar{t}_{T,max}]$ is considered important. One also might model π_{TD} as a function of (j, m), if the death rate is sufficiently high to estimate the additional parameters, although this may be unlikely in practice. With the extended model $f_{E,T,D}^+$ and utility function $U^+(y_E, y_T)$, the trial design accommodates death during follow-up.

The model assumes that the positive real valued parameters $\alpha_{E,1}, \alpha_{E,2}, \beta_{E,1}, \beta_{E,2}, \lambda_E, \alpha_{T,1}, \alpha_{T,2}, \beta_{T,1}, \beta_{T,2}, \lambda_T$ follow lognormal priors. The means were determined from the elicited values in Table 11.4 using the pseudo-sample based method. Prior variances were calibrated to obtain a design with good performance across a broad range of scenarios. It was assumed that $\zeta \sim$ beta$(1.1, 1.1)$, rescaled to have support on $(-1, +1)$. Since the schedule effects $\{\gamma_{E,1}, \cdots, \gamma_{E,M}, \gamma_{T,1}, \cdots, \gamma_{T,M}\}$ act multiplicatively on the outcome-specific standardized doses, $\gamma_{k,m} \leq 0.80$ or ≥ 1.20 may have a large effect on $d_{k,j}^\lambda$. For example, $\gamma_{k,m} = .80$ would reduce some $d_{k,j}^\lambda$ values by more than one full dose level. A more disperse prior on the $\gamma_{k,m}$'s also may cause the method to misinterpret a dose effect for a schedule effect in certain cases, especially those where a middle dose has highest utility. Consequently, the priors of the $\gamma_{k,m}$'s were specified to be highly concentrated beta distributions with domain $[0, 2]$ and parameters $(47.3, 47.3)$, which gives $\Pr[0.80 < \gamma_{k,m} < 1.20] = 0.95$. Although these priors may appear to be overly informative, in fact small changes within the subdomain $[0.80, 1.20]$ of $[0, 2]$ allow the posterior mean utility to change substantively, so that it may detect true differences between schedules. In this case, the observed data easily have the necessary effect on the posterior distributions of the $\gamma_{k,m}$'s.

TABLE 11.5: Simulations of Design 1 with sample size 72 and cohort size 3, for lognormal true event times.

	1-Day Schedule			2-Day Schedule			R_{select}
	Dose 1	Dose 2	Dose 3	Dose 1	Dose 2	Dose 3	R_{treat}
			Scenario 1				
$\bar{u}^{true}(j,m)$	52.2	57.5	62.9	52.2	57.5	62.9	
% Sel	5	8	38	5	8	35	0.82
# Pats	11.6	9.8	14.5	11.6	9.5	14.4	0.54
			Scenario 2				
$\bar{u}^{true}(j,m)$	59.0	53.7	48.1	59.0	53.7	48.1	
% Sel	39	7	4	39	6	5	0.85
# Pats	22.6	8.2	5.0	22.7	8.2	4.9	0.75
			Scenario 3				
$\bar{u}^{true}(j,m)$	53.1	58.4	63.8	56.8	62.1	67.6	
% Sel	3	5	16	6	12	58	0.81
# Pats	11.1	9.1	12.9	11.6	10.5	16.5	0.54
			Scenario 4				
$\bar{u}^{true}(j,m)$	58.6	54.6	49.7	55.4	51.4	46.5	
% Sel	54	12	5	18	5	5	0.80
# Pats	23.1	9.0	5.1	21.0	8.3	5.1	0.69
			Scenario 5				
$\bar{u}^{true}(j,m)$	52.9	63.6	50.2	52.9	63.6	50.2	
% Sel	8	34	6	9	36	6	0.74
# Pats	13.0	16.7	6.2	12.8	16.7	6.2	0.54
			Scenario 6				
$\bar{u}^{true}(j,m)$	53.5	48.1	56.5	53.5	48.1	56.5	
% Sel	21	4	23	21	4	25	0.76
# Pats	17.2	7.3	11.0	17.2	7.2	11.2	0.62

TABLE 11.6: Summary statistics for Design 1, the greedy Design 2, and the non-adaptive balanced allocation design

	Design 1		Design 2		Balanced	
Scenario	R_{select}	R_{treat}	R_{select}	R_{treat}	R_{select}	R_{treat}
1	0.82 (1)	0.54	0.78 (1)	0.45	0.85 (0)	0.50
2	0.85 (1)	0.75	0.85 (1)	0.84	0.85 (0)	0.51
3	0.81 (1)	0.54	0.78 (1)	0.48	0.83 (0)	0.50
4	0.80 (1)	0.69	0.80 (0)	0.77	0.80 (0)	0.51
5	0.74 (1)	0.54	0.65 (1)	0.48	0.77 (0)	0.40
6	0.76 (2)	0.62	0.75 (3)	0.62	0.77 (0)	0.55

The auto-SCT trial was simulated with $N_1 = 36$, $N = 72$, and $c = 3$, Y_T monitored continuously and Y_E interval censored per the evaluation schedule at 1, 3, 6, 9, 12 months. Three competing designs were studied: Design 1, the greedy Design 2, and a perfectly balanced randomized design with no interim decisions, restricting the randomization to treat exactly 12 patients at each of the six ρ pairs, with the regime maximizing $u(\rho, data)$ selected at the end. Eight simulation scenarios were considered. In Scenario 1, there is no schedule effect, Toxicity is acceptable, and Efficacy increases with dose. Scenario 2 also has no schedule effect, but Toxicity is much higher, so the lowest dose has the highest utility. In Scenario 3, the 2-day schedule is superior due to higher Efficacy. In Scenario 4, the 1-day schedule is superior. Scenario 5 has no schedule effect, but the middle dose is best. In Scenario 6, for both schedules, the utility is "V" shaped, lowest for the middle dose with the highest dose optimal. Each case was simulated 3000 times. Table 11.5 shows that Design 1 does a good job of selecting regimes with high true utilities. When all regimes are either unacceptably toxic or inefficacious (Scenarios 7 and 8, not tabled), the design stops early with no (j, m) selected with high probability.

Table 11.6 compares Design 1, the greedy Design 2, and balanced design in terms of R_{treat} and R_{select}. The main messages are that (1) compared to the greedy Design 2, the Design 1 has the same or higher R_{select} while neither design is uniformly superior to the other in terms of R_{treat}, (2) compared to the balanced design, Design 1 has nearly identical R_{select} but much higher values of R_{treat}, so is much more ethical. In summary, Design 1 has the best overall performance of the three designs and, as expected, the balanced design is ethically unacceptable.

12

Dealing with Dropouts

CONTENTS

12.1   Dropouts and Missing Efficacy 245
12.2   Probability Model 246
12.3   Dose-Finding Algorithm 248
12.4   Simulations 249

12.1   Dropouts and Missing Efficacy

In some phase I–II trials, Toxicity can be evaluated quickly but Efficacy requires a longer time period to be evaluated. For example, in oncology, particularly for cytotoxic agents, Toxicity is typically observable shortly after the treatment is administered; whereas evaluating tumor response may take many weeks or months. As a result, patient attrition often occurs, that is, patients may drop out of the study before their Efficacy outcomes are evaluated. This problem also arises in phase II trials, but is ignored by most conventional phase II designs.

As an example, Cullen et al. (1999) described two randomized trials (namely, MIC1 and MIC2 trials), designed to determine whether the addition of chemotherapy influenced duration and quality of life in patients with lung cancer. The MIC1 trial was for patients with localized, unresectable disease, and the MIC2 trial was for patients with extensive disease. In the MIC1 trial, patients were randomized to either chemotherapy followed by radical radiotherapy (CT + RT) or radiotherapy alone (RT). In the MIC2 trial, patients were randomized to chemotherapy plus palliative care (CT + PC) or palliative care alone (PC). The dropout rates were 29% and 20% for CT + RT and RT arms, respectively, in the MIC1 trial, and 22% and 24% for CT + PC and PC arms, respectively, in the MIC2 trial. Marchetti et al. (2004) reported a phase II trial to evaluate the safety and Efficacy of thalidomide in patients with myelofibrosis with myeloid metaplasia. In that trial, the dropout rate reached 51% after 6 months of treatment.

These dropouts, and the resulting missing Efficacy data, often are nonignorable, i.e., informative, in the sense that the dropout probability of a patient depends on his/her Efficacy outcome, as discussed in Chapter 5. For example, patients who do not experience Efficacy often are more likely to drop out of the study than patients who experience Efficacy. Therefore, ignoring the dropouts results in biased estimates (Little and Rubin, 2002), while the common approach of treating the dropouts as "no Efficacy" often tends to be overly conservative. In this chapter, we will assume that Toxicity is quickly evaluable, but Efficacy may be missing due to patient dropout.

An illustrative example is a phase I–II trial to find the optimal dose of plerixafor as salvage therapy for refractory or resistant AML, where Toxicity may occur at any time during the first 30 days from the start of treatment, while Efficacy is evaluated up to 90 days. Five plerixafor dose levels were investigated, 0.1, 0.3, 0.5, 0.7, 0.9 mg/kg, combined with a fixed dose of 10 mcg/kg G-CSF. Efficacy was defined as morphologic CR, or morphologic CR with incomplete blood count recovery (CRi). CR was defined as <5% blasts in bone marrow aspirate, with marrow spicules and > 200 nucleated cells, no blasts with Auer rods, no persistent extramedullary disease, absolute neutrophil account > 1,000/mm^3, and platelet count > 100,000/mm^3. CRi was defined as CR with the exception of neutropenia <1,000/mm^3 or thrombocytopenia <100,000/mm^3. Toxicity was defined as grade 4 or higher adverse events attributable to either leukostasis or tumor lysis, grade 3 toxicities attributable to leukostasis or tumor lysis that did not improve with standard supportive care measures (e.g., intravenous fluids, supplemental oxygen, leukapheresis) within 24 hours to achieve ≤ grade 2, or persistent grade 3 or higher neutropenia. The goal was to find a dose with highest Efficacy subject to the constraint $\pi_T \leq \bar{\pi}_T = .30$. Because the follow-up period for assessing Y_E was long, it was anticipated that a substantial number of patients might drop out before Y_E could be scored.

12.2   Probability Model

Assume that binary Toxicity Y_T is evaluated quickly enough so that it always is observed. For doses $d_1 < d_2 < \cdots < d_J$, Toxicity probability $\pi_T(d) = \Pr(Y_T = 1|d)$ is modeled as

$$\text{logit}\{\pi_T(d)\} = \mu_T + \beta_T d, \qquad (12.1)$$

where μ_T and β_T are unknown parameters.

Suppose that evaluation of Efficacy requires follow-up time τ, large enough so that Y_E often is subject to missingness due to patient dropout. To account for potentially non-ignorable dropout, Efficacy is treated as a time-to-event outcome, with a joint model for the Efficacy and dropout processes. While the primary interest is Efficacy, and not the dropout process, the reason for modeling them jointly is to account for nonignorable missing data caused by dropout. The dropout process can be viewed as an informative censoring process for the time to Efficacy.

For the ith patient, let $t_{E,i}$ and $t_{D,i}$ denote the times to Efficacy and dropout, respectively, and let $h_E(t_{E,i}|d_{[i]})$ and $h_D(t_{D,i}|d_{[i]})$ denote the corresponding hazard functions given that the patient received dose $d_{[i]}$. Let r_n denote the total number of dropouts at the time the $(n+1)$th patient arrives and is ready for dose assignment. The following shared-frailty proportional hazards model is assumed for $t_{E,i}$ and $t_{D,i}$,

$$h_E(t_{E,i}|d_{[i]}, \zeta_i) = \lambda \exp\{\zeta_i I(r_n > r_{\min}) + \beta_{E,1} d_{[i]} + \beta_{E,2} d_{[i]}^2\} \qquad (12.2)$$

$$h_D(t_{D,i}|d_{[i]}, \zeta_i) = \gamma \exp\{(\alpha \zeta_i + \beta_D d_{[i]}) I(r_n > r_{\min})\}, \qquad (12.3)$$

where λ and γ are baseline hazards, $\beta_{E,1}$, $\beta_{E,2}$, and β_D are regression parameters characterizing the dose effects, $I(\cdot)$ is an indicator function, and $r_{\min}$ is a prespecified positive cut-off. In equation (12.2), the quadratic term $\beta_{E,2} d_{[i]}^2$ is included to accommodate possibly unimodal or plateaued dose-Efficacy curves, e.g., for biological agents. The common frailty ζ_i shared by the two hazard functions is used to account for potentially informative censoring due to dropout, i.e., association between the times to Efficacy and dropout. We assume that $\{\zeta_i\} \sim$ iid $N(0, \sigma^2)$. To allow either positive or negative correlation, the parameter α is introduced in equation (12.3), with $\alpha > 0$ and $\alpha < 0$ corresponding to positive and negative correlation, respectively, between the times to Efficacy and dropout, and $\alpha = 0$ if they are independent.

The indicator function $I(r_n > r_{\min})$ in models (12.2) and (12.3) is used to accommodate the practical consideration that if too few (i.e., less than $r_{\min}$) patients have dropped out, there is no need to fit the dropout model because ignoring dropouts will have little impact on the design. In addition, the sparse dropout data also do not allow us to reliably estimate the dropout model. One may set $r_{\min} = 3$ or 4 so that we will not model the dropout process until there are more than 3 or 4 dropouts. Because r_n depends on n, models (12.2) and (12.3) are not the usual Cox proportional hazards regression models, but rather a sequence of conditional proportional hazards models.

Under the time-to-event model, the Efficacy of dose d, i.e., the response probability by follow-up time τ, is given by

$$\pi_E(d) = \Pr(t_{E,i} \le \tau | d).$$

The goal of the design is to find a safe dose d having largest $\pi_E(d)$ while satisfying minimum Efficacy and Toxicity requirements. For the ith patient, define the observed times $t_{E,i}^o = \min(t_{E,i}, t_{D,i}, c_i)$ and $t_{D,i}^o = \min(t_{D,i}, c_i)$, and censoring indicators $\epsilon_{E,i} = I(t_{E,i} \le \min(t_{D,i}, c_i))$ and $\epsilon_{D,i} = I(t_{D,i} \le c_i)$, where c_i is the time to administrative censoring. Note that dropout at t_D can censor t_E, but not conversely. The model parameter vector is $\theta = (\lambda, \gamma, \beta_{E,1}, \beta_{E,2}, \beta_D, \mu_T, \beta_T, \zeta_i, \sigma^2, \alpha)$. The likelihood for the ith patient with data $\mathcal{D}_{[i]} = (y_{Ti}, t^o_{E,i}, t^o_{D,i}, \epsilon_{E,i}, \epsilon_{D,i})$ is

$$\mathcal{L}(\mathcal{D}_{[i]}|\theta) = \int f(y_{T,i}|\theta) f(t^o_{E,i}, t^o_{D,i}|\zeta_i, \theta) f(\zeta_i) \mathrm{d}\zeta_i,$$

where

$$f(y_{T,i}|\theta) = \frac{\exp\{y_{T,i}(\mu_T + \beta_T d_{[i]})\}}{1 + \exp(\mu_T + \beta_T d_{[i]})},$$

and

$$\begin{aligned}
f(t^o_{E,i}, t^o_{D,i}|\theta) &= \{\lambda\exp\{\zeta_i I(r_n > r_{\min}) + \beta_{E,1}d_{[i]} + \beta_{E,2}d^2_{[i]}\}\}^{\epsilon_{E,i}} \\
&\times \exp\big(-\lambda t^o_{E,i}\exp\{\zeta_i I(r_n > r_{\min}) + \beta_{E,1}d_{[i]} + \beta_{E,2}d^2_{[i]}\}\big) \\
&\times \{\gamma\exp\{(\alpha\zeta_i + \beta_D d_{[i]})I(r_n > r_{\min})\}\}^{\epsilon_{D,i}} \\
&\times \exp(-\gamma t^o_{D,i}\exp\{(\alpha\zeta_i + \beta_D d_{[i]})I(r_n > r_{\min})\}).
\end{aligned}$$

More details on the model specification and its estimation can be found in Guo and Yuan (2015).

12.3 Dose-Finding Algorithm

The following rule-based start-up procedure is used to collect preliminary data before switching to the model-based dose-finding strategy. The trial starts by treating the first cohort of 3 patients at the lowest dose d_1. At the current dose d_j,

1. If ≥ 2 out of 3 patients experience Toxicity, then the trial switches to model-based dose finding, starting at dose d_{j-1}. If $d_j = d_1$, i.e., d_j is the lowest dose, then the trial is terminated.

2. If 1 out of 3 patients experiences Toxicity, then the trial switches to model-based dose finding, starting at dose d_j.

3. If 0 out of 3 patients experiences Toxicity, the next dose is d_{j+1}. However, if $d_j = d_J$, then the trial switches to model-based dose finding, starting at d_J.

4. Patients accrued during the start-up procedure must be followed completely to evaluate Efficacy or dropout before the model-based dose-finding algorithm is used.

The model-based dose-finding algorithm is as follows. Given $\underline{\pi}_E$ and $\bar{\pi}_T$, the admissible dose set $\mathcal{A}$ is the set of doses satisfying both the Efficacy requirement

$$\Pr(\pi_E(d) > \underline{\pi}_E|\mathcal{D}_n) > a_E + b_E n/N \tag{12.4}$$

and the Toxicity requirement

$$\Pr(\pi_T(d) < \bar{\pi}_T|\mathcal{D}_n) > a_T + b_T n/N, \tag{12.5}$$

where a_E, b_E, a_T, and b_T are non-negative tuning parameters, calibrated by simulation to achieve good design operating characteristics. Since the estimates of $\pi_T(d)$ and $\pi_E(d)$ are highly unreliable at the beginning of the trial and become more reliable as data accumulate, the posterior probability cut-offs $a_E + b_E n/N$ and $a_T + b_T n/N$ are defined to depend on the sample size n. The acceptability requirements adaptively become more stringent as more patients are enrolled into the trial.

Let d_h be the current highest tried dose, and p_c be the dose escalation cut-off. Based on the data from the k cohorts of patients who have been enrolled in the trial, the model-based dose-finding algorithm assigns a dose to the $(k+1)$th cohort as follows.

1. Based on the data obtained from the first k cohorts, if $\Pr(\pi_T(d_h) < \bar{\pi}_T|\text{data}) > p_c$ and $d_h \neq d_J$, escalate the dose and assign the $(k+1)$th cohort to d_{h+1}.

2. Otherwise, assign the $(k+1)$th cohort to the dose d in $\mathcal{A}$ with largest $\pi_E(d) = \max(\pi_E(d), d \in \mathcal{A})$. If $\mathcal{A}$ is empty, terminate the trial.

3. Once the maximum sample size is achieved, the dose in $\mathcal{A}$ with the largest estimate of $\pi_E(d)$ is selected as the final recommended dose.

12.4   Simulations

For the motivating trial, the simulations considered five doses 0.1, 0.3, 0.5, 0.7, 0.9, maximum sample size $N = 51$, and acceptability bounds $\bar{\pi}_T = 0.3$ and $\pi_E = 0.25$. The follow-up time for evaluating Efficacy was $\tau = 3$ months, and patient accrual followed a Poisson process with a rate of 3 per month. We set $\alpha = -1$, so that patients with a lower probability of experiencing Efficacy were more likely to drop out of the trial. We assumed the probability cut-offs $p_c = 0.5$, $a_T = 0.035$, $b_T = 0.095$, $a_E = 0.035$, and $b_E = 0.085$. We compared the above design, denoted as EffTox-drop, to a variant of the EffTox design described in Chapter 4. To handle dropouts, in this variant of the EffTox design, if a patient has missing Efficacy outcome due to dropout, Y_E is set as 0, i.e., no Efficacy. This strategy is commonly used in practice to handle dropouts. For the EffTox design, in the case where patients have not dropped out and their Efficacy outcomes have not yet been fully assessed, we suspended accrual to wait for their outcomes to be fully evaluated before enrolling the next new patient. The alternative approach to handling delayed Efficacy outcome is provided in Chapter 5. To make the designs comparable, the same target dose definition and dose-finding algorithm as described in Section 12.3 are used in two designs.

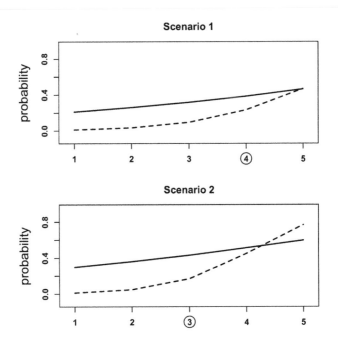

FIGURE 12.1: Dose-response curves for two scenarios in the simulation study. The solid and dashed lines are the Efficacy and Toxicity curves, respectively. Target doses are indicated by circles.

Table 12.1 shows the simulation results under two scenarios. As shown in Figure 12.1, in Scenario 1, both Toxicity and Efficacy increase with dose. The target dose is d_4, which has the highest Efficacy among the doses satisfying the acceptability criteria $\pi_T < 0.3$ and $\pi_E > 0.25$. The EffTox-drop design outperformed the EffTox design, which tended to be overly conservative and often selected d_3. This is because dropouts occurred more frequently at high doses, which are more toxic. In the EffTox design, as the dropouts were treated as no Efficacy, it tended to underestimate $\pi_E(d)$ of higher doses, which led to conservative dose escalation. In addition, the trial durations under the EffTox-drop design, 23.1 and 26.7 months under Scenarios 1 and 2, respectively, were shorter than those under the EffTox design, which were more than 32.7 and 40.2 months under Scenarios 1 and 2. This is because the EffTox-drop design eliminated the need to temporarily suspend patient accrual by modeling Efficacy as a time-to-event outcome rather than a binary outcome. In Scenario

2, Toxicity increases slowly from dose level 1 to 2 and then more rapidly after dose level 3, while Efficacy increases steadily from dose level 1 to level 5. The target dose is the third dose. When the dropout rate is 30%, the EffTox design yielded the similar selection percentage as the EffTox-drop design, but the trial duration was substantially longer. When the dropout rate is 50%, the EffTox design was conservative and more likely to select the lower dose (dose level 2). More comprehensive comparisons can be found in Guo and Yuan (2015).

TABLE 12.1: Selection percentage and the average number of patients (shown in parentheses) treated at each dose level under the EffTox-drop design and EffTox design. The bolded numbers are target doses.

	Dose level				
Design	1	2	3	4	5
			Scenario 1		
(π_E, π_T)	(0.21, 0.01)	(0.26, 0.04)	(0.32, 0.1)	**(0.38, 0.23)**	(0.46, 0.47)
		dropout rate $= 30\%$			
EffTox-drop	1.6 (3.8)	8.2 (6.4)	18.0 (10.1)	**61.8 (21.2)**	7.9 (8.7)
EffTox	1.6 (3.9)	11.2 (7.4)	26.9 (12.1)	**54.7 (18.9)**	4.0 (8.2)
		dropout rate $= 50\%$			
EffTox-drop	1.1 (3.7)	6.9 (6.1)	20.2 (10.5)	**62.9 (21.7)**	7.1 (8.5)
EffTox	3.0 (4.7)	15.0 (8.6)	29.2 (12.7)	**44.0 (17.0)**	5.2 (7.2)
			Scenario 2		
(π_E, π_T)	(0.3, 0.01)	(0.36, 0.05)	**(0.43, 0.17)**	(0.51, 0.45)	(0.6, 0.77)
		dropout rate $= 30\%$			
EffTox-drop	2.1 (4.0)	10.8 (7.9)	**74.5 (25.5)**	11.8 (12.2)	0.1 (1.2)
EffTox	2.9 (4.2)	16.4 (9.7)	**74.3 (24.1)**	5.7 (10.8)	0.0 (1.9)
		dropout rate $= 50\%$			
EffTox-drop	2.4 (4.1)	13.7 (8.8)	**71.7 (24.8)**	11.6 (11.8)	0.0 (1.2)
EffTox	4.7 (5.2)	27.9 (13.5)	**62.1 (21.5)**	4.0 (8.6)	0.0 (1.7)

To examine the design's robustness, we conducted sensitivity analyses by simulating the times to Efficacy from accelerated failure time models with a log-logistic error. Three shapes of hazard for Efficacy (increasing, decreasing, and umbrella-shaped), as shown in Figure 12.2, were considered, with the hazard for dropout increasing with the time. The marginal probabilities of Efficacy, Toxicity, and dropout were matched to the scenarios with dropout rate 30%, as shown in Table 12.1.

Figure 12.3 shows the results, which suggest that the EffTox-drop design is robust to violations of the proportional hazards assumption and is not sensitive to mis-specifications of the baseline hazards. The selection percentage of the target dose and the average number of patients treated at the target dose are similar under different shapes of hazard for Efficacy.

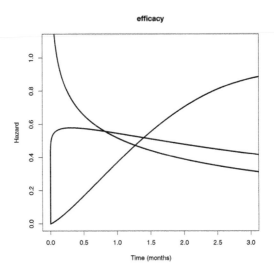

FIGURE 12.2: Three shapes of hazard for the time to Efficacy in sensitivity analysis.

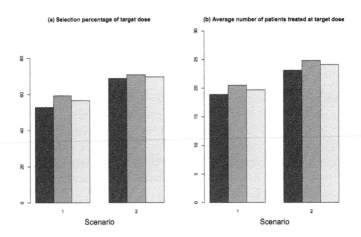

FIGURE 12.3: Results of the sensitivity analysis. Under each scenario, the bars from left to right correspond to increasing, decreasing, and hump-shaped hazards of Efficacy, respectively.

13

Optimizing Intra-Arterial tPA

CONTENTS

13.1   Rapid Treatment of Stroke 253
13.2   Probability Model 254
13.3   Decision Criteria and Trial Conduct 259
13.4   Priors 260
13.5   Simulations 261

13.1   Rapid Treatment of Stroke

Acute ischemic stroke (AIS) is a major cause of death and disability in adults (Johnston et al., 2009). Intra-arterial (IA) fibrinolytic infusion is a treatment for AIS that must be carried out within six hours of the stroke. With this treatment regime, a thrombolytic agent is delivered via two telescoping catheters directly to the site in the brain artery where the clot that caused the stroke occurred. The aim is that the agent will dissolve the clot. A supportive catheter is positioned in the carotid artery, and a smaller microcatheter within it is positioned directly into the clot. These two telescoping catheters are introduced via a sheath placed into the femoral artery and, using X-ray fluoroscopic guidance, the catheters are moved through the carotid artery leading to the site of the clot. The agent is infused via the microcatheter. Tissue plasminogen activator (tPA) is a thrombolytic agent used for intravenous (IV) treatment of AIS in adults, where its effects are well understood. In contrast, safe and efficacious concentrations of IA tPA have not been established. The design described in this chapter provides a method to optimize IA tPA for rapid treatment of AIS.

    Quantitative aspects of the IA tPA treatment regime are as follows. Let V denote a fixed maximum volume infused, and c the concentration of the tPA in mg/kg body weight. The maximum total dose thus is cV. Without loss of generality, we assume $V = 1$. Let q denote the proportion of the maximum total dose that is given as an initial bolus. The remaining proportion, $1 - q$, is given by continuous infusion at a constant rate over a fixed time period having maximum length t^*. Efficacy is defined as the time, Y_E, to dissolve the clot, including the possibility that the clot is dissolved immediately by the bolus, which implies that $\Pr(Y_E = 0) > 0$, that is, the distribution of Y_E has a point mass at 0. Infusion is stopped if it is determined that the clot is dissolved, and otherwise Y_E is right-censored at t^*. Toxicity is defined as the binary indicator Y_T of symptomatic intra-cerebral hemorrhage (SICH), which is characterized by neurological worsening compared to baseline in terms of a standardized stroke severity scale. SICH is associated with high rates of both morbidity and death. SICH is evaluated by imaging the brain using head computerized tomography (CT) scan or magnetic resonance imaging (MRI), at a fixed time, usually either 24 or 48 hours after the start of the infusion.

If the Efficacy outcome Y_E were observed continuously, each patient's outcome data would consist of Y_T and either the time Y_E if the clot is dissolved before t^* or the right-censoring time t^*. Since Efficacy is evaluated periodically, only the time interval in which Y_E occurred is known. If Efficacy is evaluated at 15-minute intervals and a patient's clot was not dissolved at the 45 minute evaluation but was dissolved at the 60 minute evaluation, then it is only known that $45 < Y_E \leq 60$. Consequently, Y_E is interval censored from 0 to t^* and administratively right-censored at t^*. Because infusion is stopped before t^* if the clot is dissolved, the amount of the agent that a patient receives is not necessarily cV, but rather depends on Y_E as well as c and q. Since Toxicity is scored after the infusion is completed, the distribution of Y_T depends on Y_E.

The following utility-based design is given in Thall et al. (2011). The goal is to construct a sequentially outcome-adaptive design to determine an optimal regime $\rho = (c, q)$, over a rectangular grid of pairs being considered. The first problem is to specify probability models for Y_E and $[Y_T | Y_E]$ that are flexible yet tractable functions of (c, q) reflecting the modes of administration and observation of (Y_E, Y_T). The second problem is to construct adaptive decision rules to choose (c, q) for successive patient cohorts.

13.2   Probability Model

Marginal models first are given for Efficacy and Toxicity, with Y_E defined in terms of standardized time, $s = t/t^*$, which has domain $0 \leq s \leq 1$. Let α denote the parameter vector of the marginal distribution of $[Y_E \mid c, q, \alpha]$. This distribution is a mixture of a discrete mass at time 0, corresponding to the bolus, and a continuous component on domain $(0, \infty)$ corresponding to the continuous infusion, defined in terms of a two-component hazard function. The first hazard component is $p_0(c, q, \alpha)$, the probability that the clot is dissolved instantly by the initial bolus at $s = 0$. The second hazard component is a continuous function, $\lambda(s, c, q, \alpha)$, defined on $s \geq 0$. Denoting the integrated continuous hazard by

$$\Lambda(s, c, q, \boldsymbol{\alpha}) = \int_0^s \lambda(y, c, q, \alpha) dy,$$

the cumulative hazard function of Y_E is

$$- \log\{1 - p_0(c, q, \boldsymbol{\alpha})\} + \Lambda(s, c, q, \alpha) \quad \text{for} \quad s \geq 0.$$

Denoting the indicator of any event A by $\mathbf{1}(A)$, this implies that the pdf of Y_E is the discrete-continuous mixture

$$
\begin{aligned}
f_E(y, c, q, \boldsymbol{\alpha}) \;=\; & p_0(c, q, \alpha) I(y = 0) \\
& + \;\{1 - p_0(c, q, \alpha)\} \lambda(y, c, q, \alpha) \, e^{-\Lambda(y, c, q, \alpha)} I(y > 0),
\end{aligned}
$$

and the cdf is

$$F_E(y, c, q, \alpha) = 1 - \{1 - p_0(c, q, \alpha)\} \, e^{-\Lambda(y, c, q, \alpha)}, \quad y \geq 0.$$

Since $\Lambda(0, c, q, \alpha) = 0$, it follows that $F_E(0, c, q, \alpha) = p_0(c, q, \alpha)$.

The parametric model given below allows both p_0 and λ to vary nonlinearly in both c and q, with these defined as functions of c^{α_1} and q^{α_2}, where $\alpha_1, \alpha_2 > 0$. To reflect clinical experience, the model is based on two key assumptions:

1) $p_0(c, q, \alpha)$ increases in c and q, and

2) the clot can dissolve instantaneously at $s = 0$ only if a bolus infusion is given.

These assumptions imply that $p_0(c, 0, \alpha) = 0$ for all $c > 0$ and $p_0(0, q, \alpha) = 0$ for all $0 \leq q \leq 1$. A simple, flexible function with these properties is

$$p_0(c, q, \alpha) = 1 - \exp(-\alpha_0 c^{\alpha_1} q^{\alpha_2}), \quad, \alpha_0 > 0. \tag{13.1}$$

The hazard function $\lambda(s, c, q, \alpha)$ for the clot dissolving during the continuous infusion must have the following properties:

1) $\lambda(s, c, q, \alpha)$ is continuous in s;

2) $\lambda(s, c, q, \alpha)$ is sufficiently flexible so that it may be monotone increasing, monotone decreasing, or non-monotone in s;

3) $\lambda(s, 0, q, \alpha) > 0$, to allow a non-zero baseline hazard if no tPA is given, $c = 0$;

4) $\lambda(s, c, 0, \alpha) > 0$ to allow the possibility that the clot is dissolved if no bolus is given;

5) $\lambda(s, c, q, \alpha)$ increases in both c and q, and the functional form may be nonlinear in either c or q.

A function λ with these properties is constructed by first defining the *cumulative delivered dose by standardized time s*,

$$d(s, c, q) = c\{q + (1 - q)s\}. \tag{13.2}$$

Note that $d(s, c, q)$ increases linearly in s with slope $c(1 - q)$ from minimum value $d(0, c, q) = cq$ at $s = 0$ to $d(1, c, q) = c$ at the last observation time $s = 1$ for Y_E. To obtain a more flexible λ, this function is elaborated as

$$d(s, c^{\alpha_1}, q^{\alpha_2}) = c^{\alpha_1}\{q^{\alpha_2} + (1 - q^{\alpha_2})s\},$$

which is the *effective cumulative delivered dose by standardized time s*. The hazard function is

$$\lambda(s, c, q, \alpha) = \alpha_3 + \frac{\alpha_4 \alpha_5 \{d(s, c^{\alpha_1}, q^{\alpha_2})\}^{\alpha_5 - 1}}{1 + \alpha_4 \{d(s, c^{\alpha_1}, q^{\alpha_2})\}^{\alpha_5}} \quad \text{for } s > 0, \tag{13.3}$$

where $\alpha_j > 0$ for all $j = 1, \cdots, 5$. The parameter α_3 is the baseline hazard of the clot dissolving if no tPA is given. The ratio added to α_3 is a log logistic hazard function with argument $d(s, c^{\alpha_1}, q^{\alpha_2})$ and shape parameter α_5. The parameter α_1 allows λ to vary nonlinearly in c while α_2 determines the relative magnitude of the contribution $c^{\alpha_1}(1 - q^{\alpha_2})s$ of the continuous infusion versus the contribution $c^{\alpha_1}q^{\alpha_2}$ of the bolus. The cumulative hazard function is

$$\Lambda(s, c, q, \alpha) = \alpha_3 s + \frac{1}{c^{\alpha_1}(1 - q^{\alpha_2})} \log\left[\frac{1 + \alpha_4\{d(s, c^{\alpha_1}, q^{\alpha_2})\}^{\alpha_5}}{1 + \alpha_4(c^{\alpha_1}q^{\alpha_2})^{\alpha_5}}\right] \quad \text{for } s > 0.$$

The distribution of Y_T is defined conditional on Y_E because Toxicity is scored by imaging at 48 hours, after Y_E has been observed, and it is a nonlinear function of c, q, and Y_E. The model accounts for the possibilities that either larger Y_E, hence a larger amount of the continuously infused agent, or failure to dissolve the clot may increase the risk of Toxicity. The following probability of Toxicity defined is a function of c, q, and Y_E has these properties. Denoting the minimum of a and b by $a \wedge b$ and $\beta = (\beta_0, \cdots, \beta_4)$, the model is

$$\pi_T(Y_E, c, q, \beta) = \Pr(Y_T = 1 \mid Y_E, c, q, \beta)$$
$$= 1 - \exp\{-\eta_T(Y_E, c, q, \beta)\}, \tag{13.4}$$

where the linear term is

$$\eta_T(Y_E, c, q, \beta) = \beta_0 + \beta_2 c^{\beta_1} q + \beta_3 c^{\beta_1}(1 - q)(Y_E \wedge 1) + \beta_4 I(Y_E > 1).$$

Since Y_E is observed at the end of each interval, as a covariate in η_T it takes on only values of the interval endpoints, given in Table 13.1, unless it appears in the indicator $I(Y_E > 1)$. If the evaluation times deviate from this planned schedule for some patients, then the likelihood can be modified easily to accommodate this, so that the actual intervals from the observation time data on Y_E are recorded during the trial. In this model, $\beta_2 c^{\beta_1} q$ is the effect of the bolus, $\beta_3 c^{\beta_1}(1-q)(Y_E \wedge 1)$ is the effect of the continuously infused portion, β_4 is the effect of failing to dissolve the clot, and $1 - e^{-\beta_0}$ is the baseline probability of Toxicity if no tPA is given. The model parameter vector $\theta = (\alpha, \beta)$ has dimension 11. Figure 13.1 illustrates how $p_0(c, q)$ and $\pi_T(c, q, .5)$ vary as highly flexible functions of c and q.

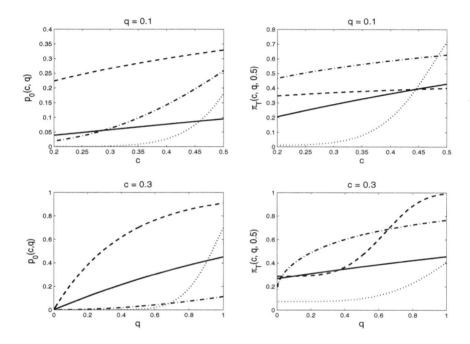

FIGURE 13.1: Illustration of the flexibility of the functions $p_0(c, q)$ and $\pi_T(c, q, 0, 5)$.

If no initial bolus is given, then $q = 0$ and the effective delivered dose at standardized time s is $d(s, c^{\alpha_1}, 0) = c^{\alpha_1} s$. In this case, α_2 is dropped from the model, the hazard function becomes

$$\lambda(s, c, 0, \alpha) = \alpha_3 + \frac{\alpha_4 \alpha_5 (c^{\alpha_1} s)^{\alpha_5 - 1}}{1 + \alpha_4 (c^{\alpha_1} s)^{\alpha_5}} \qquad \text{for } s > 0,$$

with corresponding cumulative hazard function

$$\Lambda(s, c, 0, \alpha) = \alpha_3 s + c^{-\alpha_1} \log\{1 + \alpha_4 (c^{\alpha_1} s)^{\alpha_5}\} \qquad \text{for } s > 0,$$

with $\dim(\alpha)$ reduced from 6 to 5. In this case, π_T is simplified by dropping β_2 and the linear component becomes

$$\eta_T(y_E, c, \beta) = \beta_0 + \beta_3 c^{\beta_1}(Y_E \wedge 1) + \beta_4 I(Y_E > 1),$$

and $\dim(\beta)$ is reduced from 5 to 4, so $\dim(\theta) = 9$.

We next establish a joint distribution, given $\pi_T(y_E, c, q, \beta)$ and the marginal pdf $f_E(y_E | c, q, \alpha)$ of Y_E. The joint distribution of $Y = (Y_E, Y_T)$ is

$$f_{E,T}(y_E, y_T | c, q, \theta) = f_E(y_E | c, q, \alpha) \times \Pr(Y_T = y_T | y_E, c, q, \beta)$$

for $y_T = 0, 1, y_E \geq 0$. If Y_E is observed continuously, denoting $\bar{\pi}_T = 1 - \pi_T$, each patient's likelihood is

$$\mathcal{L}(Y | c, q, \theta) = \left[p_0(c, q, \alpha) \, \pi_T(0, c, q, \beta)^{Y_T} \left\{ \bar{\pi}_T(0, c, q, \beta) \right\}^{1-Y_T} \right]^{I(Y_E=0)}$$

$$\times \left[f_E(Y_E | c, q, \alpha) \, \pi_T(Y_E, c, q, \beta)^{Y_T} \left\{ \bar{\pi}_T(Y_E, c, q, \beta) \right\}^{1-Y_T} \right]^{I(0 < Y_E \leq 1)}$$

$$\times \left[\{1 - F_E(1 | c, q, \alpha)\} \, \pi_T(1, c, q, \beta)^{Y_T} \left\{ \bar{\pi}_T(1, c, q, \beta) \right\}^{1-Y_T} \right]^{I(Y_E > 1)}.$$

The respective likelihood contributions are

    1) the probability the clot is dissolved instantaneously by the bolus,

    2) the probability the clot is dissolved during the continuous infusion, and

    3) the probability the clot is not dissolved by standardized time $s = 1$,

with each computed either with $(Y_T = 1)$ or without $(Y_T = 0)$ Toxicity.

In practice, Y_E is evaluated periodically at the ends of successive intervals, so the likelihood must account for interval censoring. For time interval $I_E = (y_E^a, y_E^b] \subset [0, 1]$, denote

$$\pi_{E,T}(I_E, y_T | c, q, \theta) = \Pr(y_E^a < Y_E \leq y_E^b, Y_T = y_T | c, q, \theta).$$

This is the probability if it is only known that $y_E^a < Y_E \leq y_E^b$. In this case, the tPA infusion is stopped at time y_E^b, the probability of Toxicity is $\pi_T(y_E^b, c, q, \beta_T)$, and

$$\pi_{E,T}(I_E, y_T | c, q, \theta) = \Pr(y_E^a < Y_E \leq y_E^b | c, q, \alpha) f_{T|E}(y_T | y_E^b, c, q, \beta)$$

$$= \{F_E(y_E^b | c, q, \alpha) - F_E(y_E^a | c, q, \alpha)\} \, \pi_T(y_E^b, c, q, \beta)^{y_T} \{1 - \pi_T(y_E^b, c, q, \beta)\}^{1-y_T}.$$

For a partition $\{I_{E,1}, \cdots, I_{E,M}\}$ of $(0, 1]$ into subintervals where Y_E may fall, the second term in the product that defines the likelihood for continuous observation of Y_E is replaced by

$$\prod_{m=1}^{M} \left[\pi_{E,T}(I_{E,m}, 1 \mid c, q, \theta)^{Y_T} \, \pi_{E,T}(I_{E,m}, 0 \mid c, q, \theta)^{1-Y_T} \right]^{I(Y_E \in I_{E,m})}. \quad (13.5)$$

13.3   Decision Criteria and Trial Conduct

Numerical elicited utilities for each combination of $Y_T = 0$ or 1 and the eight planned observation intervals for Y_E are given in Table 13.1. Given θ, the mean utility for a patient who receives the treatment combination (c, q) is

$$\bar{U}(c, q \mid \theta) = \sum_{y_T=0}^{1} \int_{y_E=0}^{\infty} U(y_E, y_T) \, f_{E,T}(y_E, y_T \mid c, q, \theta) dy_E.$$

The optimal (c, q) for each new cohort is obtained from the maximized objective function, which is the posterior mean utility

$$u(c, q, \mathcal{D}_n)^{opt} = \underset{c,q}{\mathrm{argmax}} \; E_\theta \{ \bar{U}(c, q \mid \theta) \mid \mathcal{D}_n \}$$

$$= \underset{c,q}{\mathrm{argmax}} \; E_\theta \left\{ \sum_{y_T=0}^{1} \int_{y_E=0}^{\infty} U(Y) \, f_{E,T}(Y \mid c, q, \theta) dy_E \mid \mathcal{D}_n \right\}.$$

With interval censoring due to sequential evaluation of Y_E, given the partition $\{I_{E,1}, \cdots, I_{E,M}\}$ of $[0, 1]$, a practical approach is to elicit numerical utilities for each of the $2(M + 1)$ values of Y obtained from the cross product $\{I_{E,1}, \cdots, I_{E,M}, I_{E,M+1}\} \times \{0, 1\}$, where $I_{E,M+1} = (1, \infty)$ is the outcome that the clot was not dissolved by the end of the infusion. Denote the utility of $\{Y_E \in I_{E,m}, Y_T = y_T\}$ by $U(I_{E,m}, y_T)$. This utility function accounts for the desirability of all observable Y_E, Y_T) pairs. The objective function now takes the form

$$u(c, q, \mathcal{D}_n) = \sum_{y_T=0}^{1} \sum_{m=1}^{M+1} U(I_{E,m}, y_T) \, E_\theta \left\{ \pi_{E,T}(I_{E,m}, y_T \mid c, q, \theta) \mid \mathcal{D}_n \right\}.$$

As usual, additional acceptability rules are needed to exclude (c, q) pairs that are either excessively toxic or inefficacious. Given $\mathcal{D}_n$, a pair (c, q) is *unacceptable* if either it is likely to be too toxic,

$$\Pr\{\pi_T(1, c, q, \theta) > \pi_T^* \mid \mathcal{D}_n\} > p_T, \tag{13.6}$$

or it is likely to be inefficacious,

$$\Pr\{F_E(1, c, q, \alpha) < \pi_E^* \mid \mathcal{D}_n\} > p_E, \tag{13.7}$$

where π_T^* is the maximum allowed Toxicity probability and π_E^* is the minimum allowed probability of dissolving the clot by t^*. The design also imposes the safety constraint that an untried concentration c may not be skipped when escalating, since $\pi_T(Y_E, c, q, \beta_T)$ increases in c, although it may not be monotone in q.

TABLE 13.1: Elicited utilities for the IA tPA trial

		Minutes Required to Dissolve Arterial Blood Clot							
0	1-15	16-30	31-45	46-60	61-75	76-90	91-105	106-120	> 120
No SICH									
100	95	90	85	80	75	70	60	50	30
SICH									
7	6.5	6	5	4.5	4	2	1	0	0

The clot is imaged at the start of infusion when the bolus is given, and if the clot is not dissolved immediately, then every 15 minutes up to $t^* = 120$ minutes. The observation intervals are thus $[0, 15]$, ..., $(105, 120]$ and $(120, \infty]$. A maximum of $N = 36$ patients are treated in cohorts of size 1. The goal is to choose the (c, q) pair that maximizes the posterior mean utility among the set of eight pairs obtained from $q = 0.10, 0.20$ and $c = 0.20, 0.30, 0.40, 0.50$. The admissibility limits are $\pi_T^* = 0.15$ and $\pi_E^* = 0.50$, with probability cut-offs $p_E = p_T = .90$. The starting pair is $(c, q) = (0.20, 0.10)$. If at any point in the trial, there are no (c, q) pairs then the trial is stopped. Otherwise, each next cohort is treated at the best acceptable (c, q) pair, subject to the do-not-skip rule, with $(c, q)^{opt}(\mathcal{D}_n)$ selected based on the final data.

13.4   Priors

Priors were established using the following pseudo sampling algorithm.

STEP 1: Prior means of the probabilities $p_0(c, q, \theta)$, $F_E(s, c, q, \alpha)$, and $\pi_T(y_E | c, q, \beta)$ were elicited for various values of (c, q, s, Y_E), given in Table 13.2. This was done for $s = 1/2$, corresponding to 60 minutes of infusion, and for $s = 1$, corresponding to the maximum 120 minutes. Values were elicited for the probability of Toxicity, $\pi_T(y_E, c, q, \theta)$, if the clot was dissolved instantaneously ($y_E = 0$), if it was dissolved within the 120-minute infusion ($y_E = 1$), or if it was not dissolved during the infusion ($y_E > 1$). A total of 40 prior means were elicited.

STEP 2: The elicited means were treated like the true state of nature and used to simulate 1000 pseudo samples, each of size 400 with exactly 50 patients for each (c, q) combination. Starting with a non-informative pseudo-prior on θ in which the logarithm of each entry followed a normal distribution with mean 0 and standard deviation 20, each simulated pseudo data set was used to compute a pseudo posterior. The average of the 1000 pseudo posterior means

TABLE 13.2: Elicited prior mean probabilities for each (c, q) combination studied in the IA tPA trial, in standardized time

		$c = 0.20$	$c = 0.30$	$c = 0.40$	$c = 0.50$
$q = .10$	$E\{p_0(c, q, \theta)\}$	0.10	0.15	0.15	0.25
	$E\{F_E(\frac{1}{2} \mid c, q, \theta)\}$	0.25	0.30	0.45	0.50
	$E\{F_E(1 \mid c, q, \theta)\}$	0.35	0.45	0.60	0.70
	$E\{\pi_T(0, c, q, \theta)\}$	0.02	0.03	0.03	0.03
	$E\{\pi_T(1, c, q, \theta)\}$	0.04	0.06	0.08	0.12
$q = .20$	$E\{p_0(c, q, \theta)\}$	0.15	0.20	0.25	0.30
	$E\{F_E(\frac{1}{2} \mid c, q, \theta)\}$	0.40	0.45	0.50	0.60
	$E\{F_E(1 \mid c, q, \theta)\}$	0.50	0.60	0.70	0.80
	$E\{\pi_T(0, c, q, \theta)\}$	0.02	0.03	0.03	0.03
	$E\{\pi_T(1, c, q, \theta)\}$	0.04	0.06	0.08	0.12

was used as the prior means. The pseudo sample size of 400 was chosen to be large enough so that prior means obtained in this way would not change substantively with a larger pseudo sample size.

STEP 3: Prior variances of the elements of θ were calibrated using the prior ESS of $\pi_T(s, c, q, \theta)$ and $F_E(s, c, q, \theta)$. For each of these probabilities evaluated at $s = 0$ or 1, the ESS of its prior was approximated by beta moment matching. Setting var$\{\log(\theta_j)\} = 81$ for each entry θ_j of θ gave ESS values ranging from 0.17 to 0.22 with mean 0.19.

Markov chain Monte Carlo (MCMC) with Gibbs sampling (Robert and Cassella, 1999). was used o compute posterior mean utilities and posterior probabilities used in the acceptability criteria. Sample parameters $\theta^{(1)}, \cdots, \theta^{(N)}$ distributed proportionally to the posterior integrand were generated using the two-level algorithm given by Braun et al. (2007). The Monte Carlo standard error (MCSE) was computed using the batch-means method for the values of $F_E(1, c, q)$, $\pi_T(1, c, q)$ and $u(c, q)$ of the highest and lowest (c, q) combinations. When the ratios of the MCSE to the posterior standard deviation of these quantities were $< 3\%$, this was considered to indicate MCMC convergence.

13.5 Simulations

Each simulation scenario was specified in terms of fixed values of the marginal probabilities $\pi_T(s, c, q)^{true}$ and $F_E(s, c, q)^{true}$ for $s = 0$ and 1. Interpolation was used to obtain fixed true probabilities for all s in $[0, 1]$, allowing $\pi_T(s, c, q)^{true}$ and $F_E(s, c, q)^{true}$ to take a variety of different shapes as functions of s. Details are given in Thall et al. (2011). In each scenario, the method's performance was evaluated in terms of selection percentage and number of patients treated for each (c, q), and R_{select}.

The simulation results are summarized in Table 13.3. Under each of Scenarios 1–4, the design reliably selects (c, q) pairs having higher true utilities, and the sample sizes are balanced favorably toward more desirable pairs. The results for Scenarios 5 and 6 show that if no (c, q) pair is acceptable, then the method is very likely to stop early and select no pair, with stopping percentages 91% in Scenario 5 and 83% in Scenario 6. The summary statistic R_{select} is not relevant in Scenarios 5 and 6, since in these cases the best decision is to stop the trial early and not select any pair. For Scenario 1, Figure 13.2 illustrates how the utility is obtained from the probabilities of Toxicity and Efficacy, and also gives simulation results, for all (c, q) pairs.

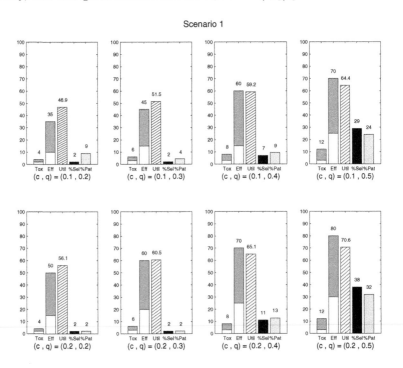

FIGURE 13.2: In Scenario 1, illustration of the utility as a function of the probabilities of Toxicity and Efficacy, with % selection and % patients treated for each (c, q) combination.

Figure 13.3 illustrates the method's sensitivity to the maximum sample size, N, in Scenarios 1–4 where an acceptable (c, q) pair exists. The figure shows that R_{select} increases with N and that, among these four cases, Scenario 2 is the easiest case and Scenario 3 is the most difficult case. Additional simulations, given in Thall et al. (2011), assessed the design's sensitivity to the

TABLE 13.3: Simulation results for the IA tPA trial design. For each (c, q) in each scenario, the true mean utility of treating a patient with that regime is u^{true}. The numerical u^{true} of the best combination is given in boldface, and utilities of unacceptable combinations have a gray background.

q		$c = 0.2$	$c = 0.3$	$c = 0.4$	$c = 0.5$	% none
Scenario 1: Prior Means						
0.1	u^{true}	46.9	51.5	59.2	64.4	6
	% Sel (n)	2% (3.2)	2% (1.6)	7% (3.4)	29% (8.7)	
0.2	u^{true}	56.1	60.5	65.1	**70.6**	
	% Sel (n)	2% (0.8)	2% (0.8)	11% (4.5)	38% (11.5)	
Scenario 2: Safe, high c and q = .20 best						
0.1	u^{true}	49.0	54.9	62.4	71.5	2
	% Sel (n)	1% (2.6)	1% (1.2)	4% (2.3)	17% (5.9)	
0.2	u^{true}	52.6	58.4	65.9	**73.8**	
	% Sel (n)	1% (0.5)	1% (0.6)	13% (5.3)	60% (16.9)	
Scenario 3: Safe, middle c and q = .10 best						
0.1	u^{true}	57.3	68.9	**70.1**	64.0	9
	% Sel (n)	3% (2.4)	8% (3.6)	33% (9.0)	33% (9.3)	
0.2	u^{true}	57.1	68.6	69.7	63.5	
	% Sel (n)	2% (0.5)	2% (0.9)	7% (5.4)	3% (2.8)	
Scenario 4: Safe, low c and q = .10 best						
0.1	u^{true}	**61.1**	58.7	51.6	48.0	12
	% Sel (n)	43% (14.4)	7% (3.3)	6% (3.4)	5% (2.8)	
0.2	u^{true}	58.2	53.9	49.5	45.0	
	% Sel (n)	22% (5.0)	3% (1.5)	2% (2.2)	1% (0.9)	
Scenario 5: Unsafe						
0.1	u^{true}	44.8	45.2	**45.2**	45.0	91
	% Sel (n)	4% (6.5)	1% (1.5)	1% (2.0)	1% (2.2)	
0.2	u^{true}	45.2	45.2	45.0	44.3	
	% Sel (n)	1% (0.9)	0% (0.4)	0% (0.8)	0% (0.6)	
Scenario 6: Safe, but no (c, q) acceptable						
0.1	u^{true}	38.2	40.0	41.9	43.3	83
	% Sel (n)	0% (2.8)	0% (1.1)	1% (1.6)	7% (5.2)	
0.2	u^{true}	39.3	41.2	43.1	**44.4**	
	% Sel (n)	0% (0.4)	0% (0.4)	1% (1.4)	7% (4.3)	

prior, cohort size, and σ. These simulations showed that, for $N = 36$, (1) there is no general pattern of either R_{select} or early stopping probability with cohort size 1, 2, 3, or for σ ranging from 7 to 20, and (2) design performance is robust to the interpolation method used to obtain $\pi_T(s, c, q)^{true}$ and $F_E(s, c, q)^{true}$.

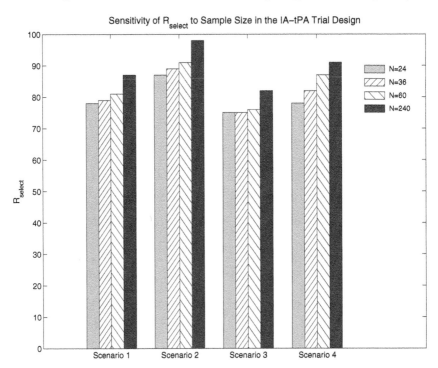

FIGURE 13.3: Sensitivity of the tPA design's overall performance to maximum sample size N, in terms of R_{select} for Scenarios 1–4.

A natural question is whether the complex model given in 13.2 may be replaced by a more parsimonious model. To address this, an alternative model was used that assumes a Weibull distribution for Y_E with hazard function $\lambda(y, c, q, \alpha) = \{\alpha_3 cq + \alpha_4 c(1 - q)\}\psi y^{\psi-1}$, and the mixture distribution simplified by fixing $\alpha_1 = \alpha_2 \equiv \beta_1 \equiv 1$ and $\beta_0 \equiv \beta_4 = 0$. This gives

$$\pi_T(y_E, c, q, \beta) = 1 - e^{-\beta_2 cq - \beta_3 c(1-q)(y_E \wedge 1)}$$

and $p_0 = 1 - e^{\alpha_0 cq}$. This model has 6 parameters, $(\alpha_0, \alpha_4, \alpha_3, \psi, \beta_2, \beta_3)$, compared to 11 for the assumed model. Simulations showed that this simpler model produces a design with very high percentages of correctly selecting the best (c, q) pairs in Scenarios 1 (96%) and 2 (99%), but also high selection percentages for unacceptable (c, q) pairs. Consequently, it has very poor performance in Scenarios 3 and 4, and much lower early stopping percentages in Scenario 5 (69% versus 91% with the more complex model) and 6 (70% versus

83% with the more complex model). The price of greater simplicity thus is a large loss of both reliability and safety.

14

Optimizing Sedative Dose in Preterm Infants

CONTENTS

14.1 Respiratory Distress Syndrome in Neonates 267
14.2 Clinical Outcomes and Probability Model 270
14.3 Prior and Likelihood 273
14.4 Decision Criteria 274
14.5 Simulations 277

14.1 Respiratory Distress Syndrome in Neonates

A severe problem seen in premature babies is respiratory distress syndrome (RDS), characterized by an inability to breathe properly. RDS is associated with the facts that the infant's lungs are not fully developed and do not have enough pulmonary surfactant, a chemical that facilitates breathing which normally is produced naturally. Without sufficient surfactant, the infant may not be able to inhale enough oxygen, which may may permanently damage the brain and other organs.

A successful procedure for preterm infants suffering from RDS is Intubation-Surfactant-Extubation (INSURE). This is carried out as soon as possible once RDS is diagnosed, when the infant is just a few hours old, to reduce the need for mechanical ventilation and the risk of bronchopulmonary dysplasia. With INSURE, the infant is intubated, surfactant is administered to the trachea via the tube, and at completion the infant is extubated. The surfactant spreads from the trachea to the lung's alveola, where it lowers surface tension and reduces alveolar collapse, thus improving lung aeration and decreasing respiratory effort. The aim is to improve the infant's ability to breathe in order to increase the probability of survival without long-term neurological or motor disabilities (Verder et al., 1994; Bohlin et al., 2007; Stevens et al., 2007). In most cases, the INSURE procedure takes at most one hour, with faster completion more desirable.

To allow the intubation to be done safely and comfortably, the infant must be sedated, most often with propofol (Ghanta et al., 2007) or remifentanyl

(Welzing et al., 2009). Although the benefits of the INSURE procedure are well-established, it also carries risks from intubation and sedation. These include adverse behavioral and emotional effects if the infant is under-sedated, while over-sedation may have adverse hemodynamic effects. Failure of the INSURE procedure may result in prolonged mechanical ventilation, a risk factor for long-term adverse pulmonary events (Stevens et al., 2007). A sedative dose must be chosen to sedate the infant sufficiently so that the INSURE procedure may be carried out, but not over-sedate. It is widely agreed that dose should be quantified by amount per kilogram (kg) of the infant's body weight, but very little is known about what an optimal sedative dose may be. Propofol doses that are too high, or given recurrently or by continuous infusion, have been associated with serious adverse effects in neonates (Murdoch and Cohen, 1999; Vanderhaegen et al., 2010; Sammartino et al., 2010). There is no established consensus regarding the dose of any sedative used with INSURE in the neonatology community. The doses used with INSURE vary widely, with neonatologists using preferred doses chosen based on personal clinical experience and consensus within their neonatal units.

The aim of the design described here is to optimize the dose of propofol given at the start of the INSURE procedure. Six doses are investigated, $\{0.5, 1.0, 1.5, 2.0, 2.5, 3.0\}$ mg/kg body weight. Difficulties in determining an optimal dose are that the probabilities of desirable and undesirable clinical outcomes are complex, possibly non-monotone functions of dose, and the outcomes are not mutually independent. Ethical concerns are especially important when treating newborn infants diagnosed with RDS. To optimize propofol dose reliably and ethically with INSURE, a clinical trial design must

1. account for complex relationships between dose and all key clinical outcomes,

2. account for risk–benefit trade-offs between Efficacy and Toxicity,

3. make sequentially adaptive decisions using the accumulating dose-outcome data during the trial, and

4. reliably choose a final, "optimal" dose for use with the INSURE procedure.

The Bayesian phase I–II design described in this chapter, given by Thall et al. (2014b), satisfies all of these requirements.

To characterize propofol dose effects in a realistic and practical way, the design uses three co-primary outcomes, including two Efficacy variables and one Toxicity variable. The design relies on utilities of the joint outcomes, elicited from neonatologists who perform the INSURE procedure. The first Efficacy outcome is that a "good sedation state," GSS, is achieved quickly. GSS is a composite event defined in terms of five established ordinal sedation assessment variables scored within five minutes of the first sedative administration. These are A_1 = Crying Irritability, A_2 = Behavior State, A_3 = Facial Expression, A_4 = Extremities Tone, and A_5 = Vital Signs. Each assessment variable takes on a value in the set {-2, -1, 0, +1, +2}, where -2 corresponds to highest sedation and +2 to highest infant discomfort. The Vital Signs score A_5 is defined in terms of four physiological variables: heart rate (HR), respiration rate (RR), blood pressure (BP), and saturated oxygen in the circulating blood (SaO_2). Figure 14.1, reproduced from Hummel et al. (2008), gives the definitions of the assessment variables.

| Assessment | Sedation | | Sedation/Pain | Pain / Agitation | |
Criteria	-2	-1	0/0	1	2
Crying Irritability	No cry with painful stimuli	Moans or cries minimally with painful stimuli	No sedation/ No pain signs	Irritable or crying at intervals Consolable	High-pitched or silent-continuous cry Inconsolable
Behavior State	No arousal to any stimuli No spontaneous movement	Arouses minimally to stimuli Little spontaneous movement	No sedation/ No pain signs	Restless, squirming Awakens frequently	Arching, kicking Constantly awake or Arouses minimally / no movement (not sedated)
Facial Expression	Mouth is lax No expression	Minimal expression with stimuli	No sedation/ No pain signs	Any pain expression intermittent	Any pain expression continual
Extremities Tone	No grasp reflex Flaccid tone	Weak grasp reflex ↓ muscle tone	No sedation/ No pain signs	Intermittent clenched toes, fists or finger splay Body is not tense	Continual clenched toes, fists, or finger splay Body is tense
Vital Signs HR, RR, BP, SaO₂	No variability with stimuli Hypoventilation or apnea	< 10% variability from baseline with stimuli	No sedation/ No pain signs	↑ 10-20% from baseline SaO₂ 76-85% with stimulation - quick recovery	↑ 20% from baseline SaO₂ ≤ 75% with stimulation - slow recovery Out of sync with vent

FIGURE 14.1: Sedation assessment score variables.

The sedation assessment score is $A = \sum_{j=1}^{5} A_j$. A good sedation score is defined as GSS = $\{-7 \leq A \leq -3\}$, with Y_G the indicator of this Efficacy event. A GSS is required to intubate the infant. If a GSS is not achieved with the initial propofol dose then an additional fixed dose of 1.0 mg/kg is given. If this still does not achieve a GSS, then another sedative may be used, at the discretion of the attending clinician. In addition to the fact that evaluating $(A_1, \cdots, A_5)$ requires many subjective decisions, because a newborn infant cannot talk to explain how it feels, reducing this vector to the binary variable Y_G was done to characterize sedation score in a meaningful yet tractable way for the purpose of dose-finding.

Because it is very desirable to complete the INSURE procedure as quickly as possible, a second Efficacy variable, Y_E, is defined as the indicator that the infant is extubated within at most 30 minutes of intubation, EXT. To account for adverse events, a composite adverse hemodynamic event, HEM, was defined. This occurs if the infant's HR falls below 80 beats per minute, SaO_2 falls below 60%, or mean BP decreases by more than 5 mm Hg from a chosen inferior limit corresponding to the infant's gestational age. This definition includes the time interval for monitoring the infant's HR, SaO_2, as the period while the infant is intubated and three hours following extubation. The indicator of HEM is Y_H.

The trinary outcome used for dose-finding is $Y = (Y_G, Y_E, Y_H)$. The design thus is very different from any adaptive dose-finding method based on one outcome, and also is more complex than phase I–II methods based on one Efficacy and one Toxicity variable.

14.2   Clinical Outcomes and Probability Model

The dose-response model uses the standardized doses obtained by dividing the raw doses by their mean, $x_1 = 0.5/1.75 = 0.286, \cdots, x_6 = 3.0/1.75 = 1.714$. Because historical data on (x, Y) are not available, the following dose-outcome model was developed based on the collective experiences and prior beliefs of the neonatologists planning the trial. The distributions of the two later outcomes, Y_E and Y_H, may depend strongly on the sedation score A. Since the definition of A includes hemodynamic events, Y_E and Y_H are not conditionally independent given A. To reflect this, the joint model for $[A, Y_G, Y_E \mid x]$ is based on the probability factorization

$$[A, Y_E, Y_H \mid x, \theta] = [A \mid x, \theta_A] [Y_E, Y_H \mid x, Y_G, \theta_{E,H}], \qquad (14.1)$$

where θ_A and $\theta_{E,H}$ are subvectors of θ. Expression (14.1) says that x may affect A, and both x and A may affect (Y_E, Y_H). To account for association between Y_E and Y_H, conditional marginals for $[Y_E \mid x, A]$ and $[Y_H \mid x, A]$ are specified, and an FGM copula is assumed to obtain a bivariate distribution. The marginals are

$$\pi_k(x, A, \theta_k) = \Pr(Y_k = 1 \mid x, A, \theta_k) = \text{logit}^{-1}\{\eta_k(x, A, \theta_k)\}, \qquad (14.2)$$

for $k = H, E$, with linear terms

$$\eta_k(x, A, \theta_k) = \theta_{k,0} + \theta_{k,1}x^{\theta_{k,4}} + \theta_{k,2}Z(A) + \theta_{k,3}(1 - Y_G), \qquad (14.3)$$

denoting $Z(A) = \{(A + 5)/15\}^2$ and $\theta_k = (\theta_{k,0}, \theta_{k,1}, \theta_{k,2}, \theta_{k,3}, \theta_{k,4})$. For each $k = E, H$, $\theta_{k,1}$ is the dose effect, $\theta_{k,2}$ is the sedation score effect, $\theta_{k,3}$ is the effect of not achieving a GSS, and x is exponentiated by $\theta_{k,4}$ to obtain flexible dose-response curves. The sedation score A is standardized as $Z(A)$ so that it does not have unduly large effects for values in its domain far away from the ideal score -5. For example, A=10 is represented by $Z(A) = 1$. The intercepts $\theta_{E,0}$ and $\theta_{H,0}$ are real-valued, with the exponents $\theta_{E,4}, \theta_{H,4} > 0$. Based on clinical experience with propofol and other sedatives used in the INSURE procedure, as reflected by the elicited prior means, it is assumed that $\theta_{E,1}, \theta_{E,2} < 0$ while $\theta_{H,1}, \theta_{H,2} > 0$. That is, given the initial sedation score, $\pi_E(x, A, \theta)$ decreases and $\pi_H(x, A, \theta)$ increases with d. Similarly, failure to achieve a GSS can only increase the probability $\pi_H(x, A, \theta)$ of an adverse hemodynamic event and decrease the probability $\pi_E(x, A, \theta)$ of extubation within 30 minutes, so $\theta_{H,3} > 0$ while $\theta_{E,3} < 0$.

Denote the joint distribution

$$\pi_{E,H}(y_E, y_H \mid x, A, \theta_k) = \Pr(Y_E = y_E, Y_H = y_H \mid x, A, \theta_k),$$

for $y_E, y_H \in \{0, 1\}$. Given the marginals $\pi_k(x, A, \theta)$, $k = E, H$, temporarily suppressing (x, A, θ), the FGM copula gives

$$
\begin{aligned}
\pi_{E,H}(y_E, y_H) \;=\; & \pi_E^{y_E}(1 - \pi_E)^{1-y_E} \pi_H^{y_H}(1 - \pi_H)^{1-y_H} \\
& + \; \phi\,(-1)^{y_E + y_H} \pi_E(1 - \pi_E)\pi_H(1 - \pi_H) \qquad (14.4)
\end{aligned}
$$

with association parameter $-1 < \phi < +1$. The joint conditional distribution of $[Y_E, Y_H \mid x, A]$ is parameterized by $\theta_{E,H} = (\theta_E, \theta_H, \psi)$, which has dimension 11, and θ_Z, described below. Denoting $\pi_A(a \mid x, \theta_A) = \Pr(A = a \mid x, \theta_A)$, the joint distribution of the observed outcome vector (A, Y_E, Y_H) is

$$\Pr(A = a, Y_E = y_E, Y_H = y_H \mid d, \theta) \;=\; \pi_A(a \mid x, \theta_A)\, \pi_{E,H}(y_E, y_H \mid x, a, \theta_{E,H}) \tag{14.5}$$

for $a = -10, -9, \cdots, +9, +10$ and $y_E, y_H \in \{0, 1\}$. The joint distribution $\pi_{G,E,H}(y \mid x, \theta)$ of $Y = (Y_G, Y_E, Y_H)$ is obtained by summing (14.5) over $a = -3, \cdots, -7$ or its complement in the A domain.

The unconditional marginals of the later event indicators, Y_E and Y_H, may be complex, non-monotone functions of x. This is because their marginals are defined in (14.2) given initial sedation score, and their unconditional marginals are obtained by averaging over the distribution of A. For $k = E, H$,

$$\bar{\pi}_k(x, \theta_k, \theta_A) \;=\; \Pr(Y_k = 1 \mid x, \theta_k, \theta_A) \;=\; \sum_{a=-10}^{+10} \pi_k(x, a, \theta_k)\, \pi_A(a \mid x, \theta_Z).$$

The unconditional joint distribution $\bar{\pi}_{E,H}(x, \theta)$ is computed similarly, from (14.4) and (14.5).

The probability $\bar{\pi}_H(x, \theta_H, \theta_A)$ of HEM plays a key role, since it determines the safety rule of the design. Overall success is defined as

$$S = (GSS \text{ and } EXT) = (-7 \le A \le -3 \text{ and } Y_E = 1).$$

This has probability $\pi_S(x, \theta)$ that depends on $\pi_A(a \mid x, \theta_A)$. A key property of the model is that, for an infant given dose x, $\bar{\pi}_H(x, \theta_H, \theta_Z)$ and $\pi_S(x, \theta)$ are averages over the initial sedation score, and they depend on θ_A.

A flexible distribution for $[A \mid x]$ is obtained by defining a beta regression model for a latent variable W with support $[0, 1]$ and mean that decreases in x, and then defining the distribution of A in terms of the distribution of W. The beta regression model for $[W \mid x]$ is formulated using the re-parameterization of the $Be(u, v)$ model in terms of its mean $\mu = u/(u+v)$ and $\psi = u+v$, where both $\mu = \mu_x$ and $\psi = \psi_x$ vary with x. The beta pdf is

$$f_W(w \mid \theta_A, x) = \frac{\Gamma(\psi_x)}{\Gamma(\mu_x \psi_x)\Gamma((1 - \mu_x)\psi_x)}\, w^{\mu_x \psi_x - 1}(1 - w)^{(1-\mu_x)\psi_x - 1}, \tag{14.6}$$

for $0 < w < 1$ (Williams, 1982; Ferrari and Cribari-Neto, 2004). Denote the indexes of doses in increasing order by $j(x) = 1, \cdots, J$. A saturated model for the mean of $[W \mid x]$ is assumed,

$$\mu_x = \left\{1 + \sum_{r=1}^{j(x)} \alpha_r\right\}^{-1}$$

where $\alpha_1, \cdots, \alpha_J > 0$. Preliminary simulations showed that the function

$$\psi_x = \{\mu_x(1 - \mu_x)\}^{1-2\gamma_1}(2 + \gamma_2 x^{\gamma_3})^2 \tag{14.7}$$

with $\gamma_1, \gamma_2 > 0$ and γ_3 real-valued gives a model that fits a wide range of simulated data quite well. This model is similar to the generalized beta regression model of Simas et al. (2010).

Denote the incomplete beta function

$$B(u, v, w) = \int_0^w p^{u-1}(1-p)^{v-1} dp, \quad \text{for } 0 < w < 1 \text{ and } u, v > 0.$$

The discrete distribution of $[A \mid x]$ is

$$\begin{aligned}
\pi_A(a \mid x, \theta_Z) &= \Pr\{(a+10)/21 \le W \le (a+11)/21 \mid x, \theta_A\} \\
&= B\left\{\frac{a+11}{21}, \mu_x\psi_x, (1-\mu_x)\psi_x\right\} \\
&\quad - B\left\{\frac{a+10}{21}, \mu_x\psi_x, (1-\mu_x)\psi_x\right\}
\end{aligned} \tag{14.8}$$

for $a = -10, -9, \cdots, +9, +10$, where

$$\theta_A = (\alpha, \gamma) = (\alpha_1, \cdots, \alpha_J, \gamma_1, \gamma_2, \gamma_3).$$

This model expresses the probability of a GSS in terms of the incomplete beta function evaluated at arguments characterized by x, the 6 dose-response parameters $\alpha = (\alpha_1, \cdots, \alpha_6)$ of μ_x, and the three parameters $\gamma = (\gamma_1, \gamma_2, \gamma_3)$ of ψ_x. While this may seem somewhat elaborate, A is a sum with 21 possible values and its distribution is a function of 6 possible doses, so a $6 \times 20 = 120$ dimensional distribution is represented by a 9-parameter model.

From (14.8), the marginal of Y_G is

$$\pi_G(x, \theta_A) = B\{8/21, \mu_x\psi_x, (1-\mu_x)\psi_x\} - B\{3/21, \mu_x\psi_x, (1-\mu_x)\psi_x\}. \tag{14.9}$$

While the beta distribution of the latent variable W is monotone in dose by construction, expressions (14.6)–(14.9) show that $\pi_G(x, \theta_A)$ is a possibly non-monotone function of dose. Figure 14.2 illustrates the flexibility of the underlying probability model for each of four different scenarios, it gives the shapes of $\Pr(GSS|x)$, $\Pr(EXT|x)$, $\Pr(HEM|x)$, and $\Pr(Success|x)$. The ranges of

$\Pr(EXT|x)$ and $\Pr(HEM|x)$ are restricted in the plots since, under scenarios in which at least one dose is acceptable, $\Pr(EXT|x)$ must be large and $\Pr(HEM|x)$ must be small. The figure shows that, depending on the true state of nature, both $\Pr(GSS|x)$, $\Pr(EXT|x)$, and $\Pr(Success|x)$ each may be monotone increasing, monotone decreasing, or inverted U-shaped in x, while $\Pr(HEM|x)$ increases with x but at a rate that may be anywhere from very small to very large. Thus, the model is sufficiently flexible to allow the observed data to determine their functional forms.

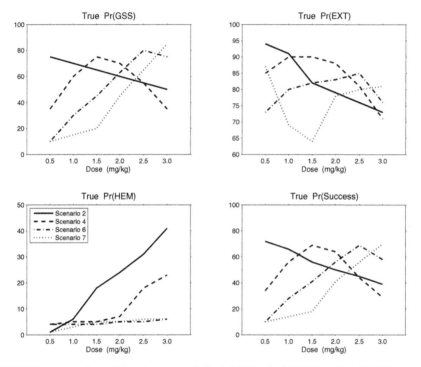

FIGURE 14.2: Possible shapes of $\Pr(GSS)$, $\Pr(EXT)$, $\Pr(HEM)$, and $\Pr(Success)$ as functions of dose.

14.3 Prior and Likelihood

Collecting terms, the model parameter vector is $\theta = (\rho, \alpha, \gamma, \theta_E, \theta_H)$, with $\dim(\theta) = 20$. To establish a prior, it was assumed that $\rho \sim Uniform[-1, +1]$. For the remaining 19 parameters, a pseudo sample-based approach was used. Details are given in Thall et al. (2014b). It was assumed that $\alpha_1, \cdots, \alpha_6$, $-\theta_{E,1}, -\theta_{E,2}, -\theta_{E,3}$, $\theta_{H,1}, \theta_{H,2}, \theta_{H,3}$ were normal truncated below at 0, γ_1,

γ_2, $\theta_{E,4}$, $\theta_{H,4}$ were lognormal, and γ_3, $\theta_{E,0}, \theta_{H,0}$ were normal. Given the prior means established by the pseudo sampling method, the prior variances were calibrated to be uninformative in the sense that effective sample size (ESS, Morita et al. (2008, 2010)) of the prior was 0.10.

For outcomes $Y_i^o = (A_i, Y_{i,E}, Y_{i,H})$ of patients $i = 1, \cdots, N$, denoting $\mathcal{Y}_n^o = (Y_1^o, \cdots, Y_n^o)$, the likelihood for the first n patients is

$$\mathcal{L}_n(\mathcal{Y}_n^o \mid \theta) = \prod_{i=1}^n \pi_A(A_i \mid x_{[i]}, \theta_A) \pi_{E,H}(Y_{i,E}, Y_{i,H} \mid x_{[i]}, A_i, \theta_{E,H}).$$

14.4   Decision Criteria

The elicited numerical utilities are given in Table 14.1. The maximum utility 100 was assigned to the best possible event (GSS = yes, EXT = yes, HEM = no), and minimum numerical utility 0 was assigned to the worst possible event (GSS = no, EXT = no, HEM = yes). The six remaining values were elicited subject to the constraints that the utility must increase as either GSS or EXT goes from "no" to "yes" and must decrease as HEM goes from "no" to "yes." This utility function formalizes the trade-offs between the INSURE procedure's risks and benefits.

For $y = (y_G, y_E, y_H)$, the mean utility of dose d given θ is

$$\overline{U}(x \mid \theta) = \sum_y U(y) \, \pi_{G,E,H}(y \mid x, \theta),$$

and the posterior mean utility of d given data $\mathcal{D}_n$ is

$$u(x \mid \mathcal{D}_n) = \int_\theta \overline{U}(x \mid \theta) \, p(\theta \mid \mathcal{D}_n) d\theta,$$

the expected payoff if the next infant is given x. Subject to the restriction that an untried dose may not be skipped when escalating, the design U^{opt} chooses each successive cohort's dose to maximize $u(x \mid \mathcal{D}_n)$ among all $x \in \{x_1, \cdots, x_6\}$.

Since Y is trinary, this leads to a complex model. A natural question is why one cannot do things much more simply, with dose-finding based on a single outcome. Given the insights obtained by establishing trinary Y and eliciting $U(y)$, it is easy to show why the common practice of using a single outcome may have very undesirable consequences. This is illustrated by the hypothetical example in Table 14.2. For the two doses 2.0 and 3.0 mg/kg, and for each of the eight possible elementary outcomes, the table gives the true outcome probability $\pi_{G,E,H}^{true}(y)$ and the probability-weighted utility $\pi_{G,E,H}^{true}(y) \times U(y)$. The criterion $\pi_G(x)$, the probability of a GSS, leads to the conclusion that 3.0

TABLE 14.1: Elicited and hypothetical utilities for the propofol trial

Elicited Consensus Utility Function

| | GSS = Yes | | GSS = No | |
	EXT = Yes	EXT = No	EXT = Yes	EXT = No
HEM = Yes	60	20	40	0
HEM = No	100	80	90	70

Hypothetical Alternative Utility Function 1: GSS given greater importance

| | GSS = Yes | | GSS = No | |
	EXT = Yes	EXT = No	EXT = Yes	EXT = No
HEM = Yes	80	60	20	0
HEM = No	100	90	45	35

Hypothetical Alternative Utility Function 2: EXT given greater importance

| | GSS = Yes | | GSS = No | |
	EXT = Yes	EXT = No	EXT = Yes	EXT = No
HEM = Yes	80	10	70	0
HEM = No	100	40	95	35

Hypothetical Alternative Utility Function 3: HEM given greater importance

| | GSS = Yes | | GSS = No | |
	EXT = Yes	EXT = No	EXT = Yes	EXT = No
HEM = Yes	30	10	20	0
HEM = No	100	90	95	85

TABLE 14.2: Hypothetical example where the two criteria $\overline{U}(x)$ based on (Y_G, Y_E, Y_H) and $\pi_G(x)$ based on Y_G alone lead to different conclusions. For each combination of $U(y)$ and dose, each tabled pair is $\pi_{G,E,H}^{true}(y)$, $\pi_{G,E,H}^{true}(y) \times U(y)$.

dose = 2.0 mg/kg	GSS = Yes		GSS = No	
	EXT = Yes	EXT = No	EXT = Yes	EXT = No
HEM = Yes	.04, 2.4	.01, 0.2	.03, 1.2	.02, 0
HEM = No	.45, 45.0	.15, 12.0	.20, 18.0	.10, 7.0

$$\overline{U}^{true} = 85.8, \quad \pi_G^{true} = .65, \quad \pi_H^{true} = .10$$

dose = 3.0 mg/kg	GSS = Yes		GSS = No	
	EXT = Yes	EXT = No	EXT = Yes	EXT = No
HEM = Yes	.14, 8.4	.08, 1.6	.04, 1.6	.04, 0
HEM = No	.40, 40.0	.18, 14.4	.06, 5.4	.06, 4.2

$$\overline{U}^{true} = 75.6, \quad \pi_G^{true} = .80, \quad \pi_H^{true} = .30$$

mg/kg is superior since $\pi_G^{true}(3.0) = .80$ while $\pi_G^{true}(2.0) = .65$. In contrast, considering the mean utility over all three outcomes leads to the opposite conclusion, since $\overline{U}^{true}(2.0) = 85.8$ versus $\overline{U}^{true}(3.0) = 75.6$. Closer inspection of the table shows that the larger mean utility for 2.0 mg/kg is due to the fact that avoiding the adverse event HEM when a GSS is not achieved contributes substantially to the overall mean utility for dose 2.0 mg/kg. Moreover, $\pi_H^{true}(2.0) = .10$ but $\pi_H^{true}(3.0) = .30$, so the higher dose is far less safe. The criterion $\pi_G(x)$ ignores these facts. While achieving a GSS is very important, consideration of all of three possible events gives a much more complete picture, and thus a more fully informed basis for choosing among doses.

As usual, a dose that is optimal in terms of the utility considered alone may be unacceptable in terms of either safety or overall success rate. In an extreme case, even if all doses have unacceptably high $\pi_H(x, \theta)$, so that no dose is acceptable, one still may compute all $u(x, \mathcal{D}_n)$ values and find the maximum. To ensure that any dose administered to an infant has both an acceptably high success rate and an acceptably low adverse event rate, the following acceptability criteria are imposed. Given physician-specified fixed upper limit $\bar{\pi}_H^*$ a dose x is *unsafe* if

$$Pr\{\bar{\pi}_H(x, \theta_H, \theta_Z) > \bar{\pi}_H^* \mid \mathcal{D}_n\} > p_{U,H} \tag{14.10}$$

for decision cut-off $p_{U,H}$. The distribution of the overall success event $S =$

$(Y_G = 1 \text{ and } Y_E = 1)$ is

$$
\begin{aligned}
\pi_S(x, \theta) &= \Pr(Y_E = 1 \text{ and } -7 \le Z \le -3 \mid x, \theta) \\
&= \sum_{a=-7}^{-3} \Pr(Y_E = 1 \mid x, A = a, \theta_E) \pi_A(a \mid x, \theta_A),
\end{aligned}
$$

parameterized by (θ_E, θ_A). Given fixed lower limit π_S^*, *a dose x has unacceptably low overall success probability* if

$$
Pr\{\pi_S(x, \theta_E, \theta_Z) < \pi_S^* \mid data\} > p_{U,S} \tag{14.11}
$$

for fixed decision cut-off $p_{U,S}$. The subset of doses that do not satisfy either (14.10) or (14.11) are *acceptable*, The upper limit $\bar{\pi}_H^* = .10$ and lower limit $\pi_S^* = .60$ are used in the trial. The modification of design U^{opt} restricted to acceptable doses is denoted by $U^{opt}(Acc)$. For trial conduct, the first cohort is treated at 1.0 mg/kg. The design chooses acceptable doses adaptively for all subsequent cohorts by maximizing posterior mean utility among the six doses, with the trial stopped early if no dose is acceptable.

14.5 Simulations

The trial was simulated with maximum sample size 60, cohort size 2, and acceptability cut-offs $p_{U,H} = p_{U,S} = 0.95$, with $p_L = 0.05$ when AR_δ is used. Figure 14.3 summarizes the simulation results for $U^{opt}(Acc)$ under four selected scenarios. This figure shows that the design has high probabilities of selecting the doses with largest true utilities, while avoiding unsafe doses.

In addition to the designs $U^{opt}(Acc)$ and U^{opt}, the following non-model-based 4-stage design also is included in the simulations, as a comparator:

1. *Stage 1*: Randomize 24 patients to the 6 doses, with 4 per dose. Select the 4 doses with highest mean utility $\overline{U}(x)$ for evaluation in stage 2.

2. *Stage 2*: Randomize 16 patients to each of the 4 selected doses, with 4 per dose, and select the 3 doses from all 6 with highest $\overline{U}(x)$ for evaluation in stage 3.

3. *Stage 3*: Randomize 12 patients to each of the 3 newly selected doses, with 4 per dose, and select the 2 doses from all 6 with highest $\overline{U}(x)$ for evaluation in stage 4.

4. *Stage 4*: Randomize 8 patients to each of the 2 remaining doses, with 4 per dose, and select the dose with highest $\overline{U}(x)$ from all 6 doses.

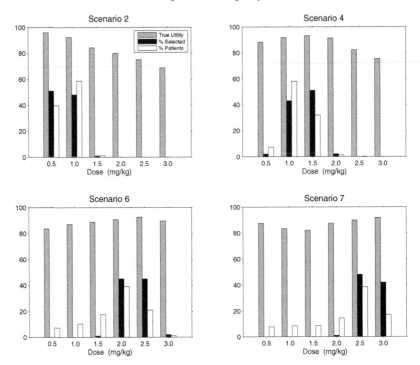

FIGURE 14.3: Selection and sub-sample size percentages for each dose in the propofol trial run using $U^{opt}(Acc)$, under four scenarios.

This non-model-based 4-stage design has a fixed sample size of 60 patients, evaluates at least 4 patients per dose, and the final selected dose has information on up to 16 patients. It interimly selects (drops) doses with higher (lower) empirical mean utilities, but it does not have rules that drop doses based on their empirical HEM or Success rates.

Table 14.3 compares the three designs under each of seven dose-outcome scenarios, given in the Supplementary Tables of Thall et al. (2014b). Scenario 1 corresponds to the elicited prior probabilities. None of the scenarios are model-based. All scenarios assume that a larger dose will shift the distribution of A toward -10, reflecting the biological effect of the sedative. The true distribution of A varies widely across the scenarios, with true $\pi_E(x)$ and $\pi_H(x)$ following the same trends as the prior in that $\pi_E(x)$ decreases and $\pi_H(x)$ increases with x given A. Since both U^{opt} and 4-*Stage* have no early stopping rules, these designs always treat 60 patients.

Compared to $U^{opt}(Acc)$, the 4-*Stage* design has R_{select} values slightly higher in Scenarios 1 and 2, with the price being many more HEM events, and in Scenarios 3–7 it also has lower R_{select} values, so even without stopping rules it is less reliable. Comparison of the model-based designs U^{opt} to $U^{opt}(Acc)$ shows the need for additional dose acceptability criteria in a sequen-

TABLE 14.3: Simulation results comparing three alternative designs for the propofol trial

Design		Scenario						
		1	2	3	4	5	6	7
$U^{opt}(Acc)$ Model Based	R_{select}	95	93	99	95	93	89	88
	R_{treat}	96	92	98	92	79	69	64
	% None	4	0	1	2	4	7	10
	# Pats	58.9	59.8	59.8	59.4	59.0	58.1	56.9
	# HEM	4.2	2.6	2.4	2.9	2.3	2.6	2.9
	# Succ	36.4	40.6	39.3	35.1	32.2	28.7	25.5
U^{opt} Model Based	R_{select}	96	93	99	90	73	49	30
	R_{treat}	96	92	98	90	64	46	21
	% None	0	0	0	0	0	0	0
	# Pats	60.0	60.0	60.0	60.0	60.0	60.0	60.0
	# HEM	4.1	2.7	2.4	2.8	2.2	2.3	2.1
	# Succ	36.7	40.8	39.6	33.0	25.7	20.2	9.2
4-Stage Non Model Based	R_{select}	97	97	92	93	89	82	84
	R_{treat}	83	65	73	76	66	63	59
	% None	0	0	0	0	0	0	0
	# Pats	60.0	60.0	60.0	60.0	60.0	60.0	60.0
	# HEM	8.8	8.9	3.2	5.0	2.7	2.9	2.7
	# Succ	34.5	35.4	33.3	31.9	29.8	28.4	23.1

tially adaptive utility-based design. These two designs have similar values of R_{select} and R_{treat} for Scenarios 1–4, but Scenarios 5–7 show the importance of dose acceptability rules. In these cases, $U^{opt}(Acc)$ has greatly superior performance. In Scenario 8, U^{opt} has a mean of 19.3 HEM events, compared to 4.9 for $U^{opt}(Acc)$. This illustrates the danger of using a design with a utility-based decision criterion without an additional rule to exclude unsafe doses or regimes. The much higher values of R_{select} and R_{treat} for $U^{opt}(Acc)$ in Scenarios 5–7 show clearly that it is both more reliable and more ethical in these cases compared to U^{opt}.

Additional scenarios, not shown in 14.3 were simulated by Thall et al. (2014b, Table 4), where either (1) all doses have true $\pi_H(x) \geq .29$, well above the upper limit .10, so no dose is safe, or (2) all doses are safe but have true $\pi_S(x) \leq .41$, well below the minimum success probability .60. In these scenarios, the $U^{opt}(Acc)$ design has probability $\geq .93$ of stopping early and not selecting any dose. Since the non-model-based 4-*Stage* design always treats 60 patients, it does not stop early in either of these two scenarios, so obviously is unethical. Moreover, across all scenarios, the 4-stage design has a much larger expected number of HEM events and much lower R_{treat} values.

The numerical limits $\pi_H(x) \leq 0.10$ and $\pi_S(x) \geq 0.60$ in the propofol trial are quite demanding, and tightly constrain the acceptable dose set. This is ethically necessary for a trial of newborn infants and, although the optimal propofol dose is not known, the INSURE procedure has been very successful. Another version of the $U^{opt}(Acc)$ design that also includes AR also was studied, to help avoid getting stuck at a sub-optimal dose. It was found that adding AR had a trivial effect on the design's behavior, and that the $U^{opt}(Acc)$ design was slightly superior. Thus may be attributed to these two very stringent dose admissibility criteria, which appear to obviate any improvement with AR. Using the utility function to reduce the three-dimensional outcome Y to a single quantity is a technical device that is ethically desirable. Comparison of U^{opt} to $U^{opt} + Acc$ shows that use of the greedy utility-based algorithm *per se* gives a design that is ethically unacceptable, but that this problem can be solved by adding dose admissibility criteria. In structurally similar clinical settings with two Efficacy events and one Toxicity event, but with less stringent numerical limits than .10 for $\pi_H(x)$ and .60 for $\pi_S(x)$), it may turn out that using AR is preferable.

Since the elicited utilities are subjective, and others may have different utilities, it is useful to carry out a sensitivity analysis in the numerical utilities. This analysis uses each the four alternative utilities in Table 14.1 to conduct the trial. One is the actual elicited utility, and each of the other three places more value on a particular outcome. The results, summarized in Figure (14.4) for R_{select} and Figure 14.5 for R_{treat}, show that the design is robust to the utility used for trial conduct.

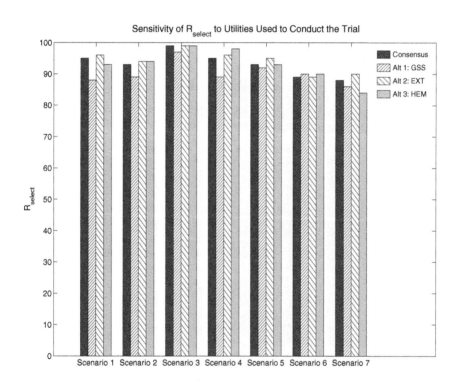

FIGURE 14.4: R_{select} values for the propofol trial conducted with $U^{opt}(Acc)$ using each of four different utilities given in Table 14.1, under each of Scenarios 1–7.

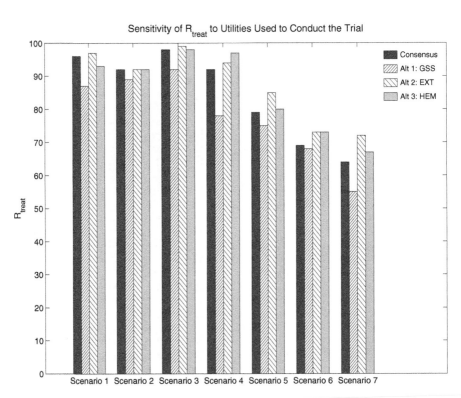

FIGURE 14.5: R_{treat} values for the propofol trial conducted with $U^{opt}(Acc)$ using each of the four different utilities given in Table 14.1, under each of Scenarios 1–7.

Bibliography

Agresti, A. (2002). Links between binary and multi-category logit item response models and quasi-symmetric loglinear models. *Annales de la Faculté des Sciences de Toulouse. Mathématiques. Série 6*, 11(4):443–454. Special issue on quasi-symmetry and categorical data analysis.

Albert, J. H. and Chib, S. (1993). Bayesian analysis of binary and polytomous response data. *Journal of the American Statistical Association*, 88:669–679.

Almirall, D., Ten Have, T., and Murphy, S. A. (2010). Structural nested mean models for assessing time-varying effect moderation. *Biometrics*, 66(1):131–139.

Anand, P. (1995). *Foundations of Rational Choice Under Risk*. Oxford University Press.

Andersson, B. S., Thall, P. F., Madden, T., Couriel, D., Wang, X., Tran, H. T., Anderlini, P., De Lima, M., Gajewski, J., and Champlin, R. E. (2002). Busulfan systemic exposure relative to regimen-related toxicity and acute graft-versus-host disease: Defining a therapeutic window for IV BuCy2 in chronic myelogenous leukemia. *Biology of Blood and Marrow Transplantation*, 8(9):477–485.

Ashford, J. R. and Sowden, R. R. (1970). Multi-variate probit analysis. *Biometrics*, 26(3):535–546.

Auer, P., Cesa-Bianchi, N., and Fischer, P. (2002). Finite-time analysis of the multiarmed bandit problem. *Machine learning*, 47(2-3):235–256.

Azriel, D., Mandel, M., and Rinott, Y. (2011). The treatment versus experimentation dilemma in dose-finding studies. *Journal of Statistical Planning and Inference*, 141:2759–2768.

Babb, J. and Rogatko, A. (2001). Patient specific dosing in a cancer phase I clinical trial. *Statistics in Medicine*, 20:2079–2090.

Babb, J., Rogatko, A., and Zacks, S. (1998). Cancer phase I clinical trials: Efficient dose escalation with overdose control. *Statistics in Medicine*, 17:1103–1120.

Barlow, R. E., Bartholomew, D. J., Bremner, J. M., and Brunk, H. D. (1972). *Statistical Inference under Order Restrictions*. John Wiley & Sons, London.

Bartroff, J. and Lai, T. (2010). Approximate dynamic programming and its applications to the design of phase I cancer trials. *Statistical Science*, 25:245–257.

Bauer, P. and Kieser, M. (1999). Combining different phases in the development of medical treatments within a single trial. *Statistics in Medicine*, 18:1833–1848.

Bedrick, E. J., Christensen, R., and Johnson, W. (1996). A new perspective on priors for generalized linear models. *Journal of the American Statistical Association*, 91:1450–1460.

Bekele, B. N. and Thall, P. F. (2004). Dose-finding based on multiple toxicities in a soft tissue sarcoma trial. *Journal of the American Statistical Association*, 99:26–35.

Bellman, R. E. (1957). *Dynamic Programming*. Princeton University Press, Princeton, NJ.

Berger, J. O. (1985). *Statistical Decision Theory and Bayesian Analysis, 2nd edition*. Springer-Verlag, New York.

Blomqvist, C., Elomaa, I., Rissanen, P., Hietanen, P., Nevasaari, K., and Helle, L. (1993). Influence of treatment schedule on toxicity and efficacy of cyclophosphamide, epirubicin, and fluorouracil in metastatic breast cancer: a randomized trial comparing weekly and every-4-week administration. *Journal of Clinical Oncology*, 11(3):467–473.

Bohlin, K., Gudmundsdottir, T., Katz-Salamon, M., Jonsson, B., and Blennow, M. (2007). Implementation of surfactant treatment during continuous positive airway pressure. *Journal of Perinatology*, 27:422–427.

Braun, T. M. (2002). The bivariate continual reassessment method: Extending the CRM to phase I trials of two competing outcomes. *Controlled Clinical Trials*, 23:240–256.

Braun, T. M. (2006). Generalizing the TiTE-CRM to adapt for early- and late-onset toxicities. *Statistics in Medicine*, 25:2071–2083.

Braun, T. M., Kang, S., and Taylor, J. M. G. (2012). A phase I/II trial design when response is unobserved in subjects with dose-limiting toxicity. *Statistical Methods in Medical Research*. doi:10.1177/0962280212464541.

Braun, T. M., Thall, P. F., Nguyen, H., and de Lima, M. (2007). Simultaneously optimizing dose and schedule of a new cytotoxic agent. *Clinical Trials*, 4:113–124.

Braun, T. M. and Wang, S. A. (2010). A hierarchical Bayesian design for phase I trials of novel combinations of cancer therapeutic agents. *Biometrics*, 66:805–812.

Bretz, F., Pinheiro, J., and Branson, M. (2005). Combining multiple comparisons and modeling techniques in dose-response studies. *Biometrics*, 61:738–748.

Bretz, F., Schmidli, H., König, F., Racine, A., and Maurer, W. (2006). Confirmatory seamless phase II/III clinical trials with hypotheses selection at interim: General concepts. *Biometrical Journal*, 48(4):623–634.

Brook, R. H., Chassin, M. R., Fink, A., Solomon, D. H., Kosecoff, J., and Park, R. E. (1986). A method for the detailed assessment of the appropriateness of medical technologies. *International Journal of Technology Assessment and Health Care*, 2:53–63.

Bryant, J. and Day, R. (1995). Incorporating toxicity considerations into the design of two-stage phase II clinical trials. *Statistics in Medicine*, 51:1372–1383.

Burnham, A. J., Viveros, R., and MacGregor, J. F. (1996). Frameworks for latent variable multivariate regression. *Journal of Chemometrics*, 10(1):31–45.

Cai, C., Liu, S., and Yuan, Y. (2014a). A bayesian design for phase ii clinical trials with delayed responses based on multiple imputation. *Statistics in medicine*, 33(23):4017–4028.

Cai, C., Yuan, Y., and Ji, Y. (2014b). A Bayesian dose finding design for oncology clinical trials of combinational biological agents. *Journal of the Royal Statistical Society: Series C (Applied Statistics)*, 63:159–173.

Carlin, B. P., Zhong, W. Z., and Koopmeiners, J. S. (2013). Discussion of Small-sample behavior of novel phase I cancer trial designs by Assaf P. Oron and Peter D. Hoff. *Clinical Trials*, 10:81–85.

Chatterjee, N. and Shih, J. (2001). A bivariate cure-mixture approach for modeling familial association in diseases. *Biometrics*, 57:779–786.

Cheung, Y. K. (2005). Coherence principles in dose-finding studies. *Biometrika*, 92:863–873.

Cheung, Y. K. (2011). *Dose Finding by the Continual Reassessment Method*. Chapman & Hall/CRC, New York.

Cheung, Y. K. and Chappell, R. (2000). Sequential designs for phase I clinical trials with late-onset toxicities. *Biometrics*, 56:1177–1182.

Chevret, S. (1993). The continual reassessment method in cancer phase I clinical trials: A simulation study. *Statistics in Medicine*, 12(12):1093–1108.

Chevret, S. (2006). *Statistical Methods for Dose-Finding Experiments*. John Wiley and Sons, England.

Chib, S. and Greenberg, E. (1998). Analysis of multivariate probit models. *Biometrika*, 85(2):347–361.

Christensen, R., Johnson, W., Branscum, A., and Hanson, T. E. (2011). *Bayesian Ideas and Data Analysis: An Introduction for Scientists and Statisticians*. CRC Press.

Clark, P., Slevin, M., Joel, S., Osborne, R., Talbot, D., Johnson, P., Reznek, R., Masud, T., Gregory, W., and Wrigley, P. (1994). A randomized trial of two etoposide schedules in small-cell lung cancer: The influence of pharmacokinetics on efficacy and toxicity. *Journal of Clinical Oncology*, 12(7):1427–1435.

Clayton, D. G. (1978). A model for association in bivariate life tables and its application in epidemiological studies of familial tendency in chronic disease incidence. *Biometrika*, 65:141–151.

Collins, L. M., Murphy, S. A., Nair, V. N., and Strecher, V. J. (2005). A strategy for optimizing and evaluating behavioral interventions. *Annals of Behavioral Medicine*, 30(1):65–73.

Conaway, M. R., Dunbar, S., and Peddada, S. D. (2004). Design for single- or multiple-agent phase I trials. *Biometrics*, 60:661–669.

Conaway, M. R. and Petroni, G. R. (1995). Bivariate sequential designs for phase II trials. *Biometrics*, 51:656–664.

Cooke, R. M. (1991). *Experts in Uncertainty: Opinion and Subjective Probability in Science*. New York, NY (United States); Oxford University Press.

Cullen, M., Billingham, L., Woodroffe, C., Chetiyawardana, A., Gower, N., Joshi, R., Ferry, D., Rudd, R., Spiro, S., Cook, J., et al. (1999). Mitomycin, ifosfamide, and cisplatin in unresectable non–small-cell lung cancer: Effects on survival and quality of life. *Journal of Clinical Oncology*, 17(10):3188–3194.

Dalkey, N. (1969). An experimental study of group opinion: the Delphi method. *Futures*, 1(5):408–426.

Dalkey, N. and Helmer, O. (1963). An experimental application of the Delphi method to the use of experts. *Management Science*, 9(3):458–467.

de Jong, S. (1993). SIMPLS: an alternative approach to partial least squares regression. *Chemometrics and Intelligent Laboratory Systems*, 18(3):251–263.

Dragalin, V. and Fedorov, V. (2006). Adaptive designs for dose-finding based on efficacy-toxicity response. *Journal of Statistical Planning and Inference*, 136:1800–1823.

Druker, B. J. (2002). Perspectives on the development of a molecularly targeted agent. *Cancer Cell*, 1(1):31–36.

Eisenhauer, E. A., Therasse, P., Bogaerts, J., Schwartz, L., Sargent, D., Ford, R., Dancey, J.and Arbuck, S., Gwyther, S. G., Mooney, M., Rubinstein, L., Shankar, L., Dodd, L., Kaplan, R., Lacombe, D., and Verweij, J. (2009). New response evaluation criteria in solid tumours: Revised RECIST guideline (version 1.1). *European Journal of Cancer*, 45:228–247.

Ellenberg, S. S. and Eisenberger, M. A. (1985). An efficient design for phase III studies of combination chemotherapies. *Cancer Treatment Reports*, 69(10):1147–1154.

Ferrari, S. L. P. and Cribari-Neto, F. (2004). Beta regression for modelling rates and proportions. *Journal of Applied Statistics*, 31:799–815.

Fleming, T. R. (1982). One-sample multiple testing procedure for phase II clinical trials. *Biometrics*, 38:143–151.

Frank, I. E. and Friedman, J. H. (1993). A statistical view of some chemometrics regression tools. *Technometrics*, 35(2):109–135.

Friedman, L. M., Furberg, C., and DeMets, D. L. (2010). *Fundamentals of Clinical Trials*, volume 4. Springer.

Gafter-Gvili, A., Leader, A., Gurion, R., Vidal, L., Ram, R., Shacham-Abulafia, A., Ben-Bassat, I., Lishner, M., Shpilberg, O., and Raanani, P. (2011). High-dose imatinib for newly diagnosed chronic phase chronic myeloid leukemia patients-systematic review and meta-analysis. *American Journal of Hematology*, 86:657–662.

Gan, H. K., Grothey, A., Pond, G. R., Moore, M. J., Siu, L. L., and Sargent, D. (2010). Randomized phase II trials: Inevitable or inadvisable? *Journal of Clinical Oncology*, 28(15):2641–2647.

Garthwaite, P. H. (1994). An interpretation of partial least squares. *Journal of the American Statistical Association*, 89(425):122–127.

Gelman, A., Jakulin, A., Pittau, M. G., and Su, Y. (2008). A weakly informative default prior distribution for logistic and other regression models. *The Annals of Applied Statistics*, 2:1360–1383.

Ghanta, S., Abdel-Latif, M. E., Lui, K., Ravindranathan, H., Awad, J., and Oei, J. (2007). Propofol compared with the morphine, atropine, and suxamethonium regimen as induction agents for neonatal endotracheal intubation: A randomized, controlled trial. *Pediatrics*, 119:1248–1255.

Gibbons, J., Egorin, M., Ramanathan, R., Fu, P., Mulkerin, D., Shibata, S., Takimoto, C., Mani, S., LoRusso, P., Grem, J., et al. (2008). Phase I and pharmacokinetic study of imatinib mesylate in patients with advanced malignancies and varying degrees of renal dysfunction: A study by the national cancer institute organ dysfunction working group. *Journal of Clinical Oncology*, 26:570–576.

Gilks, W. R., Best, N. G., and Tan, K. K. C. (1995). Adaptive rejection Metropolis sampling within Gibbs sampling. *Applied Statistics*, 44:455–472.

Gittins, J. C. (1979). Bandit processes and dynamic allocation indices. *Journal of the Royal Statistical Society. Series B (Methodological)*, 41:148–177.

Goodman, S., Zahurak, M., and Piantadosi, S. (1995). Some pratical improvements in the continual reassessment method for phase I studies. *Statistics in Medicine*, 14:1149–1161.

Gooley, T. A., Martin, P. J., Fisher, L. D., and Pettinger, M. (1994). Simulation as a design tool for phase I/II clinical trials: An example from bone marrow transplantation. *Controlled Clinical Trials*, 15:450–462.

Grieve, A. P. (1988). A Bayesian approach to the analysis of LD50 experiments. *Bayesian Statistics*, 3:617–630.

Guo, B. and Li, Y. (2014). Bayesian dose-finding designs for combination of molecularly targeted agents assuming partial stochastic ordering. *Statistics in Medicine*, 34(5):859–875.

Guo, B., Li, Y., and Yuan, Y. (2016). A dose–schedule finding design for phase I–II clinical trials. *Journal of the Royal Statistical Society: Series C (Applied Statistics)*, 65(2):259–272.

Guo, B. and Yuan, Y. (2015). A Bayesian dose-finding design for phase I/II clinical trials with nonignorable dropouts. *Statistics in Medicine*, 34(10):1721–1732.

Gyergyay, F., Nagyvanyi, K., and Bodrogi, I. (2009). Decreased toxicity schedule of suitinib in renal cell cancer: 2 weeks on/1 week off. In *ASCO Annual Meeting Proceedings*, volume 27 (15S), page e16113.

Haines, L., Perevozskaya, I., and Rosenberger, W. (2003). Bayesian optimal designs for phase I clinical trials. *Biometrics*, 59:591–600.

Hernan, M. A., Brumback, B., and Robins, J. M. (2000). Marginal structural models to estimate the causal effect of zidovudine on the survival of hiv-positive men. *Epidemiology*, 11(5):561–570.

Hobbs, B. P., Thall, P. F., and Lin, S. H. (2016). Bayesian group sequential clinical trial design using total toxicity burden and progression-free survival. *Journal of the Royal Statistical Society: Series C (Applied Statistics)*, 65(2):273–297.

Hoff, P. and Ellis, L. (2007). Targeted therapy trials: approval strategies, target validation, or helping patients? *Journal of Clinical Oncology*, 25:1639–1641.

Horiguchi, J., Rai, Y., Tamura, K., Taki, T., Hisamatsu, K., Ito, Y., Seriu, T., and Tajima, T. (2009). Phase II study of weekly paclitaxel for advanced or metastatic breast cancer in Japan. *Anticancer Research*, 29:625–630.

Houede, N., Thall, P. F., Nguyen, H., Paoletti, X., and Kramar, A. (2010). Utility-based optimization of combination therapy using ordinal toxicity and efficacy in phase I/II trials. *Biometrics*, 66:532–540.

Huang, X., Biswas, S., Oki, Y., Issa, J., and Berry, D. (2007). A parallel phase I/II clinical trial design for combination therapies. *Biometrics*, 63:429–436.

Hummel, P., Puchalski, M., Creech, S. D., and Weiss, M. G. (2008). Clinical reliability and validity of the N-Pass: Neonatal pain, agitation and sedation scale with prolonged pain. *Journal of Perinatology*, 28:55–60.

Hunink, M. M., Weinstein, M. C., Wittenberg, E., Drummond, M. F., Pliskin, J. S., Wong, J. B., and Glasziou, P. P. (2014). *Decision Making in Health and Medicine: Integrating Evidence and Values*. Cambridge University Press.

Huo, L., Yuan, Y., and Yin, G. (2012). Bayesian dose finding for combined drugs with discrete and continuous doses. *Bayesian analysis (Online)*, 7(4):1035.

Indahl, U. G., Liland, K. H., and Næs, T. (2009). Canonical partial least squares – a unified pls approach to classification and regression problems. *Journal of Chemometrics*, 23(9):495–504.

Ivanova, A. and Wang, K. (2003). Bivariate isotonic design for dose-finding with ordered groups. *Biometrics*, 25:2018–2026.

Jennison, C. and Turnbull, B. W. (1999). *Group Sequential Methods with Applications to Clinical Trials*. CRC Press.

Jin, I. H., Liu, S., Thall, P. F., and Yuan, Y. (2014). Using data augmentation to facilitate conduct of phase I–II clinical trials with delayed outcomes. *Journal of the American Statistical Association*, 109(506):525–536.

Johnston, S. C., Mendis, S., and Mathers, C. D. (2009). Global variation in stroke burden and mortality: Estimates from monitoring, surveillance, and modelling. *The Lancet Neurology*, 8:345–354.

Kato, K., Tahara, M., Hironaka, S., Muro, K., Takiuchi, H., Hamamoto, Y., Imamoto, H., Amano, N., and Seriu, T. (2011). A phase II study of paclitaxel by weekly 1-h infusion for advanced or recurrent esophageal cancer in patients who had previously received platinum-based chemotherapy. *Cancer Chemotherapy and Pharmacology*, 67:1265–1272.

Konopleva, M., Thall, P. F., Yi, C. A., Borthakur, G., Coveler, A., Bueso-Ramos, C., Benito, J., Konoplev, S., Gu, Y., Ravandi, F., Jabbour, E., Faderl, S., Thomas, D., Cortes, J., Kadia, T., Kornblau, S., Daver, N., Pemmaraju, N., Nguyen, H. Q., Feliu, J., Lu, H., Wei, C., Wilson, W. R., Melink, T. J., Gutheil, J. C., Andreeff, M., Estey, E. H., and Kantarjian, H. (2015). Phase I/II study of the hypoxia-activated prodrug PR104 in refractory/relapsed acute myeloid leukemia and acute lymphoblastic leukemia. *Haematologica*, 100(7):927–934.

Korn, E. (2004). Nontoxicity endpoints in phase I trial designs for targeted, non-cytotoxic agents. *Journal of the National Cancer Institute*, 96:977–978.

Korn, E. L., Freidlin, B., Abrams, J. S., and Halabi, S. (2012). Design issues in randomized phase II/III trials. *Journal of Clinical Oncology*, 30:667–671.

Kosorok, M. R. and Moodie, E. E. M., editors (2015). *Dynamic Treatment Regimes in Practice: Planning Trials and Analyzing Data for Personalized Medicine*. SIAM.

Kuk, A. and Chen, C. (1992). A mixture model combining logistic regression with proportional hazards regression. *Biometrika*, 79:531–541.

Lan, K. K. G. and DeMets, D. L. (1983). Discrete sequential boundaries for clinical trials. *Biometrika*, 70(3):659–663.

Lavori, P. W. and Dawson, R. (2004). Dynamic treatment regimes: practical design considerations. *Clinical Trials*, 1(1):9–20.

Le Tourneau, C., Lee, J. J., and Siu, L. L. (2009). Dose escalation methods in phase I cancer clinical trials. *Journal of the National Cancer Institute*, 101.

Lee, J., Thall, P. F., Ji, Y., and Müller, P. (2015). Bayesian dose-finding in two treatment cycles based on the joint utility of efficacy and toxicity. *Journal of the American Statistical Association*, 110(510):711–722.

Lee, J., Thall, P. F., Ji, Y., and Müller, P. (2016). A decision-theoretic phase I-II design for ordinal outcomes in two cycles. *Biostatistics*, 17(2):304–319.

Legedza, A. T. R. and Ibrahim, J. G. (2000). Longitudinal design for phase I clinical trials using the continual reassessment method. *Controlled Clinical Trials*, 21(6):574–588.

Leung, D. H. and Wang, Y. G. (2001). A Bayesian decision approach for sample size determination in phase II trials. *Biometrics*, 57:309–312.

Lim, W., Tan, E., Toh, C., Hee, S., Leong, S., Ang, P., Wong, N., and Chowbay, B. (2010). Phase I pharmacokinetic study of a weekly liposomal paclitaxel formulation (Genexol-PM) in patients with solid tumors. *Annals of Oncology*, 21:382–388.

Lipton, A., Campbell-Baird, C., Harvey, H., Kim, C., Demers, L., and Costa, L. (2010). Phase I trial of zoledronic acid+ imatinib mesylate (Gleevec) in patients with bone metastases. *American Journal of Clinical Oncology*, 33:75–78.

Little, R. J. A. and Rubin, D. B. (2002). *Statistical Analysis with Missing Data*. Wiley, New York, 2nd edition.

Liu, Q. and Pledger, G. W. (2005). Phase II and III combination designs to accelerate drug development. *Journal of the American Statistical Association*, 100:493–502.

Liu, S. and Ning, J. (2013). A Bayesian dose-finding design for drug combination trials with delayed toxicities. *Bayesian Analysis*, 8:703–722.

Liu, S., Yin, G., and Yuan, Y. (2013). Bayesian data augmentation dose finding with continual reassessment method and delayed toxicity. *The Annals of Applied Statistics*, 7(4):2138–2156.

Liu, S. and Yuan, Y. (2015). Bayesian optimal interval designs for phase I clinical trials. *Journal of the Royal Statistical Society: Series C (Applied Statistics)*, 64(3):507–523.

LoRusso, P., Boerner, S., and Seymour, L. (2010). An overview of the optimal planning, design, and conduct of phase I studies of new therapeutics. *Clinical Cancer Research*, 16:1710–1718.

Lunceford, J. K., Davidian, M., and Tsiatis, A. A. (2002). Estimation of survival distributions of treatment policies in two-stage randomization designs in clinical trials. *Biometrics*, 58:48–57.

Maller, R. A. and Zhou, X. (1996). *Survival Analysis with Long-Term Survivors*. Wiley, New York.

Mandrekar, S. J., Cui, Y., and Sargent, D. J. (2007). An adaptive phase I design for identifying a biologically optimal dose for dual agent drug combinations. *Statistics in Medicine*, 26:2317–2320.

Marchetti, M., Barosi, G., Balestri, F., Viarengo, G., Gentili, S., Barulli, S., Demory, J.-L., Ilariucci, F., Volpe, A., Bordessoule, D., et al. (2004). Low-dose thalidomide ameliorates cytopenias and splenomegaly in myelofibrosis with myeloid metaplasia: A phase II trial. *Journal of Clinical Oncology*, 22(3):424–431.

McCullagh, P. (1980). Regression models for ordinal data (with discussion). *Journal of the Royal Statistical Society: Series B (Methodological)*, 42:109–142.

Moodie, E. E. M., Richardson, T. S., and Stephens, D. A. (2007). Demystifying optimal dynamic treatment regimes. *Biometrics*, 63(2):447–455.

Morita, S., Thall, P. F., and Müller, P. (2008). Determining the effective sample size of a parametric prior. *Biometrics*, 64:595–602.

Morita, S., Thall, P. F., and Müller, P. (2010). Evaluating the impact of prior assumptions in Bayesian biostatistics. *Statistics in Biosciences*, 2:1–17.

Morita, S., Thall, P. F., and Müller, P. (2012). Prior effective sample size in conditionally independent hierarchical models. *Bayesian Analysis*, 7(3):591–614.

Murdoch, S. D. and Cohen, A. T. (1999). Propofol-infusion syndrome in children. *The Lancet*, 353:2074–2075.

Murphy, S. A. (2003). Optimal dynamic treatment regimes. *Journal of the Royal Statistical Society: Series B (Statistical Methodology)*, 65(2):331–355.

Murphy, S. A. (2005). A generalization error for Q-learning. *Journal of Machine Learning Research*, 6:1073.

Murphy, S. A. and Bingham, D. (2009). Screening experiments for developing dynamic treatment regimes. *Journal of the American Statistical Association*, 104(485):391–408.

Murphy, S. A., Collins, L. M., and Rush, A. J. (2007). Customizing treatment to the patient: Adaptive treatment strategies. *Drug and Alcohol Dependence*, 88(Suppl 2):S1.

Murphy, S. A., Van Der Laan, M. J., and Robins, J. M. (2001). Marginal mean models for dynamic regimes. *Journal of the American Statistical Association*, 96(456):1410–1423.

Nelder, J. A. and Mead, R. (1965). A simplex method for function minimization. *Computer Journal*, 7:308.

Nelsen, R. B. (2006). *An Introduction to Copulas, 2nd edition*. Springer-Verlag, New York.

Nguyen, D. V. and Rocke, D. M. (2002). Tumor classification by partial least squares using microarray gene expression data. *Bioinformatics*, 18(1):39–50.

Nieto, Y., Thall, P., Valdez, B., Andersson, B., Popat, U., Anderlini, P., Shpall, E. J., Bassett, R., Alousi, A., Hosing, C., et al. (2012). High-dose infusional gemcitabine combined with busulfan and melphalan with autologous stem-cell transplantation in patients with refractory lymphoid malignancies. *Biology of Blood and Marrow Transplantation*, 18(11):1677–1686.

O'Quigley, J. and Paoletti, X. (2003). Continual reassessment method for ordered groups. *Biometrics*, 59:430–440.

O'Quigley, J., Pepe, M., and Fisher, L. (1990). Continual reassessment method: A practical design for phase I clinical trials in cancer. *Biometrics*, 46:33–48.

O'Quigley, J., Shen, L. Z., and Gamst, A. (1999). Two-sample continual reassessment method. *Journal of Biopharmaceutical Statistics*, 9(1):17–44.

Oron, A. P. and Hoff, P. D. (2013). Small-sample behavior of novel phase I cancer trial designs. *Clinical Trials*, 10(1):63–80.

Pan, H., Zhu, C., Zhang, F., Yuan, Y., Zhang, S., Zhang, W., Li, C., Wang, L., and Xia, J. (2014). The continual reassessment method for multiple toxicity grades: A bayesian model selection approach. *PloS one*, 9(5):e98147.

Parmar, M. K. B., Barthel, F. M. S., Sydes, M., Langley, R., Kaplan, R., Eisenhauer, E., Brady, M., James, N., Bookman, M. A., Swart, A. M., Qian, W., and Royston, P. (2008). Speeding up the evaluation of new agents in cancer. *Journal of the National Cancer Institute*, 100(17):1204–1214.

Parulekar, W. and Eisenhauer, E. (2004). Phase I trial design for solid tumor studies of targeted, non-cytotoxic agents: Theory and practice. *Journal of the National Cancer Institute*, 96:990–997.

Pishvaian, M., Slack, R., Koh, E., Beumer, J., Hartley, M., Cotarla, I., Deeken, J., He, A., Hwang, J., Malik, S., et al. (2012). A phase I clinical trial of the combination of imatinib and paclitaxel in patients with advanced or metastatic solid tumors refractory to standard therapy. *Cancer Chemotherapy and Pharmacology*, 70:843–853.

Postel-Vinay, S., Arkenau, H., Ashley, S., Barriuso, J., Olmos, D., Shaw, H., Wright, M., Judson, I., De-Bono, J., and Kaye, S. (2008). Clinical benefit in phase I trials of novel molecularly targeted agents: Does dose matter? *Journal of the Royal Statistical Society: Series C (Applied Statistics)*, 26:2509.

Ramanathan, R., Egorin, M., Takimoto, C., Remick, S., Doroshow, J., LoRusso, P., Mulkerin, D., Grem, J., Hamilton, A., Murgo, A., et al. (2008). Phase I and pharmacokinetic study of imatinib mesylate in patients with advanced malignancies and varying degrees of liver dysfunction: A study by the national cancer institute organ dysfunction working group. *Journal of Clinical Oncology*, 26:563–569.

Ratain, M., Mick, R., Janisch, L., Berezin, F., Schilsky, R., Vogelzang, N., and Kut, M. (1996). Individualized dosing of amonafide based on a pharmacodynamic model incorporating acetylator phenotype and gender. *Pharmacogenetics and Genomics*, 6:93–101.

Riviere, M.-K., Yuan, Y., Dubois, F., and Zohar, S. (2015). A Bayesian dose finding design for clinical trials combining a cytotoxic agent with a molecularly targeted agent. *Journal of the Royal Statistical Society: Series C (Applied Statistics)*, 64:215–229.

Robbins, H. (1952). Some aspects of the sequential design of experiments. *Bulletin of the American Mathematical Society*, 58:527–535.

Robert, C. P. and Cassella, G. (1999). *Monte Carlo Statistical Methods*. Springer, New York.

Robertson, T., Wright, F., Dykstra, R., and Robertson, T. (1988). *Order Restricted Statistical Inference*. Wiley, New York.

Robins, J. M. (1986). A new approach to causal inference in mortality studies with a sustained exposure period - application to control of the healthy worker survivor effect. *Mathematical Modelling*, 7(9):1393–1512.

Robins, J. M. (1993). Analytic methods for estimating HIV-treatment and cofactor effects. In *Methodological Issues in AIDS Behavioral Research*, pages 213–288. Springer.

Robins, J. M. (1997). Causal inference from complex longitudinal data. In *Latent Variable Modeling and Applications to Causality*, pages 69–117. Springer.

Robins, J. M. (1998). Marginal structural models. In *Proceedings of the American Statistical Association Section on Bayesian Statistics*, pages 1–10.

Robins, J. M., Hernan, M. A., and Brumback, B. (2000). Marginal structural models and causal inference in epidemiology. *Epidemiology*, 11(5):550–560.

Rubinstein, L. V., Korn, E. L., Freidlin, B., Hunsberger, S., Ivy, S. P., and Smith, M. A. (2005). Design issues of randomized phase II trials and a proposal for phase II screening trials. *Journal of Clinical Oncology*, 23:7199–7206.

Rush, A. J., Trivedi, M., and Fava, M. (2003). Depression, IV: STAR* D treatment trial for depression. *The American Journal of Psychiatry*, 160(2):237.

Sammartino, M., Garra, R., Sbaraglia, F., and Papacci, P. (2010). Propofol overdose in a preterm baby: May propofol infusion syndrome arise in two hours? *Paediatric Anaesthesia*, 20:973–974.

Schaid, D. J., Wieand, S., and Therneau, T. M. (1990). Optimal two stage screening designs for survival comparisons. *Biometrika*, 77:507–513.

Schwarz, G. (1978). Estimating the dimension of a model. *The Annals of Statistics*, 6(2):461–464.

Shah, N. P., Kantarjian, H. M., Kim, D.-W., Réa, D., Dorlhiac-Llacer, P. E., Milone, J. H., Vela-Ojeda, J., Silver, R. T., Khoury, H. J., Charbonnier, A., et al. (2008). Intermittent target inhibition with dasatinib 100 mg once daily preserves efficacy and improves tolerability in imatinib-resistant and-intolerant chronic-phase chronic myeloid leukemia. *Journal of Clinical Oncology*, 26(19):3204–3212.

Sharma, M. R., Stadler, W. M., and Ratain, M. J. (2011). Randomized phase II trials: A long-term investment with promising returns. *Journal of the National Cancer Institute*, 103(14):1093–1100.

Simas, A. B., Barreto-Souza, W., and Rocha, A. V. (2010). Improved estimators for a general class of beta regression models. *Journal of Computational Statistics and Data Analysis*, 54:348–366.

Simon, R., Rubinstein, L., Arbuck, S. G., Christian, M. C., Freidlin, B., and Collins, J. (1997). Accelerated titration designs for phase I clinical trials in oncology. *Journal of the National Cancer Institute*, 89(15):1138–1147.

Simon, R., Wittes, R. E., and Ellenberg, S. S. (1985). Randomized phase II clinical trials. *Cancer Treatment Reports*, 69:1375–1381.

Simon, R. M. (1989). Optimal two-stage designs for phase II clinical trials. *Controlled Clinical Trials*, 10:1–10.

Sox, H. C., Blatt, M. A., Higgins, M. C., and Marton, K. I. (1988). *Medical Decision Making*. The American College of Physicians; 1st edition (November 15, 2006).

Spiegelhalter, D. J., Abrams, K. R., and Myles, J. P. (2004). *Bayesian Approaches to Clinical Trials and Health-Care Evaluation*, volume 13. John Wiley & Sons.

Stallard, N. and Friede, T. (2008). A group-sequential design for clinical trials with treatment selection. *Statistics in Medicine*, 27:6209–6227.

Stallard, N. and Todd, S. (2003). Sequential designs for phase III clinical trials incorporating treatment selection. *Statistics in Medicine*, 22:689–703.

Stevens, T. P., Harrington, E. W., Blennow, M., and Soll, R. F. (2007). Early surfactant administration with brief ventilation vs. selective surfactant and continued mechanical ventilation for preterm infants with or at risk for respiratory distress syndrome. *Cochrane Database of Systematic Reviews*, 4(4).

Stone, M. and Brooks, R. J. (1990). Continuum regression: Cross-validated sequentially constructed prediction embracing ordinary least squares, partial least squares and principal components regression. *Journal of the Royal Statistical Society. Series B (Methodological)*, 52(2):237–269. With discussion and a reply by the authors.

Sutton, R. S. and Barto, A. G. (1998). *Reinforcement Learning: An Introduction*. MIT Press, Cambridge, MA.

Swinburn, P., Lloyd, A., Nathan, P., Choueiri, T. K., Cella, D., and Neary, M. P. (2010). Elicitation of health state utilities in metastatic renal cell carcinoma. *Current Medical Research and Opinion*, 26(5):1091–1096.

Takano, M., Kikuchi, Y., Kita, T., Suzuki, M., Ohwada, M., Yamamoto, T., Yamamoto, K., Inoue, H., and Shimizu, K. (2001). Phase I and pharmacological study of single paclitaxel administered weekly for heavily pre-treated patients with epithelial ovarian cancer. *Anticancer Research*, 22:1833–1838.

Tanner, M. A. and Wong, W. H. (1987). The calculation of posterior distributions by data augmentation (with discussion). *Journal of the American Statistical Association*, 82:528–550.

Thall, P. F. (2008). A review of phase 2-3 clinical trial designs. *Lifetime Data Analysis*, 14:37–53.

Thall, P. F. (2010). Bayesian models and decision algorithms for complex early phase clinical trials. *Statistical Science*, 25:227–244.

Thall, P. F. and Cheng, S. C. (1999). Treatment comparisons based on two-dimensional safety and efficacy alternatives in oncology trials. *Biometrics*, 55(3):746–753.

Thall, P. F. and Cook, J. D. (2004). Dose-finding based on efficacy-toxicity trade-offs. *Biometrics*, 60:684–693.

Thall, P. F., Herrick, R. C., Nguyen, H. Q., Venier, J. J., and Norris, J. C. (2014a). Effective sample size for computing prior hyperparameters in Bayesian phase I-II dose-finding. *Clinical Trials*, 11:657–666.

Thall, P. F., Lee, J. J., Tseng, C. H., and Estey, E. H. (1999). Accrual strategies for phase I trials with delayed patient outcome. *Statistics in Medicine*, 18:1155–1169.

Thall, P. F., Millikan, R. E., Mueller, P., and Lee, S. J. (2003). Dose-finding with two agents in phase I oncology trials. *Biometrics*, 59:487–496.

Thall, P. F., Millikan, R. E., and Sung, H.-G. (2000). Evaluating multiple treatment courses in clinical trials. *Statistics in Medicine*, 19(8):1011–1028.

Thall, P. F. and Nguyen, H. Q. (2012). Adaptive randomization to improve utility-based dose-finding with bivariate ordinal outcomes. *Journal of Biopharmaceutical Statistics*, 22(4):785–801.

Thall, P. F., Nguyen, H. Q., Braun, T. M., and Qazilbash, M. H. (2013). Using joint utilities of the times to response and toxicity to adaptively optimize schedule-dose regimes. *Biometrics*, 69:673–682.

Thall, P. F., Nguyen, H. Q., and Estey, E. H. (2008). Patient-specific dose finding based on bivariate outcomes and covariates. *Biometrics*, 64:1126–1136.

Thall, P. F., Nguyen, H. Q., and Zinner, R. G. (2016). Parametric dose standardisation for optimising two-agent combinations in a phase I-II trial with ordinal outcomes. *Journal of the Royal Statistical Society: Series C (Applied Statistics)*. In press.

Thall, P. F., Nguyen, H. Q., Zohar, S., and Maton, P. (2014b). Optimizing sedative dose in preterm infants undergoing treatment for respiratory distress syndrome. *Journal of the American Statistical Association*, 109(507):931–943.

Thall, P. F. and Russell, K. E. (1998). A strategy for dose-finding and safety monitoring based on efficacy and adverse outcomes in phase I/II clinical trials. *Biometrics*, 54:251–264.

Thall, P. F. and Simon, R. (1990). Incorporating historical control data in planning phase II clinical trials. *Statistics in Medicine*, 9(3):215–228.

Thall, P. F. and Simon, R. (1994). A Bayesian approach to establishang sample size and monitoring criteria for phase II clinical trials. *Controlled Clinical Trials*, 15(6):463–481.

Thall, P. F., Simon, R., and Ellenberg, S. S. (1988). Two-stage selection and testing designs for comparative clinical trials. *Biometrika*, 75(2):303–310.

Thall, P. F., Simon, R. M., and Estey, E. H. (1995). Bayesian sequential monitoring designs for single-arm clinical trials with multiple outcomes. *Statistics in Medicine*, 14:357–379.

Thall, P. F. and Sung, H.-G. (1998). Some extensions and applications of a Bayesian strategy for monitoring multiple outcomes in clinical trials. *Statistics in Medicine*, 17:1563–1580.

Thall, P. F., Sung, H.-G., and Estey, E. H. (2002). Selecting therapeutic strategies based on efficacy and death in multicourse clinical trials. *Journal of the American Statistical Association*, 97(457):29–39.

Thall, P. F., Szabo, A., Nguyen, H. Q., Amlie-Lefond, C. M., and Zaidat, O. O. (2011). Optimizing the concentration and bolus of a drug delivered by continuous infusion. *Biometrics*, 67(4):1638–1646.

Thall, P. F., Wooten, L. H., Logothetis, C. J., Millikan, R. E., and Tannir, N. M. (2007). Bayesian and frequentist two-stage treatment strategies based on sequential failure times subject to interval censoring. *Statistics in Medicine*, 26(26):4687–4702.

Tseng, W. W., Zhou, S., To, C. A., Thall, P. F., Lazar, A. J., Pollock, R. E., Lin, P. P., Cormier, J. N., Lewis, V. O., Feig, B. W., et al. (2015). Phase 1 adaptive dose-finding study of neoadjuvant gemcitabine combined with radiation therapy for patients with high-risk extremity and trunk soft tissue sarcoma. *Cancer*, 121(20):3659–3667.

Tsimberidou, A., Letourneau, K., Fu, S., Hong, D., Naing, A., Wheler, J., Uehara, C., McRae, S., Wen, S., and Kurzrock, R. (2011). Phase I clinical trial of hepatic arterial infusion of paclitaxel in patients with advanced cancer and dominant liver involvement. *Cancer Chemotherapy and Pharmacology*, 68:247–253.

Tsutakawa, R. K. (1975). Bayesian inference for bioassay. Technical Report 52, University of Missouri-Columbia, Dept. of Statistics.

Tsutakawa, R. K. and Lin, H. Y. (1986). Bayesian estimation of item response curves. *Psychometrika*, 51:251–267.

Turner, T. R. and Wollan, P. C. (1997). Locating a maximum using isotonic regression. *Computational Statistics and Data Analysis*, 25:305–320.

U.S. Food and Drug Administration (2011). Guidance for Industry: Clinical Considerations for Therapeutic Cancer Vaccines.

Van Meter, E. M., Garrett-Mayer, E., and Bandyopadhyay, D. (2011). Proportional odds model for dose-finding clinical trial designs with ordinal toxicity grading. *Statistics in Medicine*, 30:2070–2080.

van Oosterom, A., Judson, I., Verweij, J., Stroobants, S., Di Paola, E., Dimitrijevic, S., Martens, M., Webb, A., Sciot, R., Van Glabbeke, M., Silberman, S., and Nielsen, O. (2001). Safety and efficacy of imatinib (STI571) in metastatic gastrointestinal stromal tumours: A phase I study. *The Lancet*, 358:1421–1423.

Vanderhaegen, J., Naulaers, G., Van Huffel, S., Vanhole, C., and Allegaert, K. (2010). Cerebral and systemic hemodynamic effects of intravenous bolus administration of propofol in neonates. *Neonatology*, 98:57–63.

Verder, H., Robertson, B., Greisen, G., Ebbesen, F., Albertsen, P., Lundstrom, K., and Jacobsen, T. (1994). Surfactant therapy and nasal continuous positive airway pressure for newborns with respiratory distress syndrome. *The New England Journal of Medicine*, 331:1051–1055.

Wages, N. A. and Conaway, M. R. (2014). Phase I/II adaptive design for drug combination oncology trials. *Statistics in Medicine*, 33(12):1990–2003.

Wahed, A. S. and Tsiatis, A. A. (2004). Optimal estimator for the survival distribution and related quantities for treatment policies in two-stage randomization designs in clinical trials. *Biometrics*, 60(1):124–133.

Wang, K. and Ivanova, A. (2005). Two-dimensional dose finding in discrete dose space. *Biometrics*, 61:217–222.

Wang, L., Rotnitzky, A., Lin, X., Millikan, R. E., and Thall, P. F. (2012). Evaluation of viable dynamic treatment regimes in a sequentially randomized trial of advanced prostate cancer. *Journal of the American Statistical Association*, 107(498):493–508.

Wathen, J. K. and Thall, P. F. (2008). Bayesian adaptive model selection for optimizing group sequential clinical trials. *Statistics in Medicine*, 27:5586–5604.

Watkins, C. J. C. H. (1989). *Learning from Delayed Rewards*. PhD thesis, Cambridge University.

Welzing, L., Kribs, A., Huenseler, C., Eifinger, F., Mehler, K., and Roth, B. (2009). Remifentanil for INSURE in preterm infants: A pilot study for evaluation of efficacy and safety aspects. *Acta Paediatrica*, 98:1416–1420.

Wijesinha, M. C. and Piantadosi, S. (1995). Dose-response models with co-variates. *Biometrics*, 51(3):977–987.

Williams, D. A. (1982). Extra binomial variation in logistic linear models. *Applied Statistics*, 31:144–148.

Wong, M. K., Mohamed, A. F., Hauber, A. B., Yang, J.-C., Liu, Z., Rogerio, J., and Garay, C. A. (2012). Patients rank toxicity against progression free survival in second-line treatment of advanced renal cell carcinoma. *Journal of Medical Economics*, 15(6):1139–1148.

Yin, G. and Yuan, Y. (2009a). Bayesian dose finding in oncology for drug combinations by copula regression. *Journal of the Royal Statistical Society: Series C (Applied Statistics)*, 58:211–224.

Yin, G. and Yuan, Y. (2009b). Bayesian model averaging continual reassessment method in phase I clinical trials. *Journal of the American Statistical Association*, 104(487):954–968.

Yin, G. and Yuan, Y. (2010). Bayesian dose finding in oncology for drug combinations by copula regression. *Appl. Statist*, 59:544–546.

Yuan, Y. and Yin, G. (2009). Bayesian dose-finding by jointly modeling toxicity and efficacy as time-to-event outcomes. *Journal of the Royal Statistical Society: Series C (Applied Statistics)*, 58:719–736.

Yuan, Y. and Yin, G. (2011). Robust EM continual reassessment method in oncology dose finding. *Journal of the American Statistical Association*, 106:818–831.

Yuan, Z. and Chappell, R. (2004). Isotonic designs for phase I cancer clinical trials with multiple risk groups. *Clinical Trials*, 1(6):499–508.

Yuan, Z., Chappell, R., and Bailey, H. (2007). The continual reassessment method for multiple toxicity grades: A Bayesian quasi-likelihood approach. *Biometrics*, 63:173–179.

Zang, Y., Lee, J. J., and Yuan, Y. (2014). Adaptive designs for identifying optimal biological dose for molecularly targeted agents. *Clinical Trials*, 11:319–327.

Zhao, Y., Zeng, D., Socinski, M. A., and Kosorok, M. R. (2011). Reinforcement learning strategies for clinical trials in nonsmall cell lung cancer. *Biometrics*, 67(4):1422–1433.

Zohar, S., Resche-Rigon, M., and Chevret, S. (2013). Using the continual reassessment method to estimate the minimum effective dose in phase II dose-finding studies: a case study. *Clinical Trials*, 10:414–421.

Index

3+3 algorithms, 5, 8–10, 11
  comparing two-cycle dose opti-
    mization approaches, 215–
    222
  example comparison with other
    designs, 10–18
  optimal biological dose finding,
    185–186
  optimal dose combination find-
    ing, 188

A

Acute ischemic stroke (AIS), 253
Acute myelogenous leukemia (AML),
  67, 69–71, 135, 246
Acute respiratory distress syndrome
  (ARDS), 77–79
Adaptive randomization (AR), 40–41,
  200
  dose and schedule optimization,
    239–240
  drug combination trials, 151–155,
    173–174
  fixed reference (FRAR), 152
  moving-reference (MRAR), 152–
    155
  neonatal sedative dose optimiza-
    tion, 280
  two-cycle dose optimization, 214–
    215
  utility-based designs, 122–125
Aranda–Ordaz link model, 160–166,
  172
Area under survival curve (AUSC),
  82–84
Attrition (dropouts), 245–252

Autologous stem cell transplantation,
  91

B

Bayesian data augmentation CRM, 7
Bayesian data augmentation for imputation, 97–99
Bayesian model averaging CRM (BMA-
  CRM), 8
Bayesian optimal interval (BOIN) de-
  sign, 144
Bayesian sequentially adaptive deci-
  sion making, 33–35
Bellman equation, 205, 209
Beta prior, 49
Biomarker-based dose finding, 129,
  137–148
  canonical partial least squares
    (CPLS) method, 139–141
  collinearity problem, 138
  comparing EffToxCovs design per-
    formance, 146–148
  dose acceptability criteria, 143–
    144
  maximum sample size, 145
Bivariate ordinal outcomes, drug-
  combination trials, 159–177,
  See also Combination trials
Bone marrow ablation, 67, 223, 231
Brain tumors, 109–110, 119–128
Breast cancer, 224
Busulfan, 223

C

Cancer therapy, 4

Canonical partial least squares (CPLS)
method, 139–141
Carboplatin, 166–168
Chronic myeloid leukemia (CML),
179, 188
Clinical outcomes
assigning utilities to, 105–111,
See also Utility-based designs
phase I-II design elements, 32–33
"Response" definitions for different scenarios, 67
Clinical trial design, conventional
dose finding paradigm, 1–5,
See also Phase I (conventional) dose finding
Clinical trial design, phase I-II designs, *See also* Phase I-II designs
Cohort size
accrual effects, 22–23
phase I (conventional) clinical
trial design, 1
Collinearity among biomarkers, 138
Combination trials, 149–150
adaptive randomization, 151–155,
173–174
Aranda-Ordaz link model, 160–
166, 172
bivariate binary outcomes, 150–
159
bivariate ordinal outcomes, 159–
177
generalized continuation ratio models, 159–160, 170–171, 177–
178
generalized proportional odds and
other alternative models, 178
illustrative application, 155–158
molecularly targeted agent combinations, 195–202
molecularly targeted and cytotoxic agent combinations,
186–195

mTOR inhibitor chemo trial,
166–168, 173–177
parametric dose standardization,
168–173
prior calibration, 164, 166
sensitivity to maximum sample
size, 176–177
Conditional mean prior (CMP), 52
Continual reassessment method (CRM),
5–8
comparing two-cycle dose optimization approaches, 215–
222
dealing with "greedy" algorithm
stickiness problem, 38
example comparison with other
designs, 10–18
superiority to 3+3 algorithms, 19
time-to-event (TITE-CRM), 71,
91
Continuation ratio (CR) models, 74–
75, 77, 159–160, 170–171,
177–178
Conventional clinical trial paradigm,
1–5, *See also* Phase I (conventional) dose finding
Cost utility, 118
Cumulative probit model, 142–143
Cyclophosphamide, 224

D

Dasatinib, 224
Decitabine, 155–158
Delphi method, 113
Dirichlet prior, 49
Dose acceptability criteria, 62–63
biomarker-based personalized dose
finding, 143–144
EffTox design with covariates
(EffToxCovs), 132–133
two-cycle dose optimization, 211–
212
Dose and schedule optimization, 223–
244

adaptive (dose, schedule)-finding
algorithm, 227–228
adaptive randomization, 239–240
Bayesian dynamic model, 225
event times outcomes, 231–244
illustrative scenarios, 228–230
maximum sample size, 227
parametric dose standardization,
235
schedule-dependent effects, 223–
224
simulation, 244
trinary outcomes, 224–231
Dose combination trials, *See also*
Combination trials
Doxorubicin, 224
Dropouts, 245–252
Drug-combination studies, *See also*
Combination trials
DTM2 methodology, 205–207
comparing two-cycle dose optimization approaches, 215–
222
Dynamic treatment regimes (DTRs),
31, 32, 204–205
adaptive randomization, 214–215
DTM2 methodology, 205–207
optimizing doses in two cycles,
203–222, *See also* Two-cycle
treatment regimes

E

Effective sample size (ESS), 46–50
computing priors from elicited
values, 51, 56, 64–65
drug combination trial, 162–163
EffTox design sensitivity to, 71–
74
Efficacy, 29–30
consequences of ignoring information, 19–22
continual reassessment method
assumptions, 7
dropout effects, 245–247

EffTox design dose admissibility
criteria, 62–63
late-onset outcomes, 22–23, *See
also* Late-onset outcomes
optimal dose combination finding, 188–193
parametric dose standardization,
169
phase II (conventional) design
evaluations, 2–3
"Response" definitions for different scenarios, 67
risk–benefit trade-offs, 35–37, *See
also* Trade-off function
schedule-dependent effects, 224
time-to-event outcomes, 79–87
trinary outcomes, 74–78
Efficacy–Toxicity (EffTox) trade-off
design, 12, 59–60
dose admissibility criteria, 62–63
dose and schedule optimization,
225
dropout handling simulation, 249–
251
example comparison with phase I
designs, 10–18
futility stopping rule, 12, 19
illustration, 69–71
late-onset design (LO-EffTox) illustration, 99–104, *See also*
Late-onset outcomes
personalized dose finding with
covariates (EffToxCovs), 129–
137
prior specification, 64–67
probability model, 60–61
sensitivity to prior effective sample size, 71–74
sensitivity to target contours, 71
simulation-based design approach,
68–69
steps for design construction, 67–
69
superiority to CRM designs, 19
time-to-event outcomes, 79–87

trade-off contours, 59–60, 63–64, 108
trade-off function, 12, 20, 36, 107
trinary outcomes, 74–78
EffToxCovs, 129–137
  comparing biomarker-based design performance, 146–148
  dose acceptability criteria, 132–133
  prior specification, 130–132
  real trial application, 135–138
  trade-off contours, 133–134
ε-information prior, 49
Epirubicin, 224
Etoposide, 224
Expansion cohorts, 2, 23–25
Exploration versus exploitation dilemma, 200

F

Fixed-reference adaptive randomization (FRAR), 152
Fluorouracil, epirubicin, cyclophosphamide (FEC), 224

G

Gamma prior, 49
Gamma regression model, 235–236
Gastrointestinal stromal tumors, 179
Gemcitabine, 223–224
Generalized continuation ratio (GCR) model, 158–160, 170–171, 177–178
Genetic alteration biomarkers, 138–139
"Greedy" decision algorithm stickiness, 37–41

I

Idarubicin (IDA), 69–71
Imatinib, 179, 186, 188, 190, 193
Imputation, 95, 97–99
Interferon, 156

Intermediate dose modeling, 168–172
Intra-arterial stroke treatment optimization, 253–265
Intubation-surfactant-extubation (INSURE) procedure, 267–270
Isotonic regression-based optimal biological dose finding, 182–183, 185–186

L

Late-onset outcomes, 20–21, 79–80, 89–90, *See also* Time-to-event outcomes
  Bayesian data augmentation, 97–99
  illustration (LO-EffTox design), 99–104
  logistical problem, 89–91
  missing data approach, 91–104, 188, *See also* Missing data approach for late-onset outcomes
Late-onset toxicities, 7, 89–90
Least squares algorithm, 54–55
Local regression-based optimal biological dose finding, 183–186
LO-EffTox design, 99–104
Logistical difficulty indexes, 90
Logistic regression models, 47, 49, 50
  optimal biological dose finding, 183–186
Long-term outcomes, *See also* Late-onset outcomes; Time-to-event outcomes
  continual reassessment method assumptions, 7
  phase III design evaluations, 3
Lung cancer, 224, 245

M

Malignant melanoma, 155–158
Markov Chain Monte Carlo (MCMC), 55, 95, 163, 174, 178, 209, 261

Maximum sample size
  dose and schedule optimization,
    227
  drug combination trials, 176–177
  EffTox design construction, 68
  personalized dose finding de-
    signs, 145
  utility-based design example, 125–
    126
Maximum tolerated dose (MTD), 2
  assumptions and expansion co-
    horts, 23–25
  combination trials, 150
  problems going from phase I to
    phase II, 18–19
Melphalan, 223, 231
Mesenchymal stem cells (MSCs), 77–
  79
Missing data approach for late-onset
    outcomes, 91–95, 188
  illustration (LO-EffTox design),
    99–104
  imputation, 95, 97–99
  probability model, 96–97
Mixture cure rate model, 80–81
Molecularly targeted agents (MTAs),
    179–180
  combining two MTAs, 195–202
  cytotoxic agent combinations, 186–
    195
  dose-Efficacy curves, 179–180,
    196–197
  Efficacy-driven minimal Toxicity
    dose finding, 180–186
  optimal biological dose defini-
    tion, 180
Moving-reference adaptive random-
    ization (MRAR), 152–155
mTOR inhibitor combination chemother-
    apy trial, 166–168, 173–177,
    195
Multiple myeloma (MM), 91, 231–234
Multi-stage treatment regimes, 31,
    204, *See also* Two-cycle treat-
    ment regimes

Myelodysplastic syndrome (MDS),
    69–71
Myelofibrosis, 245

N

Nelder-Mead algorithm, 66
Neonatal sedative dose optimization,
    267–282, *See also* Sedative
    dose optimization
Nonlinear least squares, 54–55

O

Optimal biological dose (OBD), Efficacy-
    driven dose finding, 181–
    186, *See also* Molecularly
    targeted agents
Optimal dose combination (ODC),
    See also Combination trials
  molecularly targeted agent com-
    binations, 195–202
  targeted and cytotoxic agents,
    186–195
Optimization versus exploration dilemma,
    37
Ordinal bivariate outcomes, drug-
    combination trials, 159–177,
    See also Combination trials
Ordinal Toxicity
  continual reassessment method
    extension, 8
  utility assignment example, 109–
    111

P

Paclitaxel, 166–168, 186, 188, 190, 193
Parametric dose standardization, 168–
    173, 235
Partial least squares (PLS) method,
    139–141
Pathological priors, 43–46
Patient accrual considerations, 22–
    23, 79–80, 89–91, *See also*
    Late-onset outcomes; Time-
    to-event outcomes

Patient-based utility elicitation, 112, 114

Patient dropouts, 245–252

Patient heterogeneity, 26–28, *See also* Personalized dose finding
time-to-event outcomes, 80

Pediatric brain tumors, 109–110, 119–128

Personalized dose finding, 27–28, 129
biomarker-based, 129, 137–148, *See also* Biomarker-based dose finding
canonical partial least squares (CPLS) method, 139–141
comparing EffToxCovs and biomarker-based designs performance, 146–148
cumulative probit model, 142–143
dose acceptability criteria, 132–133
EffTox design with covariates (EffToxCovs), 129–137, *See also* EffToxCovs
maximum sample size, 145
real trial application, 135–138

Phase I (conventional) dose finding, 1–2
3+3 algorithms, 5, 8–10
consequences of ignoring information, 19–22
continual reassessment method, 5–8
dealing with "greedy" algorithm stickiness problem, 38
example comparison of designs, 10–18
expansion cohorts, 2, 23–25
guessing a schedule, 25–26
late-onset outcomes, 22–23
sample size issues, 16–18
Toxicity problems in moving to phase II, 18–19

Phase I-II designs, 4, 29, *See also* Efficacy–Toxicity (EffTox) trade-off design

Efficacy and Toxicity, 29–30
"Efficacy with no Toxicity" assumption, 20–21
elements of, 30–31
example comparison with other designs, 10–18
"greedy" decision algorithm stickiness and adaptive randomization, 37–41, *See also* Adaptive randomization
patient heterogeneity considerations, 26–28, *See also* Personalized dose finding
risk–benefit trade-offs, 30, 35–37, *See also* Trade-off function
sequentially adaptive decision making, 33–35
simulation-based design approach, 41–42, 68–69
steps for design construction, 67–69
treatment regimes and clinical outcomes, 31–33
trinary outcomes, 74–78

Phase II (conventional) designs, 2–3
expansion cohorts and, 24–25

Phase II-III designs, 3

Phase III designs, 3

Physician-based utility elicitation, 111–114

Plerixafor, 246

Pool adjacent violators algorithm (PAVA), 181

PR104, 135–138

Preterm infant sedative dose optimization, 267–282, *See also* Sedative dose optimization

Prior effective sample size (ESS), *See also* Effective sample size

Prior specification
calibration for drug combination trial, 164, 166

computing from elicited values, 50–57

dose and schedule optimization, 242

effective sample size (ESS), 46–50, *See also* Effective sample size

EffTox design, 64–67

EffTox design sensitivity to, 71

inappropriately informative (pathological) priors, 43–46

least squares algorithm, 54–55

matching dimensions, 53

molecularly targeted agent combinations, 197–198

molecularly targeted and cytotoxic agent combinations, 191

neonatal sedative dose optimization, 273–274

personalized dose finding with covariates (EffToxCovs), 130–132

prior variances and covariances, 51

pseudo sampling algorithm, 45, 55–57

sequentially adaptive decision making, 33–34

simulation-based design approach and, 42

stroke treatment optimization, 260–261

subjectivity critique, 46–47

two-cycle dose optimization, 207

Progression-free survival (PFS), 22–23

continual reassessment method assumptions, 7

conventional phase I dose finding issues, 17

Propofol dose optimization, 267–282

Proportional hazards regression models, 247

Proportional odds (PO) models, 76, 178, 226

Prostate cancer, 85

Pseudo sampling algorithm, 45, 55–57, 242

Q

Q-learning functions, 205, 210

R

Radiation therapy (RT)
late-onset toxicities, 7
utility-based design example, 109–110, 119–128

Randomization, *See also* Adaptive randomization
ethical considerations, 33
phase II cancer trials and, 2, 3
SMART trial designs, 204

Reinforcement learning, 205

Remifentanil, 267

Renal cell cancer, 224

Respiratory distress syndrome, 267–270

Risk–benefit trade-offs, 30, 35–37, *See also* Trade-off function
trade-off contours, 59–60, 63–64

S

Safety rules, *See also* Stopping rules
continual reassessment method, 6–7
drug combination trial, 163
drug combination trials, 163
EffTox design, 12
inappropriately informative (pathological) priors and, 44–45
phase I-II design elements, 31
utility-based designs, 116

Sample size, *See also* Effective sample size
conventional phase I dose finding issues, 16–18

decision criterion function relia-
    bility and, 38, 40
dose and schedule optimization,
    227
drug combination trials, 176–177
EffTox design construction, 68
expansion cohorts, 23
personalized dose finding de-
    signs, 145
utility-based design example, 125–
    126
Schedule and dose optimization, 223–
    244, *See also* Dose and
    schedule optimization
Schedule-dependent effects, 223–224
Schedules, guessing for conventional
    phase I dose finding, 25–26
Sedative dose optimization, 267
    decision criteria, 274–277
    dose-outcome model, 270–273
    neonatal respiratory distress syn-
        drome, 267–270
    prior and likelihood, 273–274
    simulations, 277–282
    utilities, 268–269
Sequential, multiple assignment, ran-
    domized trial (SMART) de-
    signs, 204
Sequentially adaptive decision mak-
    ing, 33–35
    "greedy" decision algorithm stick-
        iness and adaptive random-
        ization, 37–41, *See also* Adap-
        tive randomization
    utility-based designs, 113–118,
        See also Utility-based de-
        signs
Simon's two-stage design, 2
Simulation-based design approach,
    41–42, 68–69
    dealing with dropouts, 249–251
    dose and schedule optimization,
        244
    LO-EffTox design, 102–104

neonatal sedative dose optimiza-
    tion, 277–282
personalized dose finding de-
    signs, 146
stroke treatment optimization,
    261–265
Small-cell lung cancer, 224
SMART trial designs, 204
Solid tumors, 67, 138, 186
Stem cell transplantation, 91, 99, 223,
    231–234
Stickiness of "greedy" decision algo-
    rithms, 37–41
Stopping rules, *See also* Safety rules
    3+3 designs, 9
    drug combination trials, 163
    dynamic treatment regime (DTM2),
        219–220
    EffTox design, 12, 15, 19
    inappropriately informative (patho-
        logical) priors and, 44
    phase I expansion cohorts and,
        24–25
    phase II (conventional) designs, 2
    utility-based designs, 116
Stroke treatment optimization, 253–
    265
Subjectivity, 46–47, 111–113
Sunitinib, 224

T

Targeted agents, *See also* Molecularly
    targeted agents
Thalidomide, 245
Thrombolytic agents, intra-arterial
    stroke treatment optimiza-
    tion, 253–265
Time-to-event continual reassessment
    method (TITE-CRM), 7, 91
Time-to-event outcomes, 188, *See also*
    Late-onset outcomes
    dose and schedule optimization,
        231–244
    EffTox design and, 79–87
Tissue plasminogen activator (tPA),

intra-arterial stroke treatment optimization, 253–265
Total Toxicity burden (TTB), 7
Toxicity, 29–30, *See also* Safety rules
  bounding functions for EffTox-Covs, 132–133
  consequences of ignoring information, 20–21
  definitions for different scenarios, 67
  EffTox design dose admissibility criteria, 62–63
  late-onset, 7, 89–90, *See also* Late-onset outcomes
  parametric dose standardization, 169
  problems going from phase I to phase II, 18–19
  randomized patient assignment issues, 33
  risk–benefit trade-offs, 35–37, *See also* Trade-off function
  schedule-dependent effects, 223–224
  time-to-event outcomes, 79–87
  trinary outcomes, 74–78
Toxicity and Efficacy odds ratio (TEOR), comparing two-cycle dose optimization approaches, 215–222
Trade-off contours, 59–60, 63–64
  EffTox design with covariates (EffToxCovs), 133–134
  sensitivity to target contours, 71
  utility assignment, 108
Trade-off design, *See also* Efficacy–Toxicity (EffTox) trade-off design
Trade-off function, 12, 20, 30, 35–37
  utility assignment, 107
Treatment policy, 204, *See also* Two-cycle treatment regimes
Treatment regimes
  acceptability criteria for utility-based designs, 115–116

dose-schedule regimes, *See also* Dose and schedule optimization
drug-combination studies, *See also* Combination trials
multi-cycle (dynamic treatment regimes), 31, 204, *See also* Two-cycle treatment regimes
phase I-II design elements, 31–32
SMART trial designs, 204
targeted agents, *See also* Molecularly targeted agents
utility-based design evaluation, 116–117
Trinary outcomes, 74–78, 224–231
Two-cycle treatment regimes, 32
  adaptive randomization, 214–215
  comparing DTM2 and other approaches, 215–222
  decision criteria, 209–212
  dose acceptability criteria, 211–212
  DTM2 methodology, 205–207
  illustration and simulation, 212–222
  model, 205–209
  two-cycle problem, 203–205
Type I error probability, 112–113
Type II error probability, 112–113

U

UAROET program, 128
Utility-based designs, 105–118
  adaptive randomization, 122–125
  brain tumor radiation therapy example, 109–110
  design evaluation criteria, 116–117
  mean utility computation, 107, 108, 114–115
  multiple outcomes, 118
  regime acceptability criteria, 115–116
  sensitivity analyses, 117–118

subjectivity considerations, 111–
     113
UAROET program, 128
utility assignment, 105–111
utility elicitation, 113–114

V

Valproic acid (VA), 69–71

Printed and bound by CPI Group (UK) Ltd, Croydon, CR0 4YY

17/10/2024

01775705-0002